Case Studies in Personalized Nutrition

Personalized Nutrition and Lifestyle Medicine for Healthcare Practitioners
Edited by Lorraine Nicolle, this series of accessible, evidence-based, practical guides is essential reading for practitioners and students of clinical nutrition, and all other primary and complementary healthcare professionals interested in an approach that responds to the unique health needs of every individual. Each book in the series is a powerful new tool to help practitioners achieve significant clinical improvements for their clients/patients through the cutting-edge paradigm of personalized nutrition and lifestyle medicine.

Lorraine Nicolle MSc is a Registered Nutritionist (MBANT) and an educator and author in personalized nutrition. www.lorrainenicollenutrition.co.uk

in the same series

Using Nutrigenomics within Personalized Nutrition
A Practitioner's Guide
Anne Pemberton
ISBN 978 1 84819 413 7
eISBN 978 0 85701 368 2

Mitochondria in Health and Disease
Ray Griffiths
Foreword by Lorraine Nicolle
ISBN 978 1 84819 332 1
eISBN 978 0 85701 288 3

of related interest

Biochemical Imbalances in Disease
A Practitioner's Handbook
Lorraine Nicolle and Ann Woodriff Beirne
ISBN 978 1 84819 033 7
eISBN 978 0 85701 028 5

The Functional Nutrition Cookbook
Addressing Biochemical Imbalances through Diet
Lorraine Nicolle and Christine Bailey
ISBN 978 1 78592 991 5
eISBN 978 0 85701 052 0

Case Studies in Personalized Nutrition

Part of

Personalized Nutrition and Lifestyle
Medicine for Healthcare Practitioners *series*

Angela Walker
Foreword by Lorraine Nicolle

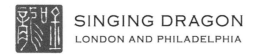
SINGING DRAGON
LONDON AND PHILADELPHIA

Figure 2.1 is adapted from Sackett 1996 with kind permission
from the Institute for Work Based Learning.
Figure 2.2 is reprinted from Murad *et al.* 2006 with kind
permission from BMJ Publishing Group Ltd.
The Functional Medicine Matrix (in the colour plate and Figure 9.4) is reprinted
from the Institute for Functional Medicine with their kind permission.

First published in 2020
by Singing Dragon
an imprint of Jessica Kingsley Publishers
73 Collier Street
London N1 9BE, UK
and
400 Market Street, Suite 400
Philadelphia, PA 19106, USA

www.singingdragon.com

Copyright © Jessica Kingsley Publishers 2020

Library of Congress Cataloging in Publication Data
A CIP catalog record for this book is available from the Library of Congress

British Library Cataloguing in Publication Data
A CIP catalogue record for this book is available from the British Library

ISBN 978 1 84819 394 9
eISBN 978 0 85701 351 4

Printed and bound by CPI Group (UK) Ltd, Croydon, CR0 4YY

Contents

Foreword

When it comes to improving chronic health conditions, the types of interventions that everyone wants are those that are tried and tested, and considered 'safe'.

In mainstream medicine, it's the large-scale population studies and randomized controlled trials that provide evidence for the interventions. But these types of studies are limited in their ability to inform the practitioner of *personalized* health care because they are designed to *minimize* variation across groups of participants.[1] In contrast to this, truly patient-centred approaches require individual variation to be embraced (n = 1).

And that's where this new text comes in – the second in our series on Personalized Nutrition and Lifestyle Medicine (PNLM). This book's aim is to arm practitioners with real-world evidence for approaches that are *patient-centred* – that is, targeted to the unique combination of needs and imbalances expressed by each individual.

The creator of this book, Angela Walker, has painstakingly pulled together patient stories from nine experienced practitioners. Each case study contributes to the evidence base for PNLM and together they drive home the types of characteristics that are common to the chronic care approaches that achieve the very best outcomes. So, on these pages, you'll witness the following:

---

1   These types of studies are also now coming under fire for other reasons, with growing numbers of scientists sounding the alarm about their reliability and validity. See Ionnidis (2018) and Archer and Lavie (2017).

- Practitioners recognizing that PNLM is equipped with the mind-blowing power to alter the behaviour of our genes, which ultimately govern our health; thus seeing the logic of drawing on this before resorting to referrals for drugs (most of which carry risks).
- Strategies that resist the urge to focus on suppressing symptoms, and instead strive to identify and tackle the underlying *causes* of those symptoms.
- Directions of travel that are dictated by each individual's functional imbalances in body systems, rather than by protocols created for named medical conditions (because different body systems may be impaired in different individuals with similar symptoms, two people with the same named disease may require very different interventions in order to improve).
- Programs designed to improve the *flexibility* of body systems to adapt continuously to environmental changes. This is done by exposing cells to levels of stress that make them more robust. Examples of such 'hormetic' practices[2] within these cases include the use of 'toxic' phytochemicals, intermittent fasting and ketogenic diets.
- Patients' dietary prescriptions being altered over time in recognition of the fact that what makes a person's diet optimal will evolve, depending on the specific biological systems that require either up- or down-regulation.
- Patients often being prescribed micronutrients at far higher levels than the standard 'recommended nutrient intakes' (RNIs). Following in the footsteps of the renowned biochemist Bruce Ames, PN does not rely on public health guidelines, preferring instead to be guided by an individual's case history and laboratory results and the scientific data to prescribe at personalized levels targeted to push specific biochemical pathways. This is controversial for those who believe that nutritional therapy

---

2   Hormesis is a dose response phenomenon in which low dose exposure to a toxin or other stressor elicits a favourable biological response, whereas high dose exposures may cause cellular inflammation and damage.

should be limited to micronutrient doses that are obtainable from diet alone. A more personal approach understands that the levels found in food may not always be sufficient to achieve optimal health. In the cases herein, the aim is to make a greater difference than would be achieved by simply bringing each individual's micronutrient intake up to the RNI benchmark.

- Collaborative relationships being built between practitioners and patients, enabling the latter to become empowered to take back responsibility for their health.

The PN reviewer Kate Neil (to whom we are grateful for reviewing this text at its final draft) has been at the vanguard of convincing practitioners that reflective practice and case study sharing are perhaps the most powerful routes to continuous learning and development. Similarly, there is growing recognition that individual cases (and the associated reflective practice) are the building blocks of a more useful evidence base in personalized health care. Chapter 2 proposes a way for this to be taken further, by incorporating validated questionnaires into the consultation that capture data on outcomes in a reliable and reproducible way.

The growing use of wearable technologies and novel applications like nutrigenomics, metabolomics and microbiota profiling will likely contribute to even more meaningful individualized data capture to enhance the evidence base of the future. (Adherence to data protection issues will be crucial here.) And thus, hopefully, a personalized approach to chronic conditions will eventually be taken more seriously and hence become more widely available to everyone who is looking to improve their long-term health.

Lorraine Nicolle MSc, MBANT, CNHC
Series Editor
www.LorraineNicolleNutrition.co.uk

References

Archer, A. and Lavie, C., 2017. Nutrition Has a 'Consensus' to Use Bad Science: An Open Letter to the National Academies. Accessed on 19/08/2019 at https://www.realclearscience.com/articles/2017/12/16/nutrition_researchers_have_a_consensus_to_use_bad_science.html.

Ionnidis, J., 2018. The challenge of re-forming nutritional epidemiologic research. *JAMA* 320, 10, 969–970. doi:10.1001/jama.2018.11025

Acknowledgements

Thank you, Kara, for the original inspiration for this book many years ago and your refreshing wisdom, expertise and infectious energy, always. I am especially thrilled and frankly flattered that together with Romilly you have contributed a case.

Jane Nodder, I hope I have done justice to what was originally a joint project and that a little of your brilliance has made it onto these pages.

A huge thank you to Lisa and everyone at Singing Dragon for having the faith in me to create this book. To Lorraine Nicolle, for going above and beyond your remit and giving so much of your time and passion to help review the manuscript. There are few more respected or knowledgeable in our field than Kate Neil, so to have you peer-review the book was an incredible honour and I know you also completely over delivered on that brief.

Of course this book would not exist without the contributors. My goal was to make it as painless for you as possible and I apologise for where I fell short on that! For your tolerance and patience as we poured over the cases and asked difficult questions, I am eternally grateful.

So many people were generous with their time and expertise for the functional testing chapter: Mark Howard, Tony Hoffman, Deirdre Nazareth, Lynn Cofer-Chase ('Lipid Lynn'), Laura Stirling, David Quig, William Shaw, Sarah Benjamin, Claire Sehinson, Helen Lynam and Anne Pemberton.

Thank you to my clients over the years who have taught me the art and science of clinical practice. Team Tignum, who gave me the mindset skills l needed. Finally, to my friends and family, thank you for giving me either space to be a hermit and write, or a distraction (usually involving ponies) to help me stay almost sane.

Angela Walker

Terminology

When referring to supplement doses, the following shorthand is used:

- QD – every day
- QOD – every other day
- BID – twice daily
- TID – three times daily
- QID – four times daily

The abbreviation mcg is used for microgram.

Client or patient?

The term *client* is used in the case studies. The term *patient* is used when part of a quotation or a discussion on a piece of research.

Antecedents, triggers and mediators

The terms *antecedents*, *mediator* and *triggers* are used to describe potential underlying factors involved in the progression of symptoms, dysfunction or progression towards diagnosed conditions:

- Antecedents are potential predisposing factors, which could be genetic or acquired.

- Triggers are provoking factors or events that may have triggered a symptom or dysfunctional response.
- Mediators are factors that contribute to symptoms and dysfunctional responses.

1

Introduction and Setting the Scene

Angela Walker

The goal of this book is to provide practitioners of personalized nutrition with clinical examples of personalized nutrition in practice to stimulate discussion of best practice and develop clinical as well as therapeutic relationship skills.

For other healthcare professionals, this book aims to demonstrate the scientific rigour applied to personalized nutrition practice. It is hoped this will inspire curiosity to explore personalized nutrition, either through collaboration and referral to an existing personalized nutrition practitioner or to develop their own skills set and education in this exciting field.

What is personalized nutrition?

Personalized nutrition takes a systems biology (see Box 1.1) approach to address the underlying imbalances in the individual that are contributing to the symptoms experienced. It goes beyond standard diet approaches on a condition or disease basis. Personalized nutrition looks at why an imbalance may have occurred through thoughtful and systematic evaluation of the individual's health history and, where possible, with the aid of laboratory test results, seeks to restore optimal function by the application of personalized diet, lifestyle and, where appropriate, tailored nutrient or supplement recommendations to address the underlying imbalances.

BOX 1.1 SYSTEMS BIOLOGY

Systems biology involves a comprehensive study of the complex interactions in a biological system. It is based on the comprehensive study of the molecular diversity of living systems and a study of the patterns and principles that reoccur in these systems.

The application of systems biology to human health involves the synthesis of information on biochemical pathways, organ systems, environmental factors such as diet and lifestyle and an evaluation of how these interactions impact on health and disease. It is one of the foundations of the scientific rationale for a personalized approach to health.

Adapted by the author from Bland et al. (2017);
Breitling (2010); Tavassoly et al. (2018)

The personalized nutrition approach identifies and implements the lifestyle factors that are most important for an individual's unique situation. The cases presented in the following chapters aim to show how simple changes, explained clearly to clients, can have a profound impact on their health and quality of life.

The application of personalized nutrition involves a combination of systems biology, nutritional science and a therapeutic relationship with the client. There is an art to personalized nutrition practice as well as a science and it is the intention of this book to showcase both. We will see how a diet change, which generally involves avoiding some foods and including other foods, will have an impact on a wide range of factors including but not limited to the microbiome, intestinal permeability, metabolic fuel, coenzymes for biochemical pathways, immune response and inflammation pathways.

We will see how empowering the client with an understanding of their health journey is an important factor in maintaining their engagement. When a client understands why they are being asked to make a change, alongside clear instructions of how to implement the change and ongoing practitioner support, the changes can often be quite straightforward to apply.

The art of practising personalized nutrition involves using coaching language and techniques to support individuals through behavioural change. While it is outside the remit of this book to discuss motivational coaching in depth, the cases include examples of how the practitioners support behavioural change through goal setting, identification of challenges and barriers, and practical mentoring support (via specific tools as well as separate coaching sessions).

The importance of case studies

Case studies provide an important role in the development of any health discipline and have a role in the evidence base for medicine (see Chapter 2). They are an important education tool, demonstrating the clinical application of a systems biology approach. They provide insight into real-life situations and how individuals respond. While case studies are used in education for personalized nutrition (at an undergraduate and professional development level), there is a paucity of *published peer-reviewed* case studies in personalized nutrition.

Case Studies in Integrative and Functional Medicine was published in 2011 (Fitzgerald and Bralley, 2011) as an accompanying text to *Laboratory Evaluations* (Bralley and Lord, 2008). It is an excellent text but is now out of print.

The context of chronic disease

Chronic health conditions are the most prevalent problems in health care, yet much of the medical systems are focused on acute disease and acute care (Holman, 2004). Chronic diseases, which are defined as diseases that are non-communicable, have replaced acute diseases as the primary issue facing most of the modern world. In 2016, non-communicable diseases, as defined by the World Health Organization (WHO), were responsible for 71% of deaths worldwide, and 89% of deaths in the UK (WHO, 2018a).

This book features eight case studies of individuals who faced a wide range of health issues. The individuals were suffering from symptoms that impacted heavily on their quality of life. The cases involve digestive disorders, autoimmunity, cardiovascular disease (CVD), obesity, chronic fatigue, endometriosis and cognitive decline – conditions that can be described as complex and multifactored, without a single aetiology. These eight individuals are representative of thousands of individuals who struggle to find a solution to their poor health and will be recognizable to anyone working as a healthcare practitioner today.

CVD (featured in Chapters 6, 7 and 8) accounts for 25% of premature deaths in men and 17% of premature deaths in women (British Heart Foundation, 2015). It was estimated that $2 billion was lost to national income in the UK due to heart disease, stroke and diabetes in 2005, a figure expected to grow in subsequent years (WHO, 2018b).

Chronic fatigue syndrome (CFS) (a diagnosis in Chapter 5 and a potential diagnosis in Chapters 9, 10 and 11) is estimated to cost at least £3.3 billion to the UK economy in lost income and support costs for the individuals involved (2020 Health, 2017).

Death rates and the economic cost of chronic disease are quantifiable. What is harder to quantify is the impact on quality of life for the individuals involved and their families and carers. Someone with CFS can expect a greater level of disability than a client with back pain/sciatica, type 2 diabetes, CVD, multiple sclerosis, lung disease and even most cancers (2020 Health, 2017).

While the impact of lifestyle factors on risk for chronic disease is broadly accepted, exactly how to implement lifestyle changes and which changes are most important for an individual is a more challenging question. There is no single diet that suits everyone. There is no single exercise programme to suit every individual. We are all biochemically unique and have a different set of life preferences and priorities. Furthermore, individuals often find it hard to make lifestyle changes. They can be confused as to which diet is right for them, and they can lack the motivation and insight on how to make changes or the support network to help. This is where personalized nutrition support can help.

The structure of the book

Is the application of personalized nutrition evidence-based? Yes, although this has been challenged by some healthcare professionals. Chapter 2 is therefore dedicated to explaining the evidence base for personalized nutrition and how evidence will be presented in each of the cases.

Functional laboratory testing is used at some level in each case study. Chapter 3 explains what is involved in functional laboratory testing, how it is used and the rationale for it. It is also an introduction for readers on how to select the most appropriate test for a clinical situation.

Chapters 4 to 11 each contain a single case study. The cases have been submitted by practitioners experienced in their own field. The practitioners contributing to the book come from Europe, the United States and Australia. While all cases are to the same structural brief, they are all a little different in terms of how they are written and presented. This was a deliberate step, to maintain the practitioner's individual style. There is always more than one way to address a personalized nutrition case, and it is helpful to understand the practitioner's individual style and approach to gain the full learning opportunity from the case. The question-and-answer section at the end of each case provides an opportunity to share some of the reflective practice that is an important clinical skill for practitioners. The final chapter is a reflection on all the cases and attempts to summarize the key elements that underpin the art and science of personalized nutrition.

The colour plate can be downloaded from www.singingdragon.com/catalogue/book/9781848193949

References

2020 Health (Ed.), 2017. *Counting the Cost: Chronic Fatigue Syndrome/Myalgic Encephalomyelitis.* Accessed on 26/05/2019 at www.meassociation.org.uk/wp-content/uploads/2020Health-Counting-the-Cost-Sept-2017.pdf

Bland, J.S., Minich, D.M., Eck, B.M., 2017. A systems medicine approach: Translating emerging science into individualized wellness. *Advances in Medicine* 2017, 1718957. https://doi.org/10.1155/2017/1718957

Bralley, J.A., Lord, R.S., 2008. *Laboratory Evaluations for Integrative and Functional Medicine,* 2nd ed. Metametrix Institute.

Breitling, R., 2010. What is systems biology? *Frontiers in Physiology* 1. https://doi.org/10.3389/fphys.2010.00009

British Heart Foundation, 2015. Cardiovascular Disease Statistics 2015. Accessed on 26/05/2019 at www.bhf.org.uk/informationsupport/publications/statistics/cvd-stats-2015

Fitzgerald, K., Bralley, J.A., 2011. *Case Studies in Integrative and Functional Medicine,* 1st ed. Metametrix Institute.

Holman, H., 2004. Chronic disease – the need for a new clinical education. *JAMA* 292, 1057–1059. https://doi.org/10.1001/jama.292.9.1057

Tavassoly, I., Goldfarb, J., Iyengar, R., 2018. Systems biology primer: The basic methods and approaches. *Essays in Biochemistry* EBC20180003. https://doi.org/10.1042/EBC20180003

WHO, 2018a. Noncommunicable diseases country profiles. Accessed on 26/05/2019 at www.who.int/nmh/publications/ncd-profiles-2018/en

WHO, 2018b. The impact of chronic disease in the United Kingdom. Accessed on 26/05/2019 at www.who.int/chp/chronic_disease_report/media/impact/en

2

The Evidence Base in Personalized Nutrition

Miguel Toribio-Mateas and Angela Walker

Clinical decisions in personalized nutrition practice must have a rational basis that is substantiated by scientific evidence. This makes professionals practising personalized nutrition evidence-based practitioners. This chapter will discuss the wider definition of evidence, including but not limited to the randomized controlled trial (RCT), and explore how practitioners can develop a comprehensive rationale for the application of food- and lifestyle-based recommendations.

Background to evidence-based medicine (EBM)

The concept of evidence-based medicine (EBM) was first discussed in a landmark paper entitled 'Evidence based medicine: what it is and what it isn't' (Sackett *et al.*, 1996). Sackett emphasized the importance of making clinical decisions based only on the best available evidence and explored the idea that not all evidence is created equal. Importantly, he advocated the use of evidence and clinical expertise concurrently in order to successfully implement the concept of EBM into clinical practice.

Good doctors use both individual clinical expertise and the best available external evidence, and neither alone is enough. (Sackett *et al.*, 1996, p.71)

A later update to the original model for EMB introduced two new considerations (Sackett, 2000). First, it stressed the importance of taking client values and preferences into account when making clinical decisions. Second, to extend the concept of clinical research beyond the restricted context of laboratories and clinical trials, Sackett encouraged medical practitioners to view themselves as researchers in their own clinical practice. This call for clinicians to become practitioner-researchers is powerful and still very much applicable to practitioners of personalized nutrition today.

Traditional hierarchy of evidence-based practice

Most practitioners of personalized nutrition are not medically trained. Therefore, the term evidence-based practice (EBP) is more appropriate in this context. EBP will be used instead of EBM for the rest of this chapter.

One of the goals of EBP is to educate clinicians in the understanding and use of published literature to optimize clinical practice (Djulbegovic and Guyatt, 2017). Not all evidence is equal. The evidence-based practitioner will take the totality of evidence into account, which means consideration of negative as well as positive evidence. Cherry-picking of evidence must be avoided.

There is a recognized hierarchy to types of evidence that informs EBP, which is shown in Figure 2.1. In this traditional pyramid, systematic reviews and meta-analysis are at the top as having highest quality, followed by randomized controlled trials, cohort studies, case-control studies and case series/reports. Expert opinion is classed as having the poorest quality.

As illustrated in Figure 2.1, unfiltered or primary sources provide evidence concerning a topic under investigation. Primary resources – for example, articles that appear in scientific journals that are indexed in databases such as PubMed – have a higher place in the hierarchy of evidence than other sources of information that have not been peer-reviewed. In the age of Instagram, it is important to realize that blogs and social media posts are classed as expert opinion and are therefore seen to have the lowest quality in an EBP hierarchy of evidence. Filtered or secondary sources are summaries and analyses of the evidence derived from and based on unfiltered primary sources. Filtered sources are useful in clinical practice as they provide an appraisal of the quality of studies and often make recommendations based on 'tried and tested' evidence.

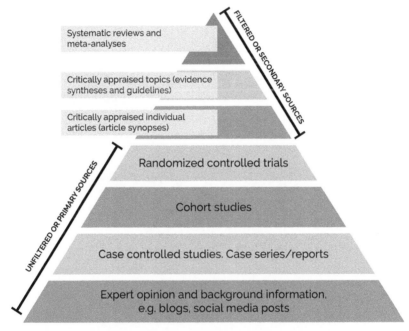

Figure 2.1 A representation of the hierarchy of evidence-based practice as a pyramid
Source: Based largely on Sackett (1996), reinterpreted by Toribio-Mateas

Modifications and critiques of the EBP model

Murad and colleagues (2016) proposed a modification to the traditional pyramid where systematic reviews are removed from the top of the pyramid and used as a lens through which other types of studies should be appraised and applied. This is depicted in Figure 2.2. Under this approach, systematic reviews (the process of selecting the studies) and meta-analyses (the statistical aggregation that produces a single effect size) are 'tools to consume and apply the evidence by stakeholders' (Murad *et al.*, 2016). This development of the EBP embraces the use of clinical insight by practitioners as initially conceived by Sackett (1996, 2000). In a clinical setting where individualization of care is paramount, and where clinicians and clients make collaborative decisions, this approach is welcomed and represents a more pragmatic and intelligent interpretation of EBP.

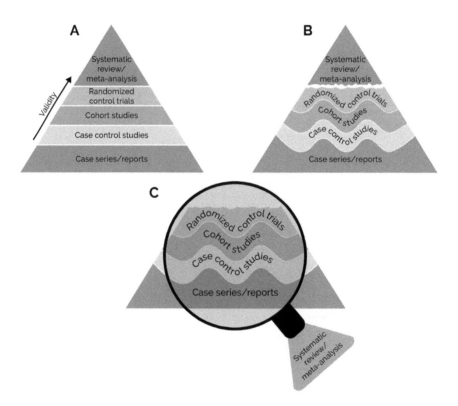

Figure 2.2 A modified evidence-based practice pyramid
Source: Reproduced with permission from Murad et al. *(2016)*

That EBM or EBP has provided a beneficial framework for the application of scientific evidence in healthcare settings is without question. However, the model is not perfect and has attracted criticism, even from some of the leading voices of the EBP movement. A noteworthy example is provided by Trisha Greenhalgh, Professor of Primary Health Sciences and leader of the Evidence-Based Medicine Renaissance Group at Oxford University. Greenhalgh has openly critiqued the fact that 'the gold standard' in the EBP model – the systematic review – has been idealized as representing a tool to remove bias from scientific research that has put it at the top of what she calls a 'spurious hierarchy of systematic over narrative reviews' (Greenhalgh, Thorne and Malterud, 2018, p.1). For many EBP proponents, qualitative research is seen as 'a poor cousin', while Greenhalgh argues that qualitative and quantitative research are equally important, but just 'different and potentially complementary form[s] of scholarship' (p.4). A full critique of EBP is beyond the scope of this chapter, but readers may be interested in the work of Rycroft-Malone *et al.* (2012) who consider the traditional systematic review approaches to be too specific and inflexible.

Complex systems or linear, cause-and-effect relationships?

The randomized controlled trial, at the heart of the EBP pyramid, is typically attempting to map and investigate a linear, cause-and effect relationship (Katerndahl, 2009; Sibbald and Roland, 1998). The human body can perhaps be more accurately described as a complex adaptive system. A study on the perception of complexity in medicine within published papers on the topic found a growing recognition that systems in nature, including those involved in the workings of the human body, involve many different components which interact in non-linear ways (Sturmberg, Martin and Katerndahl, 2014). To evaluate nutritional science in a *purely* linear fashion without consideration of synergistic and non-linear relationships risks becoming a reductionist approach.

For example, zinc is necessary as a cofactor for more than 300 enzymes (McCall, Huang and Fierke, 2000). Zinc has a structural role in plasma membranes (O'Dell, 2000) and a regulatory role in gene expression, acting as a transcription factor (Truong-Tran *et al.*, 2000). Zinc interacts with other nutrients – for example, when taken in a high dose, it can negatively affect the bioavailability of copper (Abdallah and Samman, 1993). Furthermore, the zinc ion is thought to have a regulatory role on major cellular ions including sodium (NA^+), potassium (K^+) and calcium (Ca^+) (Maret, 2017). In addition, there is a documented synergistic relationship between zinc and vitamin A whereby the antioxidant function of vitamin A is more effective when zinc levels are adequate (Matos *et al.*, 2012, 2018). An RCT measuring the impact of zinc supplementation on a single health outcome may not therefore measure the full impact on the complex and adaptive system of an individual.

Embracing complexity

Other areas of science can perhaps assist healthcare practitioners to embrace complexity. An agreement and certainty diagram is a conceptual model for complex problem solving developed in the field of organizational dynamics (Stacey, 1996). The model provides an interesting framework for considering the complexity within a practitioner/client healthcare consultation. Figure 2.3 shows a version of this model adapted from the original model and how it can be applied to the healthcare setting.

It can be said that mainstream health evidence, with a focus on testing linear relationships via randomized controlled trials, is located in the bottom left-hand corner of Figure 2.3, with high certainty and high agreement (Martin and Félix-Bortolotti, 2010).

Is that approach really appropriate when dealing with a complex system such as the human body? Could that approach be too reductive and simplistic to achieve best results when dealing with individuals who have genetic, epigenetic and lifestyle variability?

Translation of science into the context of successful personalized nutrition practice requires recognition of the non-linearity principles that characterize complex health systems. David Katerndahl is a Medicine Professor at the University of Texas Health Science Centre who studies the application of complexity science to the study of family and community medicine. According to Katerndahl, embracing complexity has the power to improve clinical practice:

Understanding the non-linear dynamics of phenomena both internal and external to our patients can (1) improve our definition of 'health'; (2) improve our understanding of patients, disease and the systems in which they converge; (3) be applied to future monitoring systems; and (4) be used to possibly engineer change.

Doctors who successfully practise the 'art' of medicine may recognize non-linear principles at work without having the jargon needed to label them. (Katerndahl, 2009, p.755)

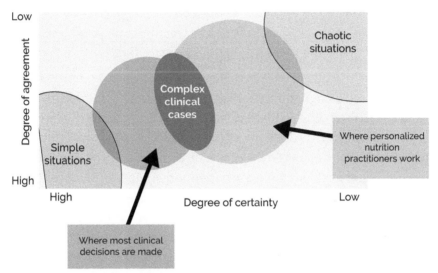

Figure 2.3 A 'certainty-agreement' diagram illustrating the context where personalized nutrition practitioners operate compared with other clinicians
The diagram aims to illustrate the context where most clinical decisions are made when following linear guidelines to tackle simple situations (e.g. supplement with vitamin B12 if B12 deficiency has been identified by means of testing) versus a situation that is chaotic in nature, typically featuring a complex set of overlapping symptoms. In this kind of unchartered territory, practitioners need to make sense of complexity by drawing from appropriate scientific evidence while using their clinical insight.
Source: Adapted from Stacey (1996) and Plsek and Greenhalgh (2001) by Toribio-Mateas

Importance of the client story

We are never illness or disease but, rather, always their sum in the world of day-to-day experience. Illness and disease are not closed systems but mutually constitutive and continuously interacting worlds. In the patient's case, it is always experience as well; we are always in contact with our own worlds of physical and emotional pain and experience – and thus identity – that cannot be reduced to the external zone of intersection between society and the men and women who constitute it. (Rosenberg, 2002, p.258)

This quotation, taken from a paper by Charles Rosenberg, Professor of the History of Science and Medicine at Harvard University, eloquently captures the role the client story. The rich texture of the client story has psychosocial and emotional aspects that are as important as the physical manifestations of disease.

Innes and colleagues (2005) propose that the narrative between client and practitioner has its own agency as a 'complex responsive process', and, further, that clients are nervous about their doctor 'reducing their story to the level of a technical description' (Innes *et al.*, 2005, p.49).

In fact, the interaction between the practitioner and client in the face of complexity and paradox can be key to tackling complex conditions such as chronic pain (Brown, 2009). The nascent nature of the personalized nutrition profession has provided the perfect environment for professionals in this field to work 'at the edge of chaos', continuously identifying patterns in their clients' narratives that enable them to make sense of reality so that they can generate recommendations that are appropriate, safe and meaningful.

A key skill needed to manage working with complexity is reflective practice. The concept of reflective practice was initially developed by Donald Schön, a visiting professor at Massachusetts Institute of Technology.

Schön claims that reflection-in-action is 'central to the "art" by which practitioners sometimes deal well with situations of uncertainty, instability, uniqueness, and value conflict' (Schön, 1983, p.50). Discussing reflection in biomedical professions, he argues that case histories are a key part of 'the physician's process of inquiry – the way in which he perceives and describes the patient, his manner of listening to the patient's descriptions of his complaints, the process by which he identifies possible explanations, conceives of strategies of diagnosis or treatment, and tests them' (Schön, 1983, p.317).

As the cases in the following chapters show, the context, narrative and sense-making between the client and practitioner is an integral part of the personalized nutrition process. The practitioners use coaching skills (active listening, targeted restatements, questioning, clarifying) combined with education to help the client implement the recommendations and achieve their health goals. The client timeline and the interpretation of tests become practical tools which help to organize, structure and inform the client's story. These tools and skills become the foundations of the developing therapeutic relationship. It is therefore proposed that the personalized nutrition clinical approach embraces many of the key elements which assist the practitioner to embrace complexity.

What does evidence look like in complex adaptive systems?

There are impressive examples of studies which aim to embrace the complexity and paradox of nutritional biochemistry in a clinical trial setting. Teams led by Dr Terry Whals have studied the impact of a multimodule approach (modified Paleolithic diet, exercise, stress reduction) to multiple sclerosis and demonstrated the effectiveness of this approach (Bisht et al., 2014; Lee et al., 2017). Dr Dale Bredesen has published case studies on an integrated personalized nutrition approach for successfully reversing Alzheimer's disease (Bredesen et al., 2016). A prospective study demonstrated proof of concept for an integrated personalized, nutrition and psychology approach to chronic fatigue (Arroll and Howard, 2012), which is currently at ethics approval stage to take into a fully randomized controlled study.

These examples illustrate that traditional clinical research *can* be conducted on a personalized nutrition approach. It is hoped these studies will pave the way for more like them. In the meantime, is it true that evidence is lacking for personalized nutrition? The absence of evidence is not the same as evidence of absence, a point that has been highlighted in discussions on evidence-based medicine (Altman and Bland, 1995; Djulbegovic, Elqayam and Dale, 2018; Sola, Dieppa and Rogido, 2007).

Furthermore, as has been discussed above, taking a more comprehensive view of evidence-based practice may lead to better solutions for complex clinical situations. In the context of personalized nutrition, there is evidence and it often needs to be collated from a wider range of sources.

Evidence from a wide range of sources

A personalized nutrition practitioner will use a wide range of sources of evidence. Let us take a specific example. The practitioner is considering whether there is evidence to support supplementing magnesium for a client.

- A starting point may be to ask, 'Are there filtered sources of evidence – a review or a meta-analysis for using magnesium in a client with similar characteristics?'
- There is a meta-analysis for magnesium use in hypertension and diabetes (Wu *et al.*, 2017).
- My client doesn't have hypertension or diabetes, but she has hypothyroidism and she is very anxious, and has some characteristics of metabolic syndrome.
- There are no primary or secondary sources for using magnesium in exactly that scenario.
- Looking from a systems biology perspective:
  - Magnesium is key for mitochondria function (Pilchova *et al.*, 2017).
  - Magnesium adenosine triphosphate (ATP) produced in the mitochondria through oxidative phosphorylation is central to any function that requires energy, plus magnesium is involved

      in iodine uptake, which is documented in a peer-reviewed article (Moncayo and Moncayo, 2017).

- Meta-analysis on the use of magnesium in anxiety found a poor quality of evidence (Boyle, Lawton and Dye, 2017). There is, however, some supportive evidence from clinical studies for the use of magnesium in anxiety (Boyle, Lawton and Dye, 2016).
- Magnesium plays an essential role in the N-methyl-d-aspartate (NMDA) receptor, serving to block the calcium channel. Via this molecular function it has a role in normalizing neurological function and avoiding neurological excitotoxicity (Kirkland, Sarlo and Holton, 2018).
- Experiential evidence from the practitioner's own clinic and discussions with peers is that magnesium is helpful for clients who have anxiety, and that some have found it to be most effective in the glycinate form.
- Is there specific evidence to substantiate magnesium glycinate? No, but experientially that seems to be the case.
- Furthermore, reviewing the client's diet, the practitioner estimates her magnesium intake from diet to be quite low. The practitioner considered testing red blood cell magnesium, but, given that magnesium has low potential for harm when used at a sensible dose, elects to supplement 300 mg magnesium as glycinate, as part of an integrated programme.

Is that evidence-based? Yes, even though some EBM practitioners may argue that the decision to supplement magnesium is based on critical thinking and not on primary research from clinical or epidemiology study designs in the hierarchy pyramid and/or filtered or secondary analysis of these. Person-centred practitioners evaluate the evidence available and use a systems biology logic, applying it to the individual case in order to make a decision. This decision is then compounded by the assessment of dietary deficiency which should also be routinely corrected in practice.

Patient-reported outcome measures (PROMS)

Patient-reported outcome measures (PROMs) such as the Measure Yourself Medical Outcome Profile (MYMOP) (Paterson, 2004, 1996; Paterson and Britten, 2000; Price, Merer and MacPherson, 2006) are useful tools in this process of clinical inquiry *and* can help a clinician gather data generated within their own practice. This client-reported data on measures of wellbeing enables the practitioner to assess client progress prior to and post-interventions, and provides an opportunity for clinicians to become practitioner-researchers and build a primary evidence base that bridges the gap where other types of evidence may not be available. PROMS have been found to be useful for capturing data describing the issues of greatest concern to clients (Sales *et al.*, 2018), thereby 'humanizing' the results of clinical trials where participants are just seen as a number.

The original model for EMP advocated that the client's own preferences should be factored into decision making (Sackett, 2000). This has been reinforced by the GRADE working group which aims to develop a common, sensible and transparent approach to grading quality (or certainty) of evidence and strength of healthcare recommendations (Andrews *et al.*, 2013). This is key to decision making in personalized nutrition. Clients typically feel more empowered when they know why the decisions they are taking about what to eat are expected to have an impact on their health. PROMS provide a structured way to keep the client's priorities central to the clinical approach.

All the cases in the following chapters use some form of PROMS. Some are fully validated tools, such as the Measure Yourself Medical Outcome Profile (MYMOP) used in Chapter 7. Some are only validated by their use in clinical practice but haven't followed the validation process of the MYMOP. An example is the Medical Symptom Questionnaire (MSQ) featured in Chapter 6, which is commonly used by functional medicine practitioners. In the rest of the cases the practitioner either asks the client to rate their top symptoms on a scale of 1 through to 10 (1 being as good as it could be, 10 being as a bad as it could be) and these scores are tracked in each appointment. Alternatively, the practitioner tracks progress through the qualitative assessment of lifestyle – for example, how much time they can spend on an activity or how frequently a symptom occurs. The advantage of using a validated tool is twofold. First, its interpretation is standardized and hence easy to understand by other practitioners who may be involved in a case. Second, its output can be used to contribute to broader research. While non-validated tools may accommodate a client's individuality, they are not suitable for research purposes as they introduce a high level of heterogeneity that can contribute to bias.

Benefit versus harm

Most rational decision making in EBM is to initiate an intervention where the expected benefits outweigh the expected harm (Djulbegovic et al., 2018). If the potential to harm is high, then the evidence to justify the use of an intervention must be much more robust. For nutrients and foods, the potential for harm is far lower than for pharmaceutical agents.

This isn't to say that practitioners shouldn't be mindful of any potential harm, particularly when recommending therapeutic foods. Could an individual make him/herself sick by drinking too much kefir, eating too much broccoli or using an excessive amount of olive oil? Potentially yes, but the risks are generally low. Examples do exist – for example, foods high in histamine (which can also be foods generally considered 'healthy') may cause a problem for someone who has difficulty with histamine. Drug–food interactions must also be considered, such as that between grapefruit juice and statins (Ando et al., 2005). Thus, when working with foods in a therapeutic manner, it is wise for practitioners to be observant of any potential risks, but to focus on benefits which, in most cases, are more likely to outweigh any serious potential harm. (Drug–nutrient interactions are described in Appendix A and are discussed in the relevant cases where medications are taken.)

Evidence presented in the case studies

In each of the eight case studies, the basis of the rationale for decisions taken is provided. This includes sharing the practitioner thinking on what the underlying factors are in a case, as well as the evidence to support the specific food- and lifestyle-based interventions.

Given the complexities involved, each of the clinical decisions taken could include hundreds of individual components. The approach to presenting the evidence is a pragmatic one. To cover the totality of evidence (positive and negative) in each and every decision would be extremely lengthy and not terribly interesting to the reader. In each case study the goal has been to provide a breadth of evidence for the approach taken. In some places a greater breadth of evidence has been discussed; in other areas evidence is presented in less depth. Importantly, it is intended to demonstrate that the clinician in each case is embracing the evidence from a wide range of sources (the full pyramid of Figures 2.1 and 2.2), that they are applying clinical expertise as well as published evidence, and that client values and preferences are taken fully into account. Finally, the way that the client narrative, reflective practice (from the Q&A) and the therapeutic relationships are used within each case demonstrates how the practitioners have learned to embrace the complexity and indeed use that to further the clinical journey.

Evolving the evidence base for personalized nutrition

Is there more that could be done to build a robust evidence base in personalized nutrition? The short answer is yes. Work is already in hand with professional bodies in the industry to develop more effective tools. Emerging technologies for data collection and analysis, such as artificial intelligence and natural language processing, as well as data sharing may facilitate the process of incorporating patient-reported outcomes into trials and routine clinical practice (Wheat *et al.*, 2018), leading to the evolution of person-centered healthcare (Perez Botero, Thanarajasingam and Warsame, 2016). With an approach that uses systematic reviews and meta-analysis as a lens through which to evaluate other types of evidence such as case studies and observational or non-randomized studies, it is hoped that this book will help to establish the role of case studies within the wider evidence base for personalized nutrition.

Acknowledgements

Angela Walker and Miguel Toribio-Mateas contributed equally to the writing of this chapter. Toribio-Mateas created Figures 2.1 and 2.3.

References

Abdallah, S.M., Samman, S., 1993. The effect of increasing dietary zinc on the activity of superoxide dismutase and zinc concentration in erythrocytes of healthy female subjects. *European Journal of Clinical Nutrition* 47, 327–332.

Altman, D.G., Bland, J.M., 1995. Statistics notes: Absence of evidence is not evidence of absence. *BMJ* 311, 485. https://doi.org/10.1136/bmj.311.7003.485

Ando, H., Tsuruoka, S., Yanagihara, H., Sugimoto, K. *et al.*, 2005. Effects of grapefruit juice on the pharmacokinetics of pitavastatin and atorvastatin. *British Journal of Clinical Pharmacology* 60, 494–497. https://doi.org/10.1111/j.1365-2125.2005.02462.x

Andrews, J.C., Schünemann, H.J., Oxman, A.D., Pottie, K. *et al.*, 2013. GRADE guidelines: 15. Going from evidence to recommendation-determinants of a recommendation's direction and strength. *Journal of Clinical Epidemiology* 66, 726–735. https://doi.org/10.1016/j.jclinepi.2013.02.003

Arroll, M.A., Howard, A., 2012. A preliminary prospective study of nutritional, psychological and combined therapies for myalgic encephalomyelitis/chronic fatigue syndrome (ME/CFS) in a private care setting. *BMJ Open* 2. https://doi.org/10.1136/bmjopen-2012-001079

Bisht, B., Darling, W.G., Grossmann, R.E., Shivapour, E.T. *et al.*, 2014. A multimodal intervention for patients with secondary progressive multiple sclerosis: Feasibility and effect on fatigue. *Journal of Alternative and Complementary Medicine* 20, 347–355. https://doi.org/10.1089/act.2014.20606

Boyle, N.B., Lawton, C., Dye, L., 2017. The effects of magnesium supplementation on subjective anxiety and stress – a systematic review. *Nutrients* 9. https://doi.org/10.3390/nu9050429

Boyle, N.B., Lawton, C.L., Dye, L., 2016. The effects of magnesium supplementation on subjective anxiety. *Magnesium Research* 29, 120–125. https://doi.org/10.1684/mrh.2016.0411

Bredesen, D.E., Amos, E.C., Canick, J., Ackerley, M. *et al.*, 2016. Reversal of cognitive decline in Alzheimer's disease. *Aging* 8, 1250–1258. https://doi.org/10.18632/aging.100981

Brown, C.A., 2009. Mazes, conflict, and paradox: Tools for understanding chronic pain. *Pain Practice* 9, 235–243. https://doi.org/10.1111/j.1533-2500.2009.00279.x

Djulbegovic, B., Elqayam, S., Dale, W., 2018. Rational decision making in medicine: Implications for overuse and underuse. *Journal of Evaluation in Clinical Practice* 24, 655–665. https://doi.org/10.1111/jep.12851

Djulbegovic, B., Guyatt, G.H., 2017. Progress in evidence-based medicine: A quarter century on. *Lancet* 390, 415–423. https://doi.org/10.1016/S0140-6736(16)31592-6

Greenhalgh, T., Thorne, S., Malterud, K., 2018. Time to challenge the spurious hierarchy of systematic over narrative reviews? *European Journal of Clinical Investigation* 48, e12931. https://doi.org/10.1111/eci.12931

Innes, A.D., Campion, P.D., Griffiths, F.E., 2005. Complex consultations and the 'edge of chaos.' *British Journal of General Practice* 55, 47–52.

Katerndahl, D.A., 2009. Lessons from Jurassic Park: Patients as complex adaptive systems. *Journal of Evaluation in Clinical Practice* 15, 755–760. https://doi.org/10.1111/j.1365-2753.2009.01228.x

Kirkland, A.E., Sarlo, G.L., Holton, K.F., 2018. The role of magnesium in neurological disorders. *Nutrients* 10. https://doi.org/10.3390/nu10060730

Lee, J.E., Bisht, B., Hall, M.J., Rubenstein, L.M. *et al.*, 2017. A Multimodal, Nonpharmacologic intervention improves mood and cognitive function in people with multiple sclerosis. *Journal of the American College of Nutrition* 36, 150–168. https://doi.org/10.1080/07315724.2016.1255160

Maret, W., 2017. Zinc in cellular regulation: The nature and significance of 'zinc signals'. *International Journal of Molecular Sciences* 18. https://doi.org/10.3390/ijms18112285

Martin, C.M., Félix-Bortolotti, M., 2010. W(h)ither complexity? The emperor's new toolkit? Or elucidating the evolution of health systems knowledge? *Journal of Evaluation in Clinical Practice* 16, 415–420. https://doi.org/10.1111/j.1365-2753.2010.01461.x

Matos, A., Souza, G., Moreira, V., Luna, M., Ramalho, A., 2018. Vitamin A supplementation according to zinc status on oxidative stress levels in cardiac surgery patients. *Nutrición Hospitalaria* 35, 767–773. https://doi.org/10.20960/nh.1666

Matos, A.C., Souza, G.G., Moreira, V., Ramalho, A., 2012. Effect of vitamin A supplementation on clinical evolution in patients undergoing coronary artery bypass grafting, according to serum levels of zinc. *Nutrición Hospitalaria* 27, 1981–1986. https://doi.org/10.3305/nh.2012.27.6.5891

McCall, K.A., Huang, C., Fierke, C.A., 2000. Function and mechanism of zinc metalloenzymes. *Journal of Nutrition* 130, 1437S–46S. https://doi.org/10.1093/jn/130.5.1437S

Moncayo, R., Moncayo, H., 2017. Applying a systems approach to thyroid physiology: Looking at the whole with a mitochondrial perspective instead of judging single TSH values or why we should know more about mitochondria to understand metabolism. *BBA Clinical* 7, 127–140. https://doi.org/10.1016/j.bbacli.2017.03.004

Murad, M.H., Asi, N., Alsawas, M., Alahdab, F., 2016. New evidence pyramid. *BMJ Evidence-Based Medicine* 21, 125–127. https://doi.org/10.1136/ebmed-2016-110401

O'Dell, B.L., 2000. Role of zinc in plasma membrane function. *Journal of Nutrition* 130, 1432S–6S. https://doi.org/10.1093/jn/130.5.1432S

Paterson, C., 2004. Seeking the patient's perspective: A qualitative assessment of EuroQol, COOP-WONCA charts and MYMOP. *Quality of Life Research* 13, 871–881. https://doi.org/10.1023/B:QURE.0000025586.51955.78

Paterson, C., 1996. Measuring outcomes in primary care: A patient generated measure, MYMOP, compared with the SF-36 health survey. *BMJ* 312, 1016–1020.

Paterson, C., Britten, N., 2000. In pursuit of patient-centred outcomes: A qualitative evaluation of the 'Measure Yourself Medical Outcome Profile'. *Journal of Health Services Research and Policy* 5, 27–36. https://doi.org/10.1177/135581960000500108

Perez Botero, J., Thanarajasingam, G., Warsame, R., 2016. Capturing and incorporating patient-reported outcomes into clinical trials: Practical considerations for clinicians. *Current Oncology Reports* 18. https://doi.org/10.1007/s11912-016-0549-2

Pilchova, I., Klacanova, K., Tatarkova, Z., Kaplan, P., Racay, P., 2017. The involvement of Mg2+ in regulation of cellular and mitochondrial functions. *Oxidative Medicine and Cellular Longevity* 2017, 6797460. https://doi.org/10.1155/2017/6797460

Plsek, P.E., Greenhalgh, T., 2001. Complexity science: The challenge of complexity in health care. *BMJ* 323, 625–628.

Price, S., Mercer, S.W., MacPherson, H., 2006. Practitioner empathy, patient enablement and health outcomes: A prospective study of acupuncture patients. *Patient Education and Counselling* 63, 239–245. https://doi.org/10.1016/j.pec.2005.11.006

Rosenberg, C.E., 2002. The tyranny of diagnosis: Specific entities and individual experience. *Milbank Quarterly* 80, 237–260.

Rycroft-Malone, J., McCormack, B., Hutchinson, A.M., DeCorby, K. *et al.*, 2012. Realist synthesis: Illustrating the method for implementation research. *Implementation Science* 7, 33. https://doi.org/10.1186/1748-5908-7-33

Sackett, D.L., 2000. The fall of 'clinical research' and the rise of 'clinical-practice research'. *Clinical Investigative Medicine* 23, 379–381.

Sackett, D.L., Rosenberg, W.M., Gray, J.A., Haynes, R.B., Richardson, W.S., 1996. Evidence based medicine: What it is and what it isn't. *BMJ* 312, 71–72.

Sales, C.M., Neves, I.T., Alves, P.G., Ashworth, M., 2018. Capturing and missing the patient's story through outcome measures: A thematic comparison of patient-generated items in PSYCHLOPS with CORE-OM and PHQ-9. *Health Expectations* 21, 615–619. https://doi.org/10.1111/hex.12652

Schön, D.A., 1983. *The Reflective Practitioner*. Basic Books.

Sibbald, B., Roland, M., 1998. Understanding controlled trials. Why are randomised controlled trials important? *BMJ* 316, 201.

Sola, A., Dieppa, F.D., Rogido, M.R., 2007. An evident view of evidence-based practice in perinatal medicine: Absence of evidence is not evidence of absence. *Jornal de Pediatria* 83, 395–414. https://doi.org/10.2223/JPED.1702

Stacey, R., 1996. *Strategic Management and Organisational Dynamics: The Challenge of Complexity to Ways of Thinking about Organisations*, 1st ed. Pearson Education.

Sturmberg, J.P., Martin, C.M., Katerndahl, D.A., 2014. Systems and complexity thinking in the general practice literature: An integrative, historical narrative review. *Annals of Family Medicine* 12, 66–74. https://doi.org/10.1370/afm.1593

Truong-Tran, A.Q., Ho, L.H., Chai, F., Zalewski, P.D., 2000. Cellular zinc fluxes and the regulation of apoptosis/gene-directed cell death. *Journal of Nutrition* 130, 1459S–66S. https://doi.org/10.1093/jn/130.5.1459S

Wheat, H., Horrell, J., Valderas, J.M., Close, J., Fosh, B., Lloyd, H., 2018. Can practitioners use patient reported measures to enhance person centred coordinated care in practice? A qualitative study. *Health and Quality of Life Outcomes* 16, 223. https://doi.org/10.1186/s12955-018-1045-1

Wu, J., Xun, P., Tang, Q., Cai, W., He, K., 2017. Circulating magnesium levels and incidence of coronary heart diseases, hypertension, and type 2 diabetes mellitus: A meta-analysis of prospective cohort studies. *Nutrition Journal* 16, 60. https://doi.org/10.1186/s12937-017-0280-3

3

Functional Laboratory Testing in Personalized Nutrition

Angela Walker

Introduction

This chapter will describe the functional laboratory tests that feature in the case studies. The goal is to provide a foundation for the clinical rationale for the selection and interpretation of these tests. There is a science and an *art* to successful use of functional testing that it is hoped this chapter and the case studies will help to convey.

What is functional laboratory testing?

The term *functional testing* is used to describe tests which look at functional imbalance in biochemistry and key body systems to help to understand the potential root cause of symptoms.

The client may arrive in the personalized nutrition practitioner's office with tests from their general practitioner (GP) or consultant. Examples of such tests include full blood count, urea and electrolytes, liver function, lipid profile, thyroid profile, iron status and glucose. Sometimes these tests will have led to a diagnosis from the GP or another physician, such as anaemia or hypothyroidism. The role of functional testing is to reveal some of the mediating factors that have led to the clients' symptoms and/or primary diagnosis and provide direction for the subsequent interventions.

Functional tests may be conducted on samples of stool, saliva, urine, plasma and whole blood, and hair. It is not a 'compulsory' element of a comprehensive personalized nutrition approach and many cases can be successfully concluded without the use of functional testing. As the case studies will show, however, they can be an extremely useful tool for the practitioner and client.

Through adding data to the client 'story' of the client's experience through the identification of imbalances, functional testing can help to empower clients and add depth to the important narrative between the client and practitioner discussed in Chapter 2. When testing results show improvements over time, this can aid client compliance and motivation. From the practitioner perspective, the more data points available, the more the practitioner is able to build a personalized and scientifically based programme.

The findings from functional testing should always be considered in clinical context. This means that a practitioner does not base a recommendation on a single functional test result but looks at the clinical presentation and how the results from a single test or selection of tests help to explain or illuminate potential underlying factors involved in the case.

Since the theme of this chapter is the clinical rationale for using functional tests, there is no detailed discussion on the technologies used, nor is there an attempt to provide an exhaustive review of the evidence for each test methodology. Where available, an overview of clinically relevant studies is briefly discussed.

Functional testing for the gastrointestinal tract forms a major part of this chapter, which is to be expected given the overall importance of gastrointestinal function. Tests that examine potential sources of inflammation within the gastrointestinal tract have been included in this section. Functional testing for advanced blood lipids, stress response and multi-panels are also covered as these all feature in the subsequent cases. There is a short discussion on the rationale for the re-evaluation of blood chemistry results. The chapter concludes with a brief introduction to genetic testing and a discussion on the logistical considerations for recommending and using functional testing.

Gastrointestinal function testing

What is tested?	Stool, urine, blood, breath
Why is it tested?	• To identify qualitative and quantitative aspects of the microbiome • To identify sources of inflammation and the presence of inflammation • To identify infections and overgrowths of yeasts, bacteria and viruses • To identify increased permeability of the gastrointestinal tract and its potential causes • To identify absorption issues • To identify potential food sensitivities and cross-reactions
Chapters used	4, 5, 6, 7, 9, 10
Routine or standard tests available*	Stool test for pathogenic bacteria and parasites *Helicobacter pylori* can be tested with urea breath test, stool antigen test, or serology Faecal calprotectin
Challenges/ issues	In comprehensive stool testing there is a choice between culture- and DNA-based methodologies. No single test covers all aspects of digestive function or all triggers and mediators or symptoms Practitioners need to prioritize and make a clinical judgement on which test or combination of tests suits each case – the case studies give examples of this in practice (especially Chapters 4, 8 and 9)
Cost**	££ to £££

*Tests routinely ordered by a medical practitioner or consultant.
** Price-to-client estimates for testing used throughout this chapter; each £ represents approximately £100 to £150.

Gastrointestinal function is central to the optimal function of the human body. Personalized nutrition practitioners are drilled from day one of their training to consider digestive function in each case. Functional testing of the gastrointestinal tract is therefore very common in personalized nutrition practice. There is, however, more than one way to assess gastrointestinal function, depending on the clinical questions being asked.

In this book, every case includes consideration of gastrointestinal function through an assessment of current and historic diet and symptoms patterns. Six of the eight cases include one or more form of gastrointestinal testing in an effort to reveal root causes for the symptoms and functional imbalances experienced by the client.

One of the challenges with gastrointestinal function testing is that no single test can measure all the functional areas on which a practitioner may hope to gain information. Tests that examine gastrointestinal function can be broad, covering a number of aspects within the gastrointestinal tract, or targeted to a specific area of interest. Table 3.1 summarizes some of the tests available and how they fit into these categories.

Table 3.1 Categories of functional gastrointestinal testing

	Broad	Targeted
Examples of tests	Comprehensive stool Organic acids	Small intestinal bacterial overgrowth (SIBO) Intestinal permeability Food sensitivity IgG4 Food cross-reactivity
Sample(s) required	Stool, urine	Urine, breathe, serum, blood spot

Comprehensive stool testing

There are two main methods available for comprehensive stool testing: culture techniques and DNA analysis. The tests used in the following case studies include both methodologies.

With culture methodologies, the sample is cultured in the laboratory and the species are identified. High-throughput techniques and proteomic analysis enable rapid, comprehensive and accurate identification of bacteria and yeasts (Croxatto, Prod'hom and Greub, 2012; van Veen, Claas and Kuijper, 2010).

A potential limitation to this method is that strict anaerobes cannot be cultured and therefore cannot be identified or measured by this methodology (Kotsilkov *et al.*, 2015). Furthermore, a certain number of vital bacteria are required to form a culture; it is possible the bacteria exist in the gastrointestinal tract but at an insufficient quantity in the sample provided.

An advantage of the culture methodology is that the species cultured can be tested for susceptibility to antimicrobials, botanical and pharmaceutical. This has definite clinical utility, giving the clinician greater insight into the most effective recommendations for that individual.

Polymerase chain reaction (PCR) is the methodology used for DNA microbial analysis. PCR is a process of exponential amplification of select segments of DNA. The method is very rapid and is becoming the method of choice in acute care settings for the identification of infectious gastrointestinal pathogens (Beal *et al.*, 2017; Goldenberg *et al.*, 2015). Studies comparing PCR with culture techniques have found PCR to be more sensitive and accurate in the detection of microbes versus culture methods (Aly *et al.*, 2012; Kotsilkov *et al.*, 2015).

The limitation of the PCR methodology is that it will only report on the specific microbial DNA used in the probes of the test design. It is answering the question 'Is microbe X present?' whereas a culture methodology asks, 'Which microbes are present?'

BOX 3.1 IS PCR TOO SENSITIVE FOR CLINICAL RELEVANCE?
When PCR methodology was introduced in stool testing, concerns were raised that it was too sensitive. Does the methodology identify microbials that don't have a clinical significance or relevance? It is true, for example, that PCR methodology will report the presence microbial DNA whether the cells are alive or dead. When a microbial cell dies, however, enzymes (DNAses) actively breakdown the cellular proteins, meaning it is less likely to be picked up in a well-designed PCR assay. If a report finds a high number of microbial cells via PCR, it can be assumed these are alive in the gastrointestinal tract. If the quantity is very low, it is possible they come from dead cells, but, of course, those cells were once alive. This is another example of how quantification helps with clinical interpretation. A higher number suggests a greater relevance or significance to the case.

PCR can target specific areas on the microbial genome and there are differences in the PCR methodologies used. Standard PCR methodologies will identify the gene of the microbe but not provide the detail at a species and strain level. Next-generation sequencing simultaneously sequences and identifies different DNA fragments (Abayasekara *et al.*, 2017). Real-time PCR can identify and quantify the microbe with more detail. For example, real-time PCR (rPCR) can identify the presence of a microbe such as *Clostridium difficile* and details such as whether the bacterium carries the gene for toxin B. What rPCR cannot report is whether the bacterium is actually expressing toxin B within that individual.

Table 3.2 summarizes the main advantages and disadvantages of PCR and culture methodologies in stool testing, and elaborates on the potential clinical implications of this via two simplified clinical scenarios. The 'real' issues from the scenario are listed in the first column. The anticipated results for each methodology are provided in a very simplified version to demonstrate that both methods have their advantages.

Table 3.2 Simplified summary of comparison between culture and PCR methodologies

	Culture methodology	PCR methodology
Main advantages	Susceptibility to an antimicrobial agent can be tested leading to clinical confidence in how to address microbes identified	Quantifiable measure from a single sample of microbe probes used in the test
Main disadvantages	Strict anaerobes cannot be measured Requires sufficient microbial cells to start the culture	No sensitivity information Microbes tested need to be defined in advance May report microbes that have minimal clinical relevance (see Box 3.1)
Scenario 1		
Yeast (*Rhodotorula mucilaginosa*)	Rhodotorula cultured from the sample with a semi-quantifiable score of +3 Susceptibility to known list of antifungals provided	Rhodotorula measured quantifiably (above normal findings)
Low commensal/ beneficial bacteria	Semi-quantified (+1) measure for bifidobacterium and lactobacillus (and other beneficial/commensals)	Quantifiable measure (below normal levels) of bifidobacterium and lactobacillus along with other expected bacteria
Interpretation	Yeast present Clinical insight on antifungal agents to use and that protective microbials are at a low level	Yeast present No insight on antifungal agents to use Know that microbials which have a protective effect are low

Scenario 2		
Pathogenic parasite (Cryptosporidium)	Negative (perhaps because cell numbers of Cryptosporidium were too low in sample)	Quantifiable measurement for Cryptosporidium, above normal range
Imbalance of commensal and beneficial bacteria	No growth for beneficial bacteria May be due to anaerobic nature *or* because numbers were too low	Quantifiable measure of bifidobacterium and lactobacillus along with other expected bacteria
Interpretation	Potential underlying factor in case is missed However, insight received that protective microbe levels are low	Identification of a potential underlying factor in the case

Which of these test findings is most useful? As Table 3.2 shows, it will to some degree depend on the individual situation and the wider clinical context. In scenario 1, the ability of the culture method to identify susceptibility to the yeast may prove favourable if the patient is very sensitive to supplements or has used an antifungal protocol in the past. Susceptibility information allows for focused use of antifungals and microbials. The lack of response to a previous protocol could have been due to resistance to the antimicrobial agent used. On the other hand, the ability of a single stool sample to provide quantifiable information on all aerobic and anaerobic microbiota may prove crucial in identifying underlying factors influencing gastrointestinal and immune function, favouring PCR methodologies (scenario 2). With experience, practitioners learn how to interpret the test in clinical context and to develop confidence about which test they feel has more clinical relevance for their clinical practice.

While both methodologies have advantages and disadvantages, it is generally accepted that DNA-based analysis will be the future of comprehensive stool testing. The challenge, as outlined in Box 3.1, is in the clinical interpretation of DNA-based information. As the case studies will show, the current information provided by both types of comprehensive stool testing can be extremely useful in clinical practice.

PCR methodology laboratories may include an algorithm to calculate a diversity index – a measure of how diverse the bacterial populations are compared with a healthy cohort. There is evidence from the American Gut study (McDonald *et al.*, 2018) and a study comparing microbiome of children in Burkino Faso and Italy using DNA sequencing that diversity responds to dietary influence (De Filippo *et al.*, 2010). A reduction of microbial diversity was seen in critically ill patients compared with healthy controls (Lankelma *et al.*, 2017). Furthermore, ageing is associated with a narrowing diversity (Dinan and Cryan, 2017), while maintaining diversity may improve biological ageing (Maffei *et al.*, 2017). From a clinical intervention perspective, a review of the current evidence for nutrition- and lifestyle-based medicine concludes that microbial diversity can be improved through dietary changes (Toribio-Mateas, 2018).

Stool tests usually include other markers. Typically, this includes information on digestive capabilities, usually pancreatic elastase and the immune response with the gut. Secretory IgA (sIgA) is a well-established marker for the innate immune response in the gastrointestinal tract. Various markers are used to reflect inflammation in the gut, including calprotectin, lactoferrin and lysozyme. A detailed discussion will not be covered here; where these arise in the case studies (Chapters 6 and 8), they are discussed in more detail.

Urinary organic acids for digestive function

Urinary organic acid testing is covered in more detail below. A urinary organic test will include metabolites of bacterial and fungal origin and therefore provide information on digestive function.

Arabinose is a metabolite which has clinical relevance as indicative of yeast overgrowth in the microbiome (Shaw, Baptist and Geenens, 2010). Twenty-three children with autism were tested for arabinose, and those with high levels of arabinose compared with controls were then treated with the antifungal Nystatin; 22 out of 23 children went forward to Nystatin intervention. This resulted in a significant reduction in the severity score of autism and normalization of arabinose levels (Shaw, Kassen and Chaves, 2000).

3-(3-hydroxyphenyl)-3-hydroxypropionic acid (HPHPA) is an organic acid found to be elevated in children with autism compared with controls and in adults with recurrent diarrhoea due to *Clostridium difficile* (Keşli *et al.*, 2014; Shaw, 2010). In a study of 62 children with autism and 62 controls, HPHPA and two other metabolites of clostridia were significantly elevated in the children with autism versus controls and normalized after antimicrobial treatment (Xiong *et al.*, 2016).

These studies show that that urinary organic acid markers can have a clinical relevance for the identification of bacterial and fungal infection or overgrowth. Chapter 6 provides an example of dysbiosis identified via organic acids testing.

Small intestinal bacterial overgrowth breath test

In a normal duodenum and jejunum the concentration of bacteria is 10^4 organisms per mL this increases to 10^5 in the ileum and exponentially grows to 10^{10-12} organisms per mL in the distal colon (Lin, 2004). If bacteria start to grow and populate in the small intestine, a situation referred to as small intestinal bacterial overgrowth (SIBO), it can lead to symptoms of irritable bowel syndrome (IBS) as well as immune activation and absorption issues. Activity in the small intestine cannot be measured in stool testing, but a SIBO breath test can be used to target this area of digestive function.

In this book, a SIBO breath test was used in Chapters 4, 9 and 10, with one positive and two negative findings.

The concept of bacterial overgrowth in the small intestine is well accepted in the context of functional gastrointestinal disorders. A SIBO breath test measures the production of different gases (hydrogen and methane) by the action of the bacteria on the substrate given. Glucose and lactulose are the two substrates used in SIBO testing. Glucose is absorbed within the first 90cm of the small intestine; hence, any gases found with a glucose breath test are indicative of a bacterial overgrowth within the proximal part of the small intestine (the first 60cm). Lactulose is not digested or absorbed by the small intestine; only bacteria have the enzyme to do so, and hence the advantage of this as a substrate is that it reflects overgrowth through to the distal end of the small intestine where is it thought to be more common (Siebecker, n.d.).

A meta-analysis in 2010 of 11 studies concluded that breath tests were abnormal in IBS subjects versus healthy controls, although heterogeneity in the substrate used was found, with lactulose being the most common (Shah *et al.*, 2010). The laboratories used for testing in the following cases all use lactulose substrate.

Interpretation of the results of functional testing should always be done in clinical context. In SIBO breath testing, the results are open to interpretation based on the symptoms presented. Two leading experts in this field take slightly different views on the reference ranges, with variability depending on whether the patient experiences constipation or not. Table 3.3 summarizes the criteria (reference ranges and presence of constipation) proposed for a positive finding of SIBO by two leading SIBO experts.

Table 3.3 Expert opinions on the criteria required for a positive identification of SIBO based on findings from a hydrogen and methane breath test

	Dr Allison Siebecker criteria	Dr Nirala Jacobi criteria
Hydrogen rise	Greater than or equal to 20 ppm in 120 mins	Greater than or equal to 20 ppm in 90–100 mins
Hydrogen rise when constipation present	Greater than or equal to 20 ppm in 140 mins	
Methane	Greater than or equal to 12 ppm in 180 mins	Greater than or equal to 20 ppm in 90–100 mins
Methane rise when constipation present	3–11 ppm in 180 mins	

Dr Allison Siebecker – www.siboinfo.com
Dr Nirala Jacobi – www.thesibodoctor.com

In an excellent review, Kolacz and Porges (2018) discuss the individual variability in the transmission and receipt of pain signals in conditions such as functional bowel disorder and chronic fatigue. Furthermore, it has been shown that pain in functional gastrointestinal disorder responds to neurological stimulation in the area of the brain relating to the location of the pain signal (Kovacic *et al.*, 2017). SIBO testing can help to remove some of the subjectivity of symptom-based analysis in this area of functional imbalance; equally, testing can help to explain to clients the underlying factors involved in their symptoms, which may also aid compliance with dietary recommendations.

The laboratories will provide a detailed protocol on what should be eaten the day prior to testing; this is to control factors which might influence the absorption and metabolism of the substrate. This can be a challenge for clients who may already be on a self-imposed restricted diet. The tests have been validated based on a patient eating the test-preparation diet, so any variation from that may affect the results and needs to be factored into interpretation.

Intestinal permeability

The digestion and absorption of nutrients is a core function of the gastrointestinal tract and requires the ability for molecules (nutrients, electrolytes, water) to pass across the gastrointestinal membrane. Antigens or toxicants, however, should remain within the gastrointestinal lumen. A dynamic barrier function is therefore required – one that will allow nutrients to pass across the intestinal membrane while regulating the passage of antigens, toxicants or other harmful, disruptive molecules. Increased intestinal permeability occurs when this dynamic barrier function is disrupted and can become a triggering or mediating factor in symptoms or dysfunction.

The most established methodology for testing for increased intestinal permeability is the polyethylene glycol (PEG) test. PEG is an inert substance containing non-toxic water-soluble molecules of known and different sizes that are not metabolized either by microbiota or other cells; they are absorbed across the gastrointestinal membrane and rapidly and easily excreted in urine (Chadwick, Phillips and Hofmann, 1977). The client consumes a controlled dose of PEG and urine is collected over a six-hour period (Lloyd, 1998; Sivakumaran et al., 1982). If the recovery rate of PEG is elevated, it indicates increased intestinal permeability.

The patient must fast for three hours before the test and limit water intake to 250 mL for the first two hours of the six-hour urine collection. Patients must not be taking medicine containing Movicol (given for constipation), which is a type of PEG. The PEG test has been used to demonstrate the role of increased permeability in eczema and food sensitivity (Jackson et al., 1981).

An alternative and newer methodology involves a serum (blood) test for evidence of zonulin and LPS and other biomarkers, depending on the laboratory. Faecal zonulin can also be measured and is included in some stool test profiles (e.g. in the profile used in Chapter 4).

Zonulin is a protein found within the tight junctions between the enterocytes, cells which regulate paracellular transport across the intestinal membrane. It is the most widely researched protein in the tight junction mechanism. Elevated levels of zonulin indicate a breakdown of the tight junctions of the intestinal enterocytes and is therefore a functional marker for increased intestinal permeability (Fasano, 2012; Fasano and Shea-Donohue, 2005; Leonard et al., 2017; Sturgeon and Fasano, 2016).

Lipopolysaccharides (LPS) are large molecules consisting of a lipid and a polysaccharide found in the membranes of gram-negative bacteria. When released from bacteria, LPS trigger the production of pro-inflammatory cytokines in the gut (Lin et al., 2015; Toribio-Mateas, 2018).

Raised levels of LPS in the blood indicate translocation of LPS through the intestinal enterocytes into systemic circulation and are therefore associated with increased gastrointestinal membrane permeability. Elevated plasma LPS is associated with a phenotype characterized by higher central obesity, insulin resistance and beta cell function impairment in overweight men (Moreira et al., 2015). The level of LPS dropped significantly compared with controls in patients who underwent bariatric surgery. It is proposed that the antidiabetic effect of bariatric surgery is due to the mechanistic reduction of translocated gut bacteria and resulting reduction in plasma LPS and associated inflammation triggers (Trøseid *et al.*, 2013).

Diamine oxidase (DAO) is the body's primary enzyme for breaking down histamine; it is primarily found in the small intestine and ascending colon. If a patient has atrophy of the villi in the small intestine, the functional area for the production of diamine oxidase can be lost or significantly reduced (Maintz and Novak, 2007). Low DAO activity can cause histamine excess and symptoms of histamine sensitivity (Manzotti *et al.*, 2016). Measuring serum DAO and histamine levels represents another way to identify the possibility of intestinal permeability or dysfunction in the area of the small intestine relating to the passage of nutrients and other substances across the gastrointestinal membrane.

Serum intestinal permeability panels usually include zonulin and LPS as either one can be elevated while the other is normal, due to a different mechanism of permeability across the gastrointestinal membrane. Additional markers such as DAO, histamine and other proteins found in the tight junctions may also be added to test profiles for further insight. It can perhaps be argued that these tests provide more insight into *why* intestinal permeability is happening than a PEG test, which is simply confirming if it is occurring or not.

In Chapters 9 and 10 we will see the use of intestinal permeability testing. Chapter 9 uses the PEG test while Chapter 10 uses zonulin and LPS.

IgG food sensitivity

Dietary components represent a potential triggering and mediating factor for over-activation of the immune system in the gastrointestinal tract. Tests for immunoglobulin G (IgG) antibodies to food can be used to identify reactions referred to as delayed sensitivity to foods. There are four subclasses of IgG, known as 1, 2, 3 and 4. IgG classes 1, 2 and 3 can form large immune complexes that bind to complement and stimulate an inflammatory response. IgG4 are functionally different from the other classes, in that they do not induce complement and immune cell activation.

The goal in the identification of IgG antibodies to food is to identify what foods, if any, are triggering inflammation; testing should therefore include IgG 1, 2 and 3 subclasses. Most IgG tests include all classes. IgG4 (note the specification of subclass 4) elevations are thought to relate to the normal immune response after prolonged exposure to foods (Carr *et al.*, 2012; Stapel *et al.*, 2008) and therefore (when used in isolation from other classes) are not clinically useful for insight into immune activation in the gastrointestinal tract or sensitivity to food.

IgG (all class) antibody tests have been used in a number of published papers, a selection of which are summarized in Table 3.4.

Table 3.4 A selection of published work using IgG (all class) antibody tests

Study	Finding	Study length	Reference
Open-label pilot 20 IBS patients (Rome II criteria) IgG and IgE antibodies to foods, (plus comprehensive stool and SIBO breath test) Elimination diet based on food antibodies test results	IgG abnormalities seen in all subjects Elimination diet led to significant improvement in stool frequency, pain and quality-of-life scores	12 months	Drisko *et al.*, 2006
150 patients with IBS (Rome II criteria) Randomized to receive elimination diet based on IgG antibody results or sham diet	True diet gave 10% reduction in symptoms Rose to 26% in fully compliant patients	12 weeks	Atkinson *et al.*, 2004

Pilot study, randomized crossover Patients with Crohn's disease (CD) given elimination diet based on IgG antibody results	Significant difference was seen in IgG antibody results of the CD compared with health controls Subjects with CD receiving diet had significant improvement in pain, stool frequency and wellbeing	6 weeks	Bentz et al., 2010
Observation 30 children with obesity versus 30 controls	Children with obesity had significantly higher number of IgG antibodies, higher C-reactive protein (CRP) and increased intima media layer of the carotid arteries compared with normal-weight children	N/A	Wilders-Truschnig et al., 2008

It is proposed that elevated IgG antibodies may represent a situation of increased gastrointestinal permeability, which allows large food molecules that would ordinarily remain within the intestinal lumen to pass across the intestinal wall and into the bloodstream (Karakuła-Juchnowicz *et al.*, 2017). Personalized nutrition practitioners may therefore implement a programme to support gastrointestinal membrane integrity based on the findings of an IgG test. Part of that programme may involve short- to medium-term elimination of the foods with high IgG antibody responses, but that is only one step of the overall approach. IgG testing was used in Chapter 6 and is discussed in Chapter 9 as the client had previously undertaken an IgG test.

Cross-reactivity of foods and other antigens

In Chapter 9 a test for cross-reactivity of dietary components to gluten was used to allow the practitioner to tailor the diet which led to the reintroduction of some foods and the avoidance of others. Cross-reactivity of dietary proteins is thought to occur due to the similarity of the molecular structure of antigens from different foods (Vojdani, 2015; Vojdani and Tarash, 2013).

Tests are also available that examine cross-reactivity between foods and body tissue proteins. Cross-reactivity between gliadin dairy and human proteins from the cerebellum have been demonstrated in autistic populations (Vojdani *et al.*, 2004). When the immune response has been disrupted and the antigen contained in a food has a similar molecular structure to the epitope within a self-protein, then antibodies can be produced that will react against the food and the body's own tissues (Vojdani, 2015). Individuals who had an antibody reactivity to food proteins tended to have a higher occurrence of autoantibodies to body tissues than those without food reactivity (Lambert and Vojdani, 2017).

Panels are available that test for the presence of antibodies to environmental chemicals bound to human tissues and pathogens. In sera from 420 patients with various autoimmune conditions, the levels of antibodies to a panel of antigens, peptides and epitopes from a range of infectious agents, food proteins and xenobiotics were significantly higher for autoimmune patients versus controls (Vojdani, 2008). The author proposed that this demonstrated a pattern whereby exposure and immune reactivity to a wide range of factors may be an early instigator of an autoimmune response. These panels were part of the intake tests shown in Chapter 10.

Which test or combination of tests to use for investigation of gastrointestinal function

Deciding which test to use becomes part of the art of clinical practice. Figure 3.1 provides a proposed flowchart for the decision-making process a clinician may use. As a general rule, if the client has a selection of gastrointestinal signs and symptoms and the clinician wants to understand digestive function at a broad level, then a comprehensive stool test will usually offer the best option. If the clinician also wants to explore other areas of function – neurotransmitters and detoxification, for example – then a urinary organic acids test may be more useful, but it will not provide the depth of insight on digestive function that a comprehensive stool test can offer.

The targeted tests will generally help to bring further insight as to *why* something is occurring. The cases in Chapters 4 and 9 show how insight from targeted tests (SIBO and intestinal permeability respectively) helped to go deeper in understanding the underlying factors. In both cases a stool test was also ordered, but that alone would not have revealed the complete picture. Food sensitivity (IgG) and cross-reactivity may help to understand the role of foods and other substances as triggers and mediators, and guide the practitioner on how to tailor the recommendations, as shown in Chapters 6, 9 and 10.

With clinical experience, practitioners become very adept at identifying signs and symptoms of SIBO and therefore knowing when to order a SIBO test. This only comes with experience. At the risk of oversimplifying, if someone has digestive symptoms, but very little is revealed in a comprehensive stool test, then running a SIBO test may well reveal the underlying issues.

Chapters 6 and 9 provide examples of how practitioners look at a pattern of results from gastrointestinal function testing in combination with symptoms and case history to make an interpretation. In Chapter 6 a pattern of low beneficial bacteria, high sIgA and high D-lactate from the organic acids test led to an interpretation of dysbiosis. In Chapter 9 a pattern of low commensal bacteria, high sIgA and modest yeast was suggestive of dysbiosis (see Box 9.2 in Chapter 9) and would provide an underlying factor for the presence of increased intestinal permeability. The point is that in neither case did the practitioner base an interpretation on a single test result but on the pattern shown within the test results.

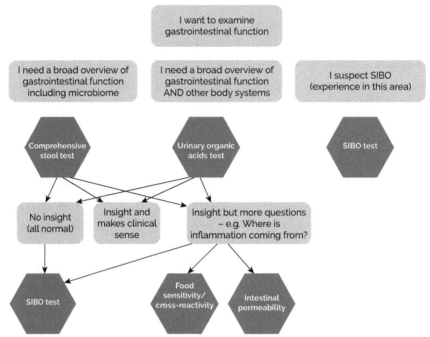

Figure 3.1 Proposed flowchart for decision making in gastrointestinal function testing

Advanced cardiovascular lipid testing

What is tested?	Whole blood, serum, plasma
Why is it tested?	For greater insight on the risk factors for cardiovascular disease
Chapters used	6, 8
Routine or standard tests available	Total cholesterol, HDL cholesterol, LDL cholesterol, triglycerides
Challenges/issues	Total cholesterol and LDL cholesterol, can over- or underestimate risk factors Additional data points potentially aid a more personalized interpretation and therefore approach
Cost	££

Advanced lipid testing extends beyond the standard total cholesterol, low-density lipoprotein cholesterol (LDL-C), high-density lipoprotein cholesterol (HDL-C) and triglycerides, and allows a look at the numbers and sizes of the lipoproteins, the cholesterol-carrying particles, as well as other atherogenic molecules (see Box 3.2).

The amount of cholesterol found in a low-density particle is variable and related to particle size, with smaller particles carrying less cholesterol than larger particles. This means that concentrations of LDL-C and LDL particle number can be discordant (lacking in harmony) (Otvos *et al.*, 2011).

Discordance analysis compares LDL-C and LDL particle number when they are discordant. Discordant analysis consistently shows an increased cardiovascular risk when the particle number is increased but total cholesterol concentration is not (Sniderman *et al.*, 2014). It therefore follows that insight into particle number provides a greater understanding of the risk factors for an individual.

For the personalized nutrition practitioner, advanced lipid tests offer two important roles, both of which are demonstrated in the cases where they are used (Chapters 6 and 8).

First, an understanding of the individual mediating factors may help to more finely tailor personalized diet and lifestyle recommendations than standard tests alone. This is clearly shown in Chapter 6 where advanced lipids were tracked while the patient was on a ketogenic-style diet and helped inform when to alter the diet recommendations. Second, the detailed insight is often a very effective way to engage the patient with their lifestyle changes; a detailed explanation of what the tests show can strongly aid compliance and the therapeutic relationship. While a client may know their cholesterol is high, that alone may not motivate them sufficiently to change. Seeing an expanded advanced lipids result, with high particle numbers and a smaller denser particle may be the catalyst to initiate lifestyle changes, as can be seen in Chapter 8. This is an example of how the additional data provided by functional testing, coupled with the practitioner's therapeutic and motivational skills may help empower a client to make lifestyle changes.

BOX 3.2 GLOSSARY OF MARKERS IN ADVANCED LIPID TESTING

Low-density lipoprotein (LDL) is not a single molecule but an aggregate of many molecules composed of protein and many molecules of cholesterol and other lipids. Cholesterol is the most abundant lipid in LDL. In a standard lipid panel, total cholesterol and HDL cholesterol are directly measured and LDL cholesterol concentration is estimated using a mathematical calculation (Cromwell *et al.*, 2007).

LDL particle number is a quantifiable measure of the number of particles within the LDL spectrum.

LDL particle size measures the diameter of particles within the LDL spectrum. An increased number of small dense LDL particles is associated with a higher risk of cardiovascular disease (CVD) than patterns containing mostly larger LDL (Diffenderfer and Schaefer, 2014).

High levels of lipoprotein (a) (Lpa(a)), which is genetic, are positively associated with an increase in CVD risk, especially when LDL-C is high (Jacobson, 2013).

Some experts prefer measuring apolipoprotein B (ApoB) rather than LDL particles. This is because every LDL, very low-density lipoprotein (VLDL), intermediate-density lipoprotein (IDL), lipoprotein (a) and remnant lipoprotein contains a single ApoB molecule. ApoB is therefore a comprehensive measure of the total number of atherogenic particles, not just those within the LDL spectrum, thus providing a way of evaluating the atherosclerotic burden for that individual (Jacobson, 2013).

Stress response testing

What is tested?	Saliva or urine
Why is it tested?	• To understand the hypothalamus–pituitary–adrenal axis function • To understand physiologically how the individual is responding to life stressors
Chapters used	5, 6, 7, 10
Routine or standard tests available	Spot serum cortisol or cortisol challenge test
Challenges/issues	How are the results going to change the recommendations made? The results can be helpful for client compliance and motivation to change
Cost	£

The hypothalamus–pituitary–adrenal (HPA) axis is the central axis through which the stress response system is controlled and activated. The HPA axis is self-regulating, with a negative feedback loop. Stimulation of the hypothalamus leads to secretion of corticotropin-releasing hormone (CRH), which tells the pituitary to release adrenocorticotropic hormone (ACTH) which tells the adrenal cortex to release cortisol. Salivary cortisol is easy to collect and has been used in research as a biomarker for stress response for many years (Clements, 2013).

Four-point salivary cortisol tests are among the best-known and most-used tests for personalized nutrition and lifestyle medicine practitioners. They are used in four cases in this book, in Chapters 5, 6, 7 and 10.

A meta-analysis of more than 200 clinical studies concluded that cortisol, as measured by saliva or serum, is elevated in humans in response to psychological stressors (Dickerson and Kemeny, 2004). The meta-analysis focused on psychological stressors such as cognitive tasks, public speaking tasks, marital conflict interactions, noise exposure, activities that would elicit an emotional response such as provocative music or film, rather than physical stressors. From the perspective of functional testing, this study provides a level of confidence that that salivary cortisol is a biomarker for the stress response. Physiological stressors such as blood glucose fluctuations, medications, nicotine, caffeine and exercise are also potential triggers for the activation of the stress response (Kudielka, Hellhammer and Wüst, 2009).

Cortisol has a circadian rhythm, as well as an ultradian rhythm (a rhythm shorter than one day but longer than one hour); furthermore, it peaks in response to a stressor, so a single measure is like aiming at a moving target. A four-point cortisol test will provide more information, but it still cannot accurately reflect smaller ultradian peaks and troughs. Although salivary cortisol is a useful biomarker for stress, there are sources of psychological and biological variation, such as age, adrenal sensitivity, adrenal capacity and cortisol binding (Hellhammer, Wüst and Kudielka, 2009). Furthermore, there are complex neurobiology mechanisms involved in how we sense and respond to stress, which allow us to detect and interpret events as either real or potential threats (stressors). Depending on whether these are physical or psychological, different networks will be engaged. Identification of a stressor activates both the sympathetic adrenomedullary (SAM) axis, secreting noradrenaline and norepinephrine, and the HPA axis, secreting cortisol. Once activated, these axes have a coordinated response that starts within seconds and can last for days (Godoy et al., 2018). In a review of salivary cortisol testing in developmental research, Clements (2013) acknowledged that cortisol, as an end product of the HPA response, is a biological indicator of stress. Variability and error can, however, arise through collection methodology and time of collection, and these need to be controlled in a research setting. What does this mean for the use of salivary cortisol testing in personalized nutrition?

In a personalized nutrition and lifestyle medicine setting, there is much greater opportunity to look at the results within clinical context. The clinician is able to ask what happened to the client on the day of the test. It is important to consider how the results support the individual's experience of over-responding to stressors or of feeling fatigued and lacking in resources to deal with day-to-day activities. This supports the imperative for the practitioner to interpret any result in clinical context. To always consider: 'How do the findings build the narrative of the client's story?'

There are newer tests, such as those using dried urine samples, that look at the relationship between cortisol and cortisone, their metabolites, and the metabolites of different catecholamines in combination with a salivary cortisol awakening response. This can be more useful in understanding the individuality of the patient's stress response, and, when used together with the organic acid markers, can include an evaluation of cofactor need. As these were not used in any of the case studies in this book, they will not be discussed here but the interested practitioner can use the resources section to explore further.

Multi-panel testing: urinary organic acids

What is tested?	Urine
Why is it tested?	• Overview of functional biochemistry • Very broad in scope of systems covered
Chapters used	4, 6
Routine or standard tests available	N/A
Challenges/issues	A lot of information gathered from the test which needs to be interpreted in clinical context
Cost	££

Organic acids are metabolic intermediates that are produced in pathways of central energy production (Krebs cycle), carbohydrate metabolism, ketone body metabolism, fatty acid beta oxidation, neurotransmitter turnover and protein metabolism.

They were originally used to identify inborn errors of metabolism (IEM) in neonates where an organic acid may be seen at a hundred- or a thousand-fold increase in comparison with those of healthy subjects.

In personalized nutrition and functional medicine, they are used to help identify functional imbalances. For example, a metabolic pathway will involve enzymatic steps which rely on micronutrient cofactors. If an organic acid is found at an elevated level, working backwards through the metabolic pathway that produces that organic acid, a blockage, potentially due to functional deficiency of a cofactor, can be the reason (Tsoukalas *et al.*, 2017).

From a single urine specimen, patterns can be identified which provide the clinician with an overview of the areas where functional imbalances may exist. An organic acids test can be expected to give clues about the following areas:

- functional vitamin and mineral status
- amino acid insufficiencies such as carnitine and N-acetyl-L-cysteine (NAC)
- oxidative damage and antioxidant need
- phase I and phase II detoxification capacity
- neurotransmitter metabolites
- mitochondrial energy production
- methylation sufficiency
- lipoic acid and coenzyme Q_{10} (CoQ_{10}) status
- functional markers for bacterial and yeast overgrowth.

Published research on organic acids

An excellent summary of the biochemical evidence linking each organic acid to nutrition, diet and lifestyle factors can be found in chapter 6 of *Laboratory Evaluations for Integrative and Functional Medicine* (Bralley and Lord, 2008). The book was written by a laboratory company and the text provides the original research sources used to compile one of the original organic acid profiles used by practitioners. Although the book is no longer in print, published papers on the profiles by the same authors (Lord and Bralley, 2008a, 2008b) are available.

Studies in autistic children have shown significant differences in levels of urinary organic acids between those with autism and neurologically normal children (Kałużna-Czaplińska, 2011; Kałużna-

Czaplińska *et al.*, 2014; Kałużna-Czaplińska, Socha and Rynkowski, 2010; Puig-Alcaraz, Fuentes-Albero and Cauli, 2016). Furthermore, supplementation of the cofactors involved in the metabolic pathways causing the elevated organic acids has been shown to lower their excretion (Kałużna-Czaplińska *et al.*, 2011).

The practitioner must remember that these types of tests are to help understand, prove or disprove the clinical questions they have surrounding a case. They are not about finding frank deficiencies but about the identification of patterns. This is shown in the way the insight from urinary organic acids testing is used in Chapters 4 and 6.

Blood chemistry tests

Although the focus of this chapter is on functional testing, it is worth mentioning that a personalized nutrition practitioner may also review conventional blood chemistry tests. Such tests may be requested from a client's medical practitioner or the client may bring these to the initial appointment.

The reference ranges used by conventional pathology laboratories typically represent where 95% of the population are placed.

> Reference ranges are valuable guides for the clinician, but they should not be regarded as absolute indicators of health and disease. Reference ranges should be used with caution, since values for healthy individuals often overlap significantly with persons afflicted with disease. (Wu, 2006, p.xvii)

The above is written in the introduction to the *Teitz Clinical Guide to Laboratory Tests*, 4th edition (Wu, 2006) which is considered an authority on laboratory testing.

As will be seen in a number of the cases in this book, where unexplained symptoms exist, the application of tighter reference ranges may be justified. Proposed reference ranges for re-evaluation of blood chemistry have been documented (Weatherby and Ferguson, 2002).

Genetic testing

The type of genetic testing most relevant to personalized nutrition is single nucleotide polymorphisms or SNPs (pronounced 'snips'). These will not be discussed in detail in this chapter, but because they feature in some of the case studies, a short introduction to the terminology used and the context for their use will be provided here.

SNPs refers to a variation of a single nucleotide base occurring at a specific position that forms the code sequence for each gene. We inherit two versions of the same gene (one from each parent). These versions are known as *alleles*. The combination of alleles determines an individual trait or characteristic (such as eye colour).

If two alleles are identical, this is known as homozygous. In test reporting, this is denoted as ++. If the two alleles are different, this is known as heterozygous, or + –. The allele that codes for the most popular version of a trait in a given population is called the 'wild type' allele. All SNPs are compared to the wild type.

SNPs are the most common form of genetic variation among individuals. Although the majority of SNPs have limited impact on an individual's overall health, some SNPs may influence how an individual will respond to dietary and lifestyle interventions, tolerance of medication and toxins, or susceptibility to developing certain diseases. An individual may carry the SNP but it may not be expressed. Furthermore, SNPs do not operate in isolation; they operate in a symphony of numerous other SNPs and it is likely that other SNPs are expressed to stabilize the overall biochemistry. For these reasons, it is very important to review the potential impact of SNPs in the context of a full case history.

SNPs are reported and discussed in Chapters 6, 7 and 10. In these cases, functional tests have also been used which help the practitioner to understand the wider potential implication of a SNP, whether it is expressed and/or is being stabilized by other factors. The interpretation is made using the findings of the functional tests as well as a wider consideration of the case history. Chapters 7 and 10 in particular contain discussions on the caution needed in the interpretation and consideration of SNPs within the wider clinical context.

Although it can be empowering for individuals in terms of knowledge and insights for personalizing their diet and lifestyle, such knowledge also has the potential to cause worry and anxiety if one learns that one has a SNP which has a potential association with an increased risk for a disease. Clients may also bring results of genetic tests that they have carried out independently with them to a personalized nutrition consultation. Potential strengths and limitations of genetic tests are best explored with clients prior to undertaking them and to gain their informed consent.

The topic of genetic testing is covered extensively in the sister publication of this series *Using Nutrigenomics within Personalized Nutrition* (2020).

Logistical considerations of testing

Cost

The cost implications of functional testing cannot be ignored. There are examples throughout the cases where practitioners considered a particular test or follow-up but did not go ahead with it due to cost implications.

Financial restraints can add to the complexity of decision making for practitioners. Financial limitations are also a real factor for many clients, especially when their health is impacting on their ability to earn. Practitioners can liaise with the client's primary medical practitioner, presenting a rationale which may facilitate free-to-client access to tests. This approach was used in Chapters 4 and 11.

It is important for the practitioner to remain neutral and to avoid making assumptions as to the affordability of testing for an individual. Practitioners can present the case for testing, explaining how they will inform decision making and case management.

What if that test unlocks a clue that helps resolve the client's health issue in two months rather than three years? An individual with chronic fatigue syndrome (CFS) costs the UK economy just under £17,000 per year (2020 Health, 2017), without taking into account the intangible costs of that person's loss of independence and quality of life. In that context asking them to spend £300 to £500 or more on testing may represent a good return on their investment.

This is not intended to diminish the very real financial challenges faced by patients who have poor health. It is, however, important to fully evaluate the potential that functional testing can bring with regard to resolving health when it is used intelligently and strategically by practitioners.

Fear

Clients may be fearful of completing tests. Many individuals find the injections involved in blood samples unpleasant. Meanwhile, the concept of collecting a sample of stool, urine or saliva may strike many individuals as unusual. This is where the therapeutic relationship between the client and practitioner becomes important. The practitioner's coaching or mentoring style and the rational case they present to the client can ease these fears or uncertainties.

Liaising with medical practitioners

There may be cases where functional testing identifies factors that warrant further medical investigations. Examples would be blood found in a stool sample that could indicate a serious pathology or a blood test that identifies a thyroid autoimmunity disorder. In such cases it is important to communicate effectively with the client's primary medical practitioners. In such cases, data protection issues meet professional ethical issues. A practitioner's professional body will typically provide guidance on how to manage this process.

Sharing test findings with other practitioners is good practice from the perspective of integrative and collaborative client case. Chapter 8 provides an example of how this can be effectively managed.

Explaining test results

It is important to explain the context of test results to clients rather than simply share the data of the results. The practitioner can help the client understand the overall story of their health through explaining what the tests mean in context. Why did this occur? What are the likely triggers and mediators? How might this relate to symptoms? These are all valid questions that help put test results in context for the client. The language used to share this information is important – a style that is neutral, non-judgemental, informative, clear and open. It is important for practitioners to develop the skills required to present functional testing to clients in a meaningful way. The cases presented in this book will help the practitioner to develop these important skills that are fundamental to the art of practice introduced in Chapter 1.

Questions to ask of a laboratory

Many of the laboratories offering functional testing are distributing tests that are processed in another country. Accreditation as a medical laboratory is therefore not always available to them (and is not necessarily compulsory). A practitioner who asks for information on a laboratory's quality control procedures and practices can reassure themselves that the laboratory is conducting testing to an appropriate standard in lieu of formal accreditation.

References

2020 Health, 2017. *Counting the Cost: Chronic Fatigue Syndrome/Myalgic Encephalomyelitis.* Accessed on 26/05/2019 at www.meassociation.org.uk/wp-content/uploads/2020Health-Counting-the-Cost-Sept-2017.pdf

Abayasekara, L.M., Perera, J., Chandrasekharan, V., Gnanam, V.S. *et al.*, 2017. Detection of bacterial pathogens from clinical specimens using conventional microbial culture and 16S metagenomics: A comparative study. *BMC Infectious Diseases* 17. https://doi.org/10.1186/s12879-017-2727-8

Aly, B.H., Hamad, M.S., Mohey, M., Amen, S., 2012. Polymerase chain reaction (PCR) versus bacterial culture in detection of organisms in otitis media with effusion (OME) in children. *Indian Journal of Otolaryngology and Head and Neck Surgery* 64, 51–55. https://doi.org/10.1007/s12070-011-0161-6

Atkinson, W., Sheldon, T.A., Shaath, N., Whorwell, P.J., 2004. Food elimination based on IgG antibodies in irritable bowel syndrome: A randomised controlled trial. *Gut* 53, 1459–1464. https://doi.org/10.1136/gut.2003.037697

Beal, S.G., Tremblay, E.E., Toffel, S., Velez, L., Rand, K.H., 2017. A gastrointestinal PCR panel improves clinical management and lowers health care costs. *Journal of Clinical Microbiology* 56. https://doi.org/10.1128/JCM.01457-17

Bentz, S., Hausmann, M., Piberger, H., Kellermeier, S. *et al.*, 2010. Clinical relevance of IgG antibodies against food antigens in Crohn's disease: A double-blind cross-over diet intervention study. *Digestion* 81, 252–264. https://doi.org/10.1159/000264649

Bralley, J.A., Lord, R.S., 2008. *Laboratory Evaluations for Integrative and Functional Medicine,* 2nd ed. Metametrix Institute.

Carr, S., Chan, E., Lavine, E., Moote, W., 2012. CSACI Position statement on the testing of food-specific IgG. *Allergy, Asthma and Clinical Immunology* 8, 12. https://doi.org/10.1186/1710-1492-8-12

Chadwick, V.S., Phillips, S.F., Hofmann, A.F., 1977. Measurements of intestinal permeability using low molecular weight polyethylene glycols (PEG 400). I. Chemical analysis and biological properties of PEG 400. *Gastroenterology* 73, 241–246.

Clements, A.D., 2013. Salivary cortisol measurement in developmental research: Where do we go from here? *Developmental Psychobiology* 55, 205–220. https://doi.org/10.1002/dev.21025

Cromwell, W.C., Otvos, J.D., Keyes, M.J., Pencina, M.J. *et al.*, 2007. LDL particle number and risk of future cardiovascular disease in the Framingham Offspring Study – implications for LDL management. *Journal of Clinical Lipidology* 1, 583–592. https://doi.org/10.1016/j.jacl.2007.10.001

Croxatto, A., Prod'hom, G., Greub, G., 2012. Applications of MALDI-TOF mass spectrometry in clinical diagnostic microbiology. *FEMS Microbiology Reviews* 36, 380–407. https://doi.org/10.1111/j.1574-6976.2011.00298.x

De Filippo, C., Cavalieri, D., Di Paola, M., Ramazzotti, M. *et al.*, 2010. Impact of diet in shaping gut microbiota revealed by a comparative study in children from Europe and rural Africa. *Proceedings of the National Academy of Sciences of the United States of America* 107, 14691–14696. https://doi.org/10.1073/pnas.1005963107

Dickerson, S.S., Kemeny, M.E., 2004. Acute stressors and cortisol responses: A theoretical integration and synthesis of laboratory research. *Psychological Bulletin* 130, 355–391. https://doi.org/10.1037/0033-2909.130.3.355

Diffenderfer, M.R., Schaefer, E.J., 2014. The composition and metabolism of large and small LDL. *Current Opinion in Lipidology* 25, 221–226. https://doi.org/10.1097/MOL.0000000000000067

Dinan, T.G., Cryan, J.F., 2017. Gut instincts: Microbiota as a key regulator of brain development, ageing and neurodegeneration. *Journal of Physiology* 595, 489–503. https://doi.org/10.1113/JP273106

Drisko, J., Bischoff, B., Hall, M., McCallum, R., 2006. Treating irritable bowel syndrome with a food elimination diet followed by food challenge and probiotics. *Journal of the American College of Nutrition* 25, 514–522.

Fasano, A., 2012. Intestinal permeability and its regulation by zonulin: Diagnostic and therapeutic implications. *Clinical Gastroenterology and Hepatology* 10, 1096–1100. https://doi.org/10.1016/j.cgh.2012.08.012

Fasano, A., Shea-Donohue, T., 2005. Mechanisms of disease: The role of intestinal barrier function in the pathogenesis of gastrointestinal autoimmune diseases. *Nature Clinical Practice Gastroenterology and Hepatology* 2, 416–422. https://doi.org/10.1038/ncpgasthep0259

Godoy, L.D., Rossignoli, M.T., Delfino-Pereira, P., Garcia-Cairasco, N., de Lima Umeoka, E.H., 2018. A comprehensive overview on stress neurobiology: Basic concepts and clinical implications. *Frontiers in Behavioral Neuroscience* 12, 127. https://doi.org/10.3389/fnbeh.2018.00127

Goldenberg, S.D., Bacelar, M., Brazier, P., Bisnauthsing, K., Edgeworth, J.D., 2015. A cost benefit analysis of the Luminex xTAG Gastrointestinal Pathogen Panel for detection of infectious gastroenteritis in hospitalised patients. *Journal of Infection* 70, 504–511. https://doi.org/10.1016/j.jinf.2014.11.009

Hellhammer, D.H., Wüst, S., Kudielka, B.M., 2009. Salivary cortisol as a biomarker in stress research. *Psychoneuroendocrinology* 34, 163–171. https://doi.org/10.1016/j.psyneuen.2008.10.026

Jackson, P.G., Lessof, M.H., Baker, R.W., Ferrett, J., MacDonald, D.M., 1981. Intestinal permeability in patients with eczema and food allergy. *Lancet* 1, 1285–1286.

Jacobson, T.A., 2013. Lipoprotein(a), cardiovascular disease, and contemporary management. *Mayo Clinic Proceedings* 88, 1294–1311. https://doi.org/10.1016/j.mayocp.2013.09.003

Kałużna-Czaplińska, J., 2011. Noninvasive urinary organic acids test to assess biochemical and nutritional individuality in autistic children. *Clinical Biochemistry* 44, 686–691. https://doi.org/10.1016/j.clinbiochem.2011.01.015

Kałużna-Czaplińska, J., Socha, E., Rynkowski, J., 2011. B vitamin supplementation reduces excretion of urinary dicarboxylic acids in autistic children. *Nutrition Research* 31, 497–502. https://doi.org/10.1016/j.nutres.2011.06.002

Kałużna-Czaplińska, J., Socha, E., Rynkowski, J., 2010. Determination of homovanillic acid and vanillylmandelic acid in urine of autistic children by gas chromatography/mass spectrometry. *Medical Science Monitor* 16, CR445–450.

Kałużna-Czaplińska, J., Żurawicz, E., Struck, W., Markuszewski, M., 2014. Identification of organic acids as potential biomarkers in the urine of autistic children using gas chromatography/mass spectrometry. *Journal of Chromatography B* 966, 70–76. https://doi.org/10.1016/j.jchromb.2014.01.041

Karakuła-Juchnowicz, H., Szachta, P., Opolska, A., Morylowska-Topolska, J. *et al.*, 2017. The role of IgG hypersensitivity in the pathogenesis and therapy of depressive disorders. *Nutritional Neuroscience* 20, 110–118. https://doi.org/10.1179/147683051 4Y.0000000158

Keşli, R., Gökçen, C., Buluğ, U., Terzi, Y., 2014. Investigation of the relation between anaerobic bacteria genus clostridium and late-onset autism etiology in children. *Journal of Immunoassay and Immunochemistry* 35, 101–109. https://doi.org/10.1080/15321819.2013.792834

Kolacz, J., Porges, S.W., 2018. Chronic diffuse pain and functional gastrointestinal disorders after traumatic stress: Pathophysiology through a polyvagal perspective. *Frontiers in Medicine* 5. https://doi.org/10.3389/fmed.2018.00145

Kotsilkov, K., Popova, C., Boyanova, L., Setchanova, L., Mitov, I., 2015. Comparison of culture method and real-time PCR for detection of putative periodontopathogenic bacteria in deep periodontal pockets. *Biotechnology and Biotechnological Equipment* 29, 996–1002. https://doi.org/10.1080/13102818.2015.1058188

Kovacic, K., Hainsworth, K., Sood, M., Chelimsky, G. *et al.*, 2017. Neurostimulation for abdominal pain-related functional gastrointestinal disorders in adolescents: A randomised, double-blind, sham-controlled trial. *Lancet Gastroenterology and Hepatology* 2, 727–737. https://doi.org/10.1016/S2468-1253(17)30253-4

Kudielka, B.M., Hellhammer, D.H., Wüst, S., 2009. Why do we respond so differently? Reviewing determinants of human salivary cortisol responses to challenge. *Psychoneuroendocrinology* 34, 2–18. https://doi.org/10.1016/j.psyneuen.2008.10.004

Lambert, J., Vojdani, A., 2017. Correlation of tissue antibodies and food immune reactivity in randomly selected patient specimens. *Journal of Clinical and Cellular Immunology* 8, 1–10. https://doi.org/10.4172/2155-9899.1000521

Lankelma, J.M., van Vught, L.A., Belzer, C., Schultz, M.J. *et al.*, 2017. Critically ill patients demonstrate large interpersonal variation in intestinal microbiota dysregulation: A pilot study. *Intensive Care Medicine* 43, 59–68. https://doi.org/10.1007/s00134-016-4613-z

Leonard, M.M., Sapone, A., Catassi, C., Fasano, A., 2017. Celiac disease and nonceliac gluten sensitivity: A review. *JAMA* 318, 647. https://doi.org/10.1001/jama.2017.9730

Lin, H.C., 2004. Small intestinal bacterial overgrowth: A framework for understanding irritable bowel syndrome. *JAMA* 292, 852–858. https://doi.org/10.1001/jama.292.7.852

Lin, R., Zhou, L., Zhang, J., Wang, B., 2015. Abnormal intestinal permeability and microbiota in patients with autoimmune hepatitis. *International Journal of Clinical and Experimental Pathology* 8, 5153–5160.

Lloyd, J.B., 1998. Intestinal permeability to polyethyleneglycol and sugars: A re-evaluation. *Clinical Science* 95, 107–110.

Lord, R.S., Bralley, J.A., 2008a. Clinical applications of urinary organic acids. Part 1: Detoxification markers. *Alternative Medicine Review* 13, 205–215.

Lord, R.S., Bralley, J.A., 2008b. Clinical applications of urinary organic acids. Part 2. Dysbiosis markers. *Alternative Medicine Review* 13, 292–306.

Maffei, V.J., Kim, S., Blanchard, E., Luo, M. *et al.*, 2017. Biological aging and the human gut microbiota. *Journals of Gerontology Series A* 72, 1474–1482. https://doi.org/10.1093/gerona/glx042

Maintz, L., Novak, N., 2007. Histamine and histamine intolerance. *American Journal of Clinical Nutrition* 85, 1185–1196. https://doi.org/10.1093/ajcn/85.5.1185

Manzotti, G., Breda, D., Di Gioacchino, M., Burastero, S.E., 2016. Serum diamine oxidase activity in patients with histamine intolerance. *International Journal of Immunopathology and Pharmacology* 29, 105–111. https://doi.org/10.1177/0394632015617170

McDonald, D., Hyde, E., Debelius, J.W., Morton, J.T. *et al.*, 2018. American Gut: An open platform for citizen science microbiome research. *mSystems* 3. https://doi.org/10.1128/mSystems.00031-18

Moreira, A.P.B., Alves, R.D.M., Teixeira, T.F.S., Macedo, V.S. *et al.*, 2015. Higher plasma lipopolysaccharide concentrations are associated with less favorable phenotype in overweight/obese men. *European Journal of Nutrition* 54, 1363–1370. https://doi.org/10.1007/s00394-014-0817-6

Otvos, J.D., Mora, S., Shalaurova, I., Greenland, P., Mackey, R.H., Goff, D.C., 2011. Clinical implications of discordance between low-density lipoprotein cholesterol and particle number. *Journal of Clinical Lipidology* 5, 105–113. https://doi.org/10.1016/j.jacl.2011.02.001

Puig-Alcaraz, C., Fuentes-Albero, M., Cauli, O., 2016. Relationship between adipic acid concentration and the core symptoms of autism spectrum disorders. *Psychiatry Research* 242, 39–45. https://doi.org/10.1016/j.psychres.2016.05.027

Shah, E.D., Basseri, R.J., Chong, K., Pimentel, M., 2010. Abnormal breath testing in IBS: A meta-analysis. *Digestive Diseases and Sciences* 55, 2441–2449. https://doi.org/10.1007/s10620-010-1276-4

Shaw, W., 2010. Increased urinary excretion of a 3-(3-hydroxyphenyl)-3-hydroxypropionic acid (HPHPA), an abnormal phenylalanine metabolite of Clostridia spp. in the gastrointestinal tract, in urine samples from patients with autism and schizophrenia. *Nutritional Neuroscience* 13, 135–143. https://doi.org/10.1179/147683010X12611460763968

Shaw, W., Baptist, J., Geenens, D., 2010. Immunodeficiency, gastrointestinal candidiasis, wheat and dairy sensitivity, abnormal urine arabinose, and autism: A case study. *North American Journal of Medicine and Science* 3, 1.

Shaw, W., Kassen, E., Chaves, E., 2000. Assessment of antifungal drug therapy in autism by measurement of suspected microbial metabolites in urine with gas chromatography-mass spectrometry. *Clinical Practice of Alternative Medicine* 1, 15–26.

Siebecker, A., n.d. SIBO Testing. Accessed on 26/05/2019 at www.siboinfo.com/testing1.html

Sivakumaran, T., Jenkins, R.T., Walker, W.H., Goodacre, R.L., 1982. Simplified measurement of polyethylene glycol 400 in urine. *Clinical Chemistry* 28, 2452–2453.

Sniderman, A.D., Lamarche, B., Contois, J.H., de Graaf, J., 2014. Discordance analysis and the Gordian Knot of LDL and non-HDL cholesterol versus apoB. *Current Opinion in Lipidology* 25, 461–467. https://doi.org/10.1097/MOL.0000000000000127

Stapel, S.O., Asero, R., Ballmer-Weber, B.K., Knol, E.F. *et al.*, 2008. Testing for IgG4 against foods is not recommended as a diagnostic tool: EAACI Task Force Report. *Allergy* 63, 793–796. https://doi.org/10.1111/j.1398-9995.2008.01705.x

Sturgeon, C., Fasano, A., 2016. Zonulin, a regulator of epithelial and endothelial barrier functions, and its involvement in chronic inflammatory diseases. *Tissue Barriers* 4, e1251384. https://doi.org/10.1080/21688370.2016.1251384

Toribio-Mateas, M., 2018. Harnessing the power of microbiome assessment tools as part of neuroprotective nutrition and lifestyle medicine interventions. *Microorganisms* 6. https://doi.org/10.3390/microorganisms6020035

Trøseid, M., Nestvold, T.K., Rudi, K., Thoresen, H., Nielsen, E.W., Lappegård, K.T., 2013. Plasma lipopolysaccharide is closely associated with glycemic control and abdominal obesity: Evidence from bariatric surgery. *Diabetes Care* 36, 3627–3632. https://doi.org/10.2337/dc13-0451

Tsoukalas, D., Alegakis, A., Fragkiadaki, P., Papakonstantinou, E. *et al.*, 2017. Application of metabolomics: Focus on the quantification of organic acids in healthy adults. *International Journal of Molecular Medicine* 40, 112–120. https://doi.org/10.3892/ijmm.2017.2983

van Veen, S.Q., Claas, E.C.J., Kuijper, E.J., 2010. High-throughput identification of bacteria and yeast by matrix-assisted laser desorption ionization-time of flight mass spectrometry in conventional medical microbiology laboratories. *Journal of Clinical Microbiology* 48, 900–907. https://doi.org/10.1128/JCM.02071-09

Vojdani, A., 2015. Molecular mimicry as a mechanism for food immune reactivities and autoimmunity. *Alternative Therapies in Health and Medicine* 21 Suppl 1, 34–45.

Vojdani, A., 2008. Antibodies as predictors of complex autoimmune diseases. *International Journal of Immunopathology and Pharmacology* 21, 267–278. https://doi.org/10.1177/039463200802100203

Vojdani, A., O'Bryan, T., Green, J.A., Mccandless, J. *et al.*, 2004. Immune response to dietary proteins, gliadin and cerebellar peptides in children with autism. *Nutritional Neuroscience* 7, 151–161. https://doi.org/10.1080/10284150400004155

Vojdani, A., Tarash, I., 2013. Cross-Reaction between gliadin and different food and tissue antigens. *Food and Nutrition Sciences* 4, 20. https://doi.org/10.4236/fns.2013.41005

Weatherby, D., Ferguson, S., 2002. *Blood Chemistry and CBC Analysis: Clinical Laboratory Testing from a Functional Perspective*. Bear Mountain Publishing.

Wilders-Truschnig, M., Mangge, H., Lieners, C., Gruber, H.-J., Mayer, C., März, W., 2008. IgG antibodies against food antigens are correlated with inflammation and intima media thickness in obese juveniles. *Experimental and Clinical Endocrinology and Diabetes* 116, 241–245. https://doi.org/10.1055/s-2007-993165

Wu, A.H.B., 2006. *Tietz Clinical Guide to Laboratory Tests*, 4th ed. Saunders.

Xiong, X., Liu, D., Wang, Y., Zeng, T., Peng, Y., 2016. Urinary 3-(3-Hydroxyphenyl)-3-hydroxypropionic acid, 3-Hydroxyphenylacetic acid, and 3-Hydroxyhippuric acid are elevated in children with autism spectrum disorders. *BioMed Research International* 2016, 9485412. https://doi.org/10.1155/2016/9485412

4

Recurrent Urinary Tract Infections (UTIs) with Antibiotic Dependency

Practitioner: Lorraine Nicolle

Setting the scene

In this case there was a clearly expressed aim: to be rid of a seemingly entrenched vulnerability to urinary tract infections (UTIs). The case shows that, rather than simply 'treating the condition', the use of a *personalized*, systems-based approach brought about resolution of the longer-term vulnerability to the infections, as well as improvements in many other health issues that the client had hitherto come to accept as 'just part of getting older'. These included other medical diagnoses, namely irritable bowel syndrome with constipation (IBS-C), sinusitis, arthralgia and gastro-oesophageal reflux. Medical investigations had found no organic pathologies within the colon, stomach or oesophagus.

A UTI is a microbial infection that can affect any part of the urinary tract, including the bladder (cystitis), urethra (urethritis) or kidneys (pyelonephritis). The cause is usually cross-contamination of microbes in the faeces (most commonly *Escherichia coli*). The lining of the urethra and bladder become irritated as a result.

Factors increasing vulnerability include pregnancy, kidney stones, urinary catheters, constipation (if it compromises bladder emptying), diabetes and a weakened immune system.

National Health Service (NHS) advice on reducing risk includes tips on faecal hygiene, drinking plenty of fluids, urinating regularly and fully emptying the bladder, showering instead of bathing, wearing loose cotton underwear rather than tight, synthetic clothing and avoiding spermicidal lubricants or perfumed personal care products (NHS, 2017).

Medical treatment usually comprises antibiotics and painkillers. Antibiotics courses may span anything from three days to six months in recurrent cases and may also include agents to acidify the urine, in order to help prevent reinfection. Prescriptions may be preceded by urine analysis for bacteria, red cells or pus, and possibly a urine culture to identify the bacterial species.

Initial case presentation

TT is a 52-year-old professional female presenting with a 13-year history of recurrent UTIs. The UTIs cause debilitating symptoms: frequent attacks of painful, 'stinging' urination, bladder urgency, throbbing pain in the urethra, lower abdominal discomfort and general fatigue, weakness, irritability, apathy and 'brain fog'.

She felt reliant on repeat courses of antibiotics (trimethoprim, nitrofurantoin and, more recently, methenamine hippurate and ciprofloxacin) from which she experienced 'exhausting' side effects, yet UTI symptoms resurged if medication was stopped. Paracetamol was taken regularly during attacks.

Recently, the UTI attacks have appeared to trigger sinus pain and nasal congestion, and to worsen her gastro-oesophageal reflux and IBS-C symptoms.

The initial consultation was undertaken one month after TT finished the last antibiotic course. She was again suffering UTI and sinus symptoms. She had decided not to take more medications in the immediate future and was keen to gain insight into the underlying causes of her problems.

Her primary goal was to be free of recurrent UTIs. The lack of progress over many years left her overwhelmed with stress, pessimism and confusion about how to improve her situation.

In-depth interviewing elicited the following key points from her timeline:

- Family history of asthma, allergies, alcoholism and cardiovascular disease (CVD).
- Normal birth, breastfed for six weeks, normal childhood illnesses and immunizations.
- IBS-C symptoms from age 13. She was prescribed a 'high-fibre' diet, which helped somewhat but symptoms recurred intermittently during her 20s and 30s.
- Stress in her late 20s from her divorce and the death of her father.
- Age 32, moved to Egypt for work (management consultant). Gastroenteritis (approximately four episodes). Sometimes treated with antibiotics, other times no treatment sought. Occasional painful sinus symptoms started – usually self-limiting but antibiotics taken on two occasions. (She still had occasional flare-ups to the present day, more recently coinciding with UTI symptoms.)
- Age 36, moved back to the UK. Developed appendicitis and had appendectomy.
- Age 36–40, worked in a global role – worldwide travel. Age 39 started to develop UTIs and embarked on repeated courses of antibiotics.
- Age 45, stress from second divorce. Since then, increasing stress load from bereavements, loss of job and worsening health.
- Age 51, diagnosis (via biopsy) of chronic infection within the urothelium. Prescribed a three-month course of ciprofloxacin that TT was unable to complete due to side effects of leg pains, poor appetite, nausea, diarrhoea, anxiety and insomnia. Severe pain in bladder after stopping the antibiotics. Prescribed methenamine hippurate but after six weeks there was no improvement, so she decided to stop. TT reported that medics have said her ongoing symptoms could either be due to a bacterial infection within the

urothelium or due to compromised structure of the urothelium, secondary to long-term antibiotic use.

TT believed she was post-menopausal (last menstruation age 50). At interview, she reported being unaware of any associated symptoms. However, she had recently experienced abdominal weight gain and vaginal dryness.

Current symptoms
Painful, 'stinging' urination, bladder urgency, chronic bladder and urethral pain, lower abdominal discomfort, now coinciding with sinus pain and itchy, watery eyes and nose, general fatigue, weakness, irritability, apathy and 'brain fog'. Ongoing gastro-oesophageal reflux, abdominal distention after eating (TT cannot associate this with any particular foods), constipation, straining on defecation, belching, odorous flatulence, muscular and joint stiffness and aches (arthralgia), low mood, anxiety, often tearful, feels run down and often overwhelmed with stress, frequent headaches (three days out of seven), vaginal dryness, prone to swollen lymph nodes and hayfever, bruxism (dentist has prescribed a mouth guard), cravings for sugars and starches, occasional episodes of uncontrolled (binge) eating, and dizziness and irritability if a meal is skipped, abdominal weight gain (waist-to-hip ratio of 1).

Current diet
TT's diet was consciously low in gluten and processed foods (believing this may help her symptoms), and unconsciously low in oily fish and red meat (taste aversion). A typical day comprised:

- 7am: porridge with semi-skimmed milk and stewed apple or honey.
- Midday: baked beans on gluten-free (GF) toast; or shop-bought soup and GF roll; apple or pear and 70% chocolate (approx. 35g).
- Snack: oatcakes or rice cakes and hummus or avocado or cottage cheese; or a commercial nut-seed-cereal bar; or a handful mixed nuts; or crisps (vegetable crisps where possible).

- GF pasta with tomato and vegetable sauce with cheese; or fish or chicken with mixed vegetables and sweet potatoes/squash, brown rice or GF pasta.
- Yogurt and stewed seasonal fruit (plums, apples, pears, rhubarb, etc.).
- 3 pints (1.7 litres) water and three teas with semi-skimmed milk.
- No alcohol (due to family history of alcoholism).

Following her own research, she had self-prescribed probiotics (various strains of *Lactobacilli* and *Bifidobacteria*) and peppermint oil (for the IBS), D-mannose (for the UTIs) and glucosamine sulphate (for the arthralgia). She reported no improvement in her symptoms after three months of taking these, and that she feels her health is continually declining.

Investigations

- Recent full blood count, haematology and biochemistry bloods, including haemoglobin, alpha 1 (HbA1c) (glycated haemoglobin), showed nothing out of range.
- The practitioner made a referral to TT's GP requesting markers for immune function and inflammation, namely serum vitamin D, CRP (C-reactive protein), ESR (erythrocyte sedimentation rate) and ferritin; and also to discuss the post-menopausal vaginal discomfort. A key question the practitioner had in mind was whether menopausal vaginal atrophy is present. Any such diagnosis would signal the possibility that structural support may be lacking for mucous membranes generally, including the urothelium. Might this potentiate TT's vulnerability to UTIs? (Following this referral, the client was prescribed a vaginal pessary delivering localized oestrogen but TT took the decision not to proceed with this.)
- The following functional laboratory tests were ordered (see Chapter 3 for a fuller discussion on functional testing):
  - Lactulose breath test to identify the presence of any small intestine bacterial overgrowth (SIBO). This was due to TT's many symptoms associated with excessive GI gas production.

- Stool analysis of the microbiome (plus zonulin levels). This was primarily to identify any microbial infection in the large intestine, given TT's history of gastroenteritis and international travel, and because of her history of antibiotics, which can disrupt the microbiota, enabling opportunistic microbes to proliferate.
- Urinary organic acids, as a relatively cost-effective way to assess multiple body systems and functional nutrient deficiencies that may affect immune system function and the propensity to recurrent infections. For this client, the practitioner was also interested in markers relating to neurotransmitter and stress hormone metabolites, mitochondrial energy production, glycaemic control and detoxification.
- Plasma homocysteine, given the history of toxicity-related (medications and infections) and stress-related burdens on the methylation system, the family history of CVD and the symptoms of poor cognition and low mood.

Case interpretation and analysis

The practitioner used a functional matrix (based on the Institute of Functional Medicine model) to identify possible underlying contributory factors to TT's compromised health, which would in turn help to inform decision making about potential interventions.

Digestion and assimilation

- Symptoms indicated functional gastrointestinal imbalances such as possible dysbiosis, microbial infection, intestinal hyperpermeability, insufficient digestive secretions, immune system reactivity (loss of 'immune tolerance') and/or gut–brain neurological disruption.
- History of international travel, stress, gastroenteritis and antibiotics may predispose TT to such dysfunctions.

Communication: hypothalamus–pituitary–ovarian (HPO) axis

The practitioner hypothesized that a sharp drop in circulating oestrogen levels (post-menopausal) may be contributing to:

- reduced collagen integrity (vaginal dryness, vulnerable urothelium, arthralgia) (Powell, Dhaher and Szleifer, 2015; Thornton, 2013)
- diminished serotonin levels and receptor function (low mood and anxiety) (Ryan and Ancelin, 2012)
- transient inflammation (arthralgia, immune system reactivity re. itchy, watery eyes, sinusitis, UTI symptoms and associated malaise, low mood and anxiety) (Kiecolt-Glaser, Derry and Fagundes, 2015; McCormick, 2007).

Communication: hypothalamus–pituitary–adrenal (HPA) axis

- A history of stress inputs and the numerous symptoms of stress and fatigue indicate a possible dysregulated pattern of catecholamine and cortisol output.
- Could oestrogen-deficiency symptoms be exacerbated by possible suboptimal dehydroepiandrosterone (DHEA) levels from adrenal stress? (Post-menopause, DHEA is aromatized locally within tissues for oestrogen synthesis.)
- Could possible hyper-cortisol production be suppressing the immune response in relation to the recurrent UTIs?

Communication: glucose and insulin metabolism

- Some of TT's symptoms indicate possible fluctuations in blood glucose.
- The interplay between glucose metabolism and HPA function means that any dysfunctions within these systems could be driving each other. For example, hypoglycaemia triggers adrenaline, which in turn promotes elevated cortisol production.

Structure

- The lack of dietary omega-3 fatty acids (a taste aversion to oily fish) may be affecting the structure and function of cellular membranes. Could poor omega-3 status be contributing to low mood, anxiety (Grosso *et al.*, 2014) and/or to possible inflammation (arthralgia, sinusitis, UTIs, itchy nose and eyes) (Calder, 2017)?
- There is a likely need to support the integrity of the epithelial lining of both the gastrointestinal and urogenital tracts, due to likely oestrogen diminution and microbial dysbiosis in these areas.
- Could some of TT's systemic symptoms be driven in part by intestinal hyperpermeability? Such a situation, commonly known as 'leaky gut', has been associated with systemic inflammatory symptoms (Bischoff *et al.*, 2014).
- TT's arthralgia is a sign that her largest structural system, the musculoskeletal system, may be compromised.

Hepatic biotransformation (detoxification)

Certain issues in TT's case history suggest the likely presence of a heavy toxicant load:

- Potential malabsorption of detoxification conjugates, methyl donors and cofactor nutrients (amino acids, B vitamins and magnesium), due to gastrointestinal issues.
- A long history of prescription drugs and paracetamol, the latter being known to devour glutathione stores. Glutathione is one of the most important endogenous antioxidant and detoxification molecules.
- Possible hypomethylation, given the history of stress and prescription drugs and a heightened need for ongoing tissue repair (due to sinusitis, UTIs and possible increased intestinal permeability). All of these processes (stress hormone metabolism, drug metabolism and the healing and maintenance of body tissues) require methylation. Thus, a greater need for these may be

putting pressure on TT's methylation efficiency. The practitioner hypothesized that TT's mood, cognition and tissue repair (within the musculoskeletal system, the urinary tract, the gut and the sinuses) may be compromised by suboptimal methylation.

- It is worth remembering that TT also has a family history of CVD. Elevated blood levels of homocysteine, a marker of hypomethylation, has been associated with CVD: homocysteine may compromise arterial structure and function due to its adverse effects on the cardiovascular endothelium and smooth-muscle cells (Ganguly and Alam, 2015; Lai and Kan, 2015; Wang and Jin, 2017).

Immune system

Aspects of TT's case history indicating a need to regulate the immune system included:

- Inflammatory symptoms (sinusitis, UTIs, arthralgia, low mood).
- A lack of dietary omega-3 fatty acids EPA and DHA, which act as precursors to anti-inflammatory eicosanoids.
- The possible presence of intestinal hyperpermeability and dysbiosis (gastrointestinal and urogenital) which promote systemic inflammation (Bischoff *et al.*, 2014).
- The presence of abdominal visceral adiposity, which promotes inflammatory adipokine synthesis.
- The practitioner also hypothesized that TT's vitamin D status may be poor, given her geographical location and lifestyle. Active vitamin D is an immune-regulating, anti-inflammatory hormone.

Mitochondrial function and redox

- Is TT sufficient in the micronutrients required for mitochondrial health for optimal energy production from foods (B vitamins, omega-3 fatty acids especially DHA, magnesium, antioxidants)?
- There is evidence that many of the environmental inputs present in TT's life history can compromise mitochondrial function, leading to poor energy production and increased free-radical

activity. Such inputs include inflammation, antibiotics, visceral adiposity (especially from excessive carbohydrate intake) and sedentary living (Griffiths, 2018).

- Might TT also be more prone to oxidative stress because of her history of paracetamol use, which can deplete glutathione levels?

Initial management plan

This plan was prescribed prior to the results of the functional laboratory investigations.

Diet

A diet based on the low-FODMAP[3] principles was prescribed. For further information on the evidence for this diet in IBS and other conditions, see www.monashfodmap.com.

Rather than following the full diet, TT was advised to avoid the high-FODMAP foods that she was eating most frequently and to replace these with low-FODMAP alternatives. It was explained to TT that her existing diet appeared to be particularly high in lactose (from dairy), fructose (from honey and certain fruits), fructans (onions, garlic and cashews) and galactooligosaccharides (from beans/pulses and cashews).

The rationale for using low-FODMAPs as a basis for TT's diet was to reduce the intake of sugars and starches that are easily fermentable and that therefore act as substrates for dysbiotic bacteria in the gut (the likely presence of which is indicated by the excessive gastrointestinal gas production). The diet is well evidenced for relieving TT's types of gastrointestinal symptoms (Nanayakkara et al., 2016) and is also well supported with practical resources and user communities.

An initial focus on gastrointestinal health was agreed not only because TT's IBS symptoms are so debilitating, but also because the presence of a gastrointestinal microbial imbalance may theoretically limit the resolution of her UTIs and other symptoms. Preliminary

---

3   The term 'FODMAP' is an acronym, derived from Fermentable Oligo-, Di-, Mono-saccharides And Polyols.

research indicates that gut dysbiosis may be implicated in problems elsewhere in the body, such as inflammation, arthralgia, sinusitis, low mood and poor cognition (Nayan *et al.*, 2015; Thevaranjan *et al.*, 2017; Wang, Braun and Enck, 2018).

Videos were recommended for TT to view, in order to help her understand the potential influence of gastrointestinal function on certain of her symptoms ('Food for thought: How your belly controls your brain' – TEDx Talk by Ruairi Robertson).

TT also agreed to remove dietary inputs that tend to relax the cardiac sphincter and therefore contribute to oesophageal reflux: caffeine, alcohol and peppermint.

Supplements

TT was advised to stop all self-prescribed supplements, the rationale being her reported lack of improvement after having taken them for three months. Moreover:

- **Probiotic bacteria:** Given TT's symptoms and long history of antibiotics and stress, the presence of a small intestinal bacterial overgrowth (SIBO) is possible. Although probiotics have a long history of use in supporting gut and immune health, they may potentially worsen symptoms of gastrointestinal gas, bloating and brain fogginess in some individuals with SIBO (Rao *et al.*, 2018). In addition, TT has agreed to test for SIBO and this requires abstinence from supplements that alter the microbiome.
- **Peppermint oil:** The smooth-muscle relaxant properties of peppermint oil can make it helpful in cases of bowel spasms involved in IBS. But these same properties may also be contributing to the reflux, by relaxing the cardiac sphincter.
- **Glucosamine sulphate:** This is a mucopolysaccharide, which can feed bacterial overgrowths.
- **D-mannose:** Although a monosaccharide, D-mannose is poorly absorbed. Some expert opinions maintain that it therefore remains in the small intestine for long enough to become a substrate for bacterial overgrowths (Siebecker, n.d.). TT was not sufficiently confident to remove this supplement without clear

evidence of the presence of SIBO, so it was agreed to maintain this until the results were available.

During this initial phase, TT was gently steered away from her current *modus operandi* of trialling supplements to treat individual symptoms, and more towards the goal of identifying the deeper causes. This is elaborated upon in the discussion and conclusion below.

Management at six weeks

Results of the laboratory investigations

Below are the results that were reported to be outside the 'normal' reference range:

- ESR slightly raised (19 mm/hr – reference range 0–15 mm/hr).
- Vitamin D deficiency (35 nmol/L – reference range 75–200 nmol/L).
- Significant SIBO (methane-producing) – shown in Figure 4.1. An overgrowth of certain additional bacteria in the large intestine – shown in Figure 4.2. Although classed as non-pathogenic, any microbes found at abnormally elevated levels can contribute to gastrointestinal symptoms. (See Box 9.2 in Chapter 9 for a definition of dysbiosis.) Moreover, the relative abundance of the *Euryarchaeota* phylum was found to be significantly higher than that of the lab's healthy cohort (see Figure 4.3). *Euryarchaeota* comprises methanogenic archaea (Horz and Conrads, 2010) and, as seen, elevated methane levels were found on TT's lactulose breath test. Methanogens are thought to be involved in both IBS and obesity, both of which affect TT. (A waist-to-hip ratio of greater than 0.85 in women is classed as abdominal obesity (World Health Organization, 2011).
- Increased faecal zonulin indicating possible intestinal hyperpermeability. Although the stool level of zonulin is not considered a definitive diagnosis of increased intestinal permeability, this condition has been associated with SIBO in

the literature, especially in cases of post-infectious IBS (Lin, 2004). TT's IBS symptoms became apparent following a history of gastroenteritis and her lactulose breath test result indicated the presence of a SIBO.

- Elevations in certain urinary organic acids (OA). As discussed in Chapter 3, the practitioner primarily looks at patterns of OA rather than individual makers. For TT, the results were suggestive of functionally low levels of B vitamins, and other cofactors required for the processes of methylation and mitochondrial energy production. There are some specific markers on an OA test that are clinically useful. In this case, methylamalonate was elevated, indicating that functional levels of vitamin B12 may be low (Langan and Goodbred, 2017; McMullin *et al.*, 2001). (Test results not shown.)
- Elevated urinary levels of the catecholamine metabolite vanilmandelic acid, which may indicate HPA hyperfunction. (Test result not shown.)
- Raised homocysteine (13 umol/L – reference range 5–12 umol/L; 7–8 umol/L is considered optimal by many practitioners). Elevated homocysteine can be related to methylation imbalance.

Protocol: 10 gm of lactulose diluted in 200 ml of water
Method: Hydrogen and methane values measured every 20 minutes for 180 minutes

Basal levels: Hydrogen = 0 ppm Methane = 55 ppm

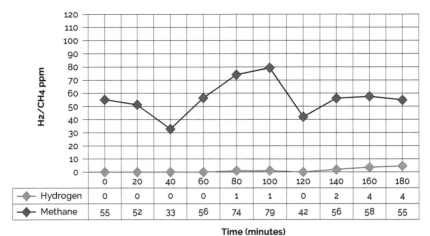

	0	20	40	60	80	100	120	140	160	180
Hydrogen	0	0	0	0	1	1	0	2	4	4
Methane	55	52	33	56	74	79	42	56	58	55

Time (minutes)

Figure 4.1 SIBO test result (see online colour plate)

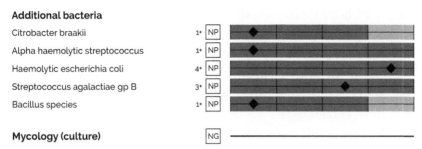

Additional bacteria

Citrobacter braakii	1⁺ NP	
Alpha haemolytic streptococcus	1⁺ NP	
Haemolytic escherichia coli	4⁺ NP	
Streptococcus agalactiae gp B	3⁺ NP	
Bacillus species	1⁺ NP	

Mycology (culture) NG

Figure 4.2 Excerpt from comprehensive stool test results (see online colour plate)

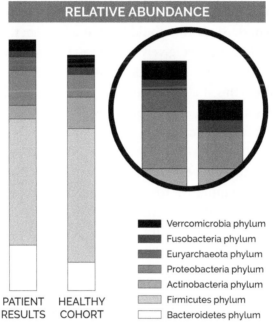

Figure 4.3 Excerpt from the comprehensive stool test results (see online colour plate)

Diet

- TT reported a powerful response to the reduction of FODMAPs in her diet, with a marked improvement in gastrointestinal gas, bloating, flatulence, churning, belching and reflux. But her need for snacking between meals had increased, as had her symptoms of sugar cravings, feeling shaky and irritable between meals and night waking.

- A 24-hour dietary recall revealed that TT had been following the guidelines of the full low-FODMAP diet more stringently than the practitioner had intended. Consequently, as the diet in its off-the-shelf form allows many types of refined sugars and starches, TT's diet had become higher in these foods and lower in vegetables, as she was now avoiding many of the vegetables she had previously eaten. This may have started to compromise blood glucose control mechanisms, contributing to her hypoglycaemic-like symptoms. Interestingly, TT's constipation had not worsened despite the inadvertent reduction in dietary fibre. It was hypothesized this could be due to the methane-lowering potential of the diet, given that excessive methane production can be a cause of constipation (Kunkel *et al.*, 2011).

- To address this, TT's diet was modified to reduce the sugars and starches normally allowed on a low-FODMAP diet. These were replaced with more protein, fat and vegetables, specifically 8–10 vegetable portions/day, one portion being 80 g. Practical tips included to weigh her vegetable portions until she had gained sufficient familiarity to gauge portion sizes visually, and to challenge herself to try every one of the 'green light' vegetables on the Monash University app and in this way aim to eat 30+ plant foods a week. This latter recommendation has been found to be a potent driver of gastrointestinal microbial diversity, which is linked to improved systemic health (McDonald *et al.*, 2018).

- With these changes, TT's diet remained low in FODMAPs, as her lab results indicated the presence of a significant SIBO and colonic dysbiosis. Although evidence is lacking for this way of eating *resolving* such imbalances, it can help to support quality of life during an intervention plan, as TT had already discovered, with such significant improvement in her IBS symptoms. It was decided not to move TT to a more SIBO-specific diet, as this would have been more restrictive; also, such diets are not as well-resourced with client/patient apps, recipe books and online communities. It was important that TT maintained motivation in the face of so many dietary changes.

- There is some opinion that the low-FODMAP diet should be used for as short a time as possible (Hill, Muir and Gibson, 2017). However, this practitioner has experienced improved efficacy when used for longer periods (of up to several months) in circumstances where SIBO tests reveal exceptionally high results. As seen, care is taken to ensure that within the key dietary restrictions a wide range of plant foods is consumed. Practitioner-supplied menu plans and recipes can make this more possible.

Supplements

- Herbal antimicrobials:
  - Berberine: 5000 g QD in three divided doses with meals. As an antimicrobial, berberine may improve microbiota balance, while reducing gut inflammation and improving gut barrier integrity, all of which are potentially important targets for TT (Siebecker, n.d.). Berberine may also increase levels of the commensal bacterium *Akkermansia muciniphila* (Zhu *et al.*, 2018), which has been associated with leanness and with better gut barrier integrity (Derrien, Belzer and de Vos, 2017; Naito, Uchiyama and Takagi, 2018).
  - Allicin (rather than whole garlic, which contains fermentable oligosaccharides): 2700 mg QD in three divided doses with meals. Allicin has been found specifically to reduce *methanogenic* microbial overgrowths (Ma *et al.*, 2016; Siebecker, n.d.).
- Oligomeric proanthocyanidins (OPCs) and anthocyanins: 160 mg BID. These pigmented flavonoids (found naturally in many blue, purple and red plants) were prescribed to support collagen integrity that may be compromised by the low oestrogen state. Collagen supports structural tissues within the sinuses, musculoskeletal joints, bladder, vagina and gastrointestinal tract, all of which are symptomatic in this case. OPCs and anthocyanins help to inhibit enzymes (matrix metalloproteases) that degrade collagen in inflammatory situations, such as can arise from the sharp drop in oestrogen levels at menopause. What's more,

cranberry extract is often used in UTIs and it is thought to be cranberry's OPC and anthocyanin content that provides its anti-adhesion activity within the bladder against *Escherichia coli* (Feliciano, Krueger and Reed, 2015; Micali *et al.*, 2014; Vostalova *et al.*, 2015). This knowledge, together with the positive SIBO test result, motivated TT to trial a break from using the D-mannose.

- Fish oil: combined EPA+DHA at a dose of 1000 mg QD due to the historic poor dietary intake, inflammatory symptoms and family history of cardiovascular disease.

- A methylated B complex QD (see formula in Appendix 4.1) to help address the functionally low levels indicated by the OA results, as well as to support the aim of reducing homocysteine levels (by supporting methylation), low mood and anxiety (Bender, Hagan and Kingston, 2017; Kennedy, 2016; Lewis *et al.*, 2013; Mikkelsen, Stojanovska and Apostolopoulos, 2016).

- Vitamin D: 4000 IU QD, reducing to 2000 IU QD after three months to address the serum deficiency and to support improved immune function and tolerance (Hewison, 2012), arthralgia (Heidari, Heidari and Tilaki, 2014) and mood (Bičíková *et al.*, 2015).

- Magnesium: 390 mg QD elemental provided as citrate, bisglycinate and taurate, to help address the functionally low levels indicated by the OA test and to support the aims of reducing TT's possible hyperactive HPA response and associated symptoms of stress and anxiety (Boyle, Lawton and Dye, 2017; Wienecke and Nolden, 2016). Like the B vitamins (particularly folate and B12), magnesium is essential for optimal methylation. While folate (once metabolized to 5-methyltetrahydrofolate) acts a methyl donor to recycle homocysteine back to methionine, B12 is a crucial cofactor for the enzyme methionine synthase that catalyzes this reaction. Magnesium is just as important but acts as a cofactor elsewhere in the cycle, namely in the metabolism of methionine to SAMe – S-adenosylmethionine – which is the body's and brain's primary methyl donor. In TT's case, optimal methylation is particularly required for structural support, including of the epithelial linings of the gastrointestinal tract, vagina, bladder and sinuses; as well as for the synthesis and breakdown of neurotransmitters involved in mood, cognition, stress response, sleep and gut motility; appropriate response of the adaptive immune system; the production of energy coenzymes like Q_{10}; and detoxification processes, including of toxic metabolic products from microbial overgrowths.

- *Rhodiola rosea*: 300 mg extract standardized to 3% rosavins twice a day before 2 pm. *Rhodiola* may help the body adapt to stress and improve stress-related symptoms of low mood, fatigue and anxiety (Lekomtseva, Zhukova and Wacker, 2017).

Case management

Looking back after nine months, it was clear that the gut dysbiosis plan had proved to be a key point of leverage. All IBS symptoms had resolved, including the constipation, as had the UTI symptoms, sinus pain, fatigue, mood, brain fog and arthralgia.

TT had remained on herbal antimicrobials for four months in total, with berberine being alternated with oil of oregano (100 mg TID after meals, standardized to 65% carvacrol) every six weeks. The allicin was maintained for the full four months. Once the herbal antimicrobials were successfully stopped, she was able to gradually broaden the diet to introduce most foods, by trialling them one at a time. This structured reintroduction process enabled the identification of certain key foods that seemed to trigger symptoms and she continued to avoid these (onions, cauliflower, lactose-containing dairy products).

At nine months, TT's key area of concern was her tendency towards sugar cravings and uncontrolled eating when under stress (mainly from work). When this occurred, the binge-eating would trigger her IBS symptoms to return and this would start the UTI symptoms (and associated low mood and anxiety). UTI symptoms during these flares were very much milder than they had been in the past, however. As the initiating input appeared to be stress, the programme evolved to focus on further strategies to support adrenal function, including optimizing sleep and making referrals for exercise, relaxation, psychological support and 'brain training'. The new programme also included 'rescue' mini-programmes, where necessary. These included short periods of returning to a lower-FODMAP way of eating plus herbal antimicrobials to rebalance the gut microbiome, where indicated by symptom relapses.

Far from being steady and linear in nature, TT's rate of progress was somewhat iterative and included challenges that required directional changes at times. For example:

- At first the herbal antimicrobials caused side effects (a worsening of bladder symptoms, joint pain, headaches, fatigue and mood). Thus, the programme was altered to be 'longer and thinner'. Such side effects can be caused where an anti-dysbiotic programme causes increased toxic load, albeit transient (Pound and May, 2005). TT started on a significantly lower dose of the herbal antimicrobials and gradually increased this, reducing it again to a tolerable dose whenever symptoms worsened.
- Later in the programme, the client's UTI, gut, sinus and mood symptoms returned following a bout of heavy flu. At this point she was recommended to go back to the antimicrobial programme for a short period. This had the additional advantage of the allicin being immune-supportive (Majewski, 2014).
- Following the antimicrobial programme, the experiential use of a probiotic supplement (multiple strains of *Lactobacilli* and *Bifidobacteria*), trialled at TT's request, was found to correlate with a return of the gastrointestinal bloating and reflux within two weeks of starting the supplement. This triggered anxiety about a potential return of the UTI symptoms. The probiotics were therefore stopped and the symptoms calmed down after a few days.

Throughout, TT had remained on a low-GL (glycaemic load), wholefoods diet, avoiding her key triggers (above) and continuing to take the methylated B complex, vitamin D, magnesium and anthocyanins/OPCs. Rhodiola was reduced to symptomatic, occasional use only.

Intermittent fasting (IF) was introduced by starting with a 12-hour fast every night and gradually increasing this to 14 hours (by skipping breakfast). TT felt extremely well on this schedule. IF may be helpful in

SIBO prevention because it supports the functioning of the migrating motor complex (MMC), which helps to keep the small intestine free of microbial overgrowths (Deloose and Tack, 2016). Ginger was also included in the diet as a prokinetic spice (Ghayur and Gilani, 2005)

There is also growing evidence that IF may promote healthy ageing by helping to control inflammation, glucose and insulin metabolism, cardiovascular health and mood and cognition, all of which have been cited by the client as concerns/aims (Kelly *et al.*, 2015; Patterson *et al.*, 2015).

TT was now generally symptom-free and described feeling healthier and 'younger' than she did 15 years earlier. She also recognized that she could not have tolerated her current healthy regime (low-GL, IF) without first having made the preliminary steps of resolving her functional gastrointestinal issues, improving immune tolerance and working on blood glucose control, adrenal gland function, neurochemistry and the other imbalances found.

The latest laboratory tests showed many markers to be back within the normal range: ESR (9 mm/hr), vitamin D (85 nmol/L), homocysteine (7.8 umol/L). A repeat lactulose breath test confirmed that there was no evidence of SIBO. Other markers were not remeasured, due to lack of funds and the client maintaining a feeling of wellbeing. Most importantly, TT had achieved her primary goal of resolving the symptoms of recurrent UTIs and had been able to break her dependency on antibiotics.

Discussion and conclusion

The catalyst that brought this client to the attention of a personalized nutrition practitioner was the seemingly entrenched situation of chronic UTIs. However, this case is far from a demonstration of a nutritional protocol for chronic UTIs. Rather, it has been included here to illustrate that a personalized, systems-based model of chronic health care can reveal new opportunities for interventions that would otherwise not have been brought to light. It shows that a single health issue can be caused by multiple underlying factors, and that addressing these factors not only improves the symptoms but brings longer-term prevention. This then has the domino effect of improving other long-standing signs and symptoms of poor health not previously considered by the client to be related to the key concern of the recurrent UTIs.

Biochemical systems in the human body work together in a complex network of influence. For example, improving the structural issues affecting the urothelium, the gastrointestinal epithelium and the musculoskeletal system involved addressing imbalances in the microbiome, inflammation, methylation, adrenal function (which may also support better sex hormone balance) and blood glucose metabolism. Nutritional approaches can lack efficacy if they remain allopathic. Our client TT had diligently self-prescribed nutritional supplements that are widely used in specific health symptoms and which may have a documented logical mechanism of effect (e.g. D-mannose for UTI symptoms, probiotics for gastrointestinal symptoms and glucosamine for arthralgia). But, as this case shows, simply taking 'a pill for an ill', even if that pill is a nutritional supplement rather than a pharmaceutical drug, can be useless in the absence of consideration of the complex network of body system dysfunctions that is driving the symptoms.

A further illustration of this concept is the issue of constipation in this case. A symptom-led nutritional approach may be to prescribe more dietary fibre. But that was not the route taken here because it was identified that one of the likely drivers of the constipation was the methanogenic SIBO, methane being a gas that can slow transit time. Many of the types of fibre typically given for constipation such as psyllium husk, wheat bran, inulin, FOS (fructo-oligosaccharides) and GOS (galacto-oligosaccharides) can promote SIBO and this in theory could worsen constipation symptoms. So, in this case, the resolution of the methanogenic SIBO became the point of leverage, and this involved reducing, rather than increasing, some types of fibre, especially those that are more fermentable. Improving the constipation seemed to help improve the UTIs, perhaps partly by taking some physical pressure off the bladder.

Off-the-shelf therapeutic diets are best personalized for maximum efficacy. In this case, a low-FODMAP diet proved to be powerful for the client's gastrointestinal issues, but further recommendations were given in order to better support blood glucose metabolism, adrenal health and gastrointestinal microbial diversity. One particular challenge here was that of achieving dietary plant diversity while remaining low in dietary fermentable fibres. Such personalization is a key area in which practitioners can add value. A low-FODMAP diet done without such expert input may lead to diminished diversity of the gut microbiota, which is generally associated with poorer health outcomes.

The evidence used to justify interventions should not be limited to randomized controlled trials. Such studies are designed to minimize variation across groups of participants, rather than to embrace the uniqueness of the individual client. The use of probiotics, for example, is evidenced in IBS trials and in UTIs (Beerepoot *et al.*, 2012), but this does not dictate that such an intervention would necessarily be helpful in any one individual case. Far more enlightening may be data about mechanisms – namely, which mechanisms are going wrong within the individual client's biochemistry, and which nutritional agents have been reported to alter such mechanisms. This sort of data is elucidated through cell studies, animal studies and, to a certain extent, case reports (n = 1). All these types of data constitute 'evidence', as discussed in Chapter 2.

Another value of case reports in an evidence base is their ability to enlighten on how different biological systems may be impaired in different individuals with the same disease. This is another reason that people with exactly the same symptoms may require very different interventions. Not everybody with recurrent UTIs is going to have weaknesses in the same body systems as TT. Each individual case is an opportunity for building practitioner knowledge and evidence.

Medical diagnoses are not necessarily of prime importance for giving direction. In this particular case, the issue of whether TT was suffering from interstitial cystitis (IC) was considered periodically. IC is characterized by long-term UTI symptoms but without the presence of infection. The cause is unknown, but theories include damage to the urothelium, weak pelvic floor muscles, allergies and/or autoimmune processes. Although TT had not been medically assessed for IC, the presence or not of any such diagnosis was not necessary in progressing the case. This is because a personalized, systems-based model requires the practitioner to focus on identifying and addressing the unique set of *underlying* functional imbalances that exist within the client, no matter what labels have been attached to the collection of symptoms.

It is also worth noting that IC diagnoses are usually made in the absence of identifying a microbial driver. TT's medical investigations appeared to acknowledge a microbial driver. What's more, she did respond to antibiotics. Unfortunately, these were becoming less of an option because of her diminishing ability to tolerate the antibiotics and because her symptoms would return at the end of each course.

All these inherent qualities of a systems-based, personalized approach were involved in enabling the client to reach her goals.

Ultimately, it is impossible to be sure which specific strands of the intervention programme were the real game-changers here. But such certainty is not necessary because when a personalized model of chronic care is used to its full advantage, it cannot fail to bring to light aspects in the client's biochemistry that are in need of support. And, in turn, supporting those identified dysfunctions cannot fail to improve the client's health in some way. This becomes all the more clear when we understand that most chronic illness is preceded by years of malfunction in body systems.

Moving forward, TT is likely to experience a return of certain symptoms if and when she is exposed to the types of antecedents, triggers and mediators that were identified during the therapeutic journey and, in particular, in times of stress and/or pressures on immune function. But the client is now better equipped to manage her health – she has gained an understanding of why and how the health issues to which she is vulnerable can resurface, and, more importantly, she knows when and where to turn for help, both for self-care and for input from a practitioner.

Q&A

AW: Reflecting on the case, is there anything you would do differently?

LN: In retrospect, I would like to think that at the initial stage I would have been more alert to TT's psychological issues surrounding foods and her self-perceived 'addiction' to dietary starches and sugars. Had I picked up the signs earlier on, the programme may have required fewer iterations in order to reach the diet that was the most therapeutic.

And given that side effects were experienced when the client embarked on the intensive anti-dysbiotic programme, I might have been more cautious with this stage of the programme and eased her into it more gently, by starting her on a lower dose of the herbal antimicrobial supplements.

AW: Did you consider other testing or intervention options for UTIs?

LN: Yes, indeed. In particular, I kept in mind whether it might be necessary to move the focus more towards the role of biofilms in TT's situation. There is a growing recognition that where infections are chronic, there is usually biofilm involvement. In such situations, there may be multiple microbial species at play, and these may evade standard culture tests to identify them, as they are encased in a self-produced matrix of exopolysaccharides and exoproteins, adhering to the urothelium. The easiest way to picture a biofilm is to think of dental plaque, or the visible scum on the surface of stagnant water. Biofilm bacteria and yeasts may be more resistant to antimicrobials, including those produced by probiotic organisms.

More advanced testing techniques are now available (DNA sequencing), to identify all the microorganisms within the client's urogenital tract, including the biofilm. There is evidence that this may enable more accurate identification of the urogenital dysbiosis, enabling more targeted intervention (Mouraviev and McDonald, 2018). Had this been necessary, I would also have given consideration to the use of 'biofilm disruptors', with the aim of gaining more access to the culprit microbes. Nutritional biofilm disruptors typically comprise synergistic enzymes and/or N-acetyl-L-cysteine that break down the matrix proteins and polysaccharides.

Had no success been achieved with the original approach, I would have moved on to exploring the biofilm avenue. However, as the case progressed, it became apparent that efficacy did not necessarily require more investment in scrutinizing the disease itself, as much as the application of a *holistic* look at the interconnected body systems within the client's unique biochemistry. It required consideration not only of the infection but of the host's internal terrain.

AW: I love how you talk about personalizing an off-the-shelf diet, and also the learning process TT went through – she followed low-FODMAPs very accurately but ended up including highly refined foods which you highlighted in a 24-hour diet recall. Do you have any other tips or advice on how to help guide clients with that learning process and not get frustrated?

LN: Yes, and indeed this is something that in retrospect I might have done differently. All off-the-shelf diets need tailoring to the needs of the individual client. If I had been more attuned to TT's propensity to favour high-glycaemic foods, I would have focused more on swapping these for alternatives, while explaining how to lower FODMAPs in her diet. I would also have given more practical tips on how to alter standard low-FODMAP recommendations. Creating a bank of handouts that take the best elements from different off-the-shelf diets enables clients to get more targeted support without the practitioner having to 'reinvent the wheel' each time. Guidelines comprising food lists, meal plans and recipes for adopting a low-GL, more wholefoods version of the low-FODMAP diet would likely benefit many clients, by targeting not only gut dysbiosis problems but also issues with blood glucose and insulin control, and HPA function.

AW: Did you ever get her to enjoy eating oily fish!?

LN: I did have some limited success by encouraging TT to incorporate smaller fish in a somewhat disguised fashion, such as using anchovies in a phenol-rich 'green sauce' (green leaves and herbs, whole lemon, root ginger, olive oil, olives, capers and anchovies blitzed in a high-speed blender for use over vegetables, fish, chicken or meat). She was also prepared to eat tinned sardines and pilchards if mashed well with other flavourings such as lemon juice, and she would occasionally grill salmon. However, she maintained that she did not enjoy the taste and she also became concerned about levels of toxic pollutants that can contaminate fatty fish. Sadly, in my clinical experience, clients who tend to have healthier levels of intracellular EPA and DHA (ascertained by a laboratory investigation of erythrocyte membrane fatty acid levels), also tend to ingest higher levels of mercury (as ascertained via metal levels in whole blood). One therefore wonders about the ethics of encouraging individuals to eat oily fish where they are not inclined to do so. One option would be to run these tests and then discuss the results with the client, to enable more informed and individualized decision making.

Appendix 4.1 Methylated B complex formula

Ingredient	Amount
Thiamine (vitamin B1)	25 mg
Riboflavin (vitamin B2)	25 mg
Niacin (vitamin B3)	25 mg
Vitamin B6 (P5P)	25 mg
Folate (methylfolate)	250 mcg
Vitamin B12 (methylcobalamin)	250 mcg
Biotin	200 mcg
Pantothenic acid (vitamin B5)	25 mg
Choline bitartrate	25 mg
Inositol	25 mg
PABA	25 mg
L-glycine	10 mg

References

Beerepoot, M.A.J., ter Riet, G., Nys, S., van der Wal, W.M. *et al.*, 2012. Lactobacilli vs antibiotics to prevent urinary tract infections: A randomized, double-blind, noninferiority trial in postmenopausal women. *JAMA Internal Medicine* 172, 704–712. https://doi.org/10.1001/archinternmed.2012.777

Bender, A., Hagan, K.E., Kingston, N., 2017. The association of folate and depression: A meta-analysis. *Journal of Psychiatric Research* 95, 9–18. https://doi.org/10.1016/j.jpsychires.2017.07.019

Bičíková, M., Dušková, M., Vítků, J., Kalvachová, B. *et al.*, 2015. Vitamin D in anxiety and affective disorders. *Physiological Research* 64 Suppl 2, S101–103.

Bischoff, S.C., Barbara, G., Buurman, W., Ockhuizen, T. *et al.*, 2014. Intestinal permeability – a new target for disease prevention and therapy. *BMC Gastroenterology* 14, 189. https://doi.org/10.1186/s12876-014-0189-7

Boyle, N.B., Lawton, C., Dye, L., 2017. The effects of magnesium supplementation on subjective anxiety and stress – a systematic review. *Nutrients* 9. https://doi.org/10.3390/nu9050429

Calder, P.C., 2017. Omega-3 fatty acids and inflammatory processes: From molecules to man. *Biochemical Society Transactions* 45, 1105–1115. https://doi.org/10.1042/BST20160474

Deloose, E., Tack, J., 2016. Redefining the functional roles of the gastrointestinal migrating motor complex and motilin in small bacterial overgrowth and hunger signaling. *American Journal of Physiology – Gastrointestinal and Liver Physiology* 310, G228–233. https://doi.org/10.1152/ajpgi.00212.2015

Derrien, M., Belzer, C., de Vos, W.M., 2017. Akkermansia muciniphila and its role in regulating host functions. *Microbial Pathogenesis* 106, 171–181. https://doi.org/10.1016/j.micpath.2016.02.005

Feliciano, R.P., Krueger, C.G., Reed, J.D., 2015. Methods to determine effects of cranberry proanthocyanidins on extraintestinal infections: Relevance for urinary tract health. *Molecular Nutrition and Food Research* 59, 1292–1306. https://doi.org/10.1002/mnfr.201500108

Ganguly, P., Alam, S.F., 2015. Role of homocysteine in the development of cardiovascular disease. *Nutrition Journal* 14. https://doi.org/10.1186/1475-2891-14-6

Ghayur, M.N., Gilani, A.H., 2005. Pharmacological basis for the medicinal use of ginger in gastrointestinal disorders. *Digestive Diseases and Sciences* 50, 1889–1897. https://doi.org/10.1007/s10620-005-2957-2

Griffiths, R., 2018. *Mitochondria in Health and Disease*, 1st ed. Singing Dragon.

Grosso, G., Galvano, F., Marventano, S., Malaguarnera, M. *et al.*, 2014. Omega-3 fatty acids and depression: Scientific evidence and biological mechanisms. *Oxidative Medicine and Cellular Longevity* 2014, 313570. https://doi.org/10.1155/2014/313570

Heidari, B., Heidari, P., Tilaki, K.H., 2014. Relationship between unexplained arthralgia and vitamin D deficiency: A case control study. *Acta Medica Iranica* 52, 400–405.

Hewison, M., 2012. Vitamin D and immune function: An overview. *Proceedings of the Nutrition Society* 71, 50–61. https://doi.org/10.1017/S0029665111001650

Hill, P., Muir, J.G., Gibson, P.R., 2017. Controversies and recent developments of the low-FODMAP diet. *Gastroenterology and Hepatology* 13, 36–45.

Horz, H.-P., Conrads, G., 2010. The discussion goes on: What is the role of *Euryarchaeota* in humans? *Archaea* 2010. https://doi.org/10.1155/2010/967271

Kelly, J.R., Kennedy, P.J., Cryan, J.F., Dinan, T.G., Clarke, G., Hyland, N.P., 2015. Breaking down the barriers: The gut microbiome, intestinal permeability and stress-related psychiatric disorders. *Frontiers in Cellular Neuroscience* 9, 392. https://doi.org/10.3389/fncel.2015.00392

Kennedy, D.O., 2016. B vitamins and the brain: Mechanisms, dose and efficacy – a review. *Nutrients* 8. https://doi.org/10.3390/nu8020068

Kiecolt-Glaser, J.K., Derry, H.M., Fagundes, C.P., 2015. Inflammation: Depression fans the flames and feasts on the heat. *American Journal of Psychiatry* 172, 1075–1091. https://doi.org/10.1176/appi.ajp.2015.15020152

Kunkel, D., Basseri, R.J., Makhani, M.D., Chong, K., Chang, C., Pimentel, M., 2011. Methane on breath testing is associated with constipation: A systematic review and meta-analysis. *Digestive Diseases and Sciences* 56, 1612–1618. https://doi.org/10.1007/s10620-011-1590-5

Lai, W.K.C., Kan, M.Y., 2015. Homocysteine-induced endothelial dysfunction. *Annals of Nutrition and Metabolism* 67, 1–12. https://doi.org/10.1159/000437098

Langan, R.C., Goodbred, A.J., 2017. Vitamin B12 deficiency: Recognition and management. *American Family Physician* 96, 384–389.

Lekomtseva, Y., Zhukova, I., Wacker, A., 2017. *Rhodiola rosea* in subjects with prolonged or chronic fatigue symptoms: Results of an open-label clinical trial. *Complementary Medicine Research* 24, 46–52. https://doi.org/10.1159/000457918

Lewis, J.E., Tiozzo, E., Melillo, A.B., Leonard, S. *et al.*, 2013. The effect of methylated vitamin B complex on depressive and anxiety symptoms and quality of life in adults with depression. *ISRN Psychiatry* 2013, 621453. https://doi.org/10.1155/2013/621453

Lin, H.C., 2004. Small intestinal bacterial overgrowth: A framework for understanding irritable bowel syndrome. *JAMA* 292, 852–858. https://doi.org/10.1001/jama.292.7.852

Ma, T., Chen, D., Tu, Y., Zhang, N., Si, B., Deng, K., Diao, Q., 2016. Effect of supplementation of allicin on methanogenesis and ruminal microbial flora in Dorper crossbred ewes. *Journal of Animal Science and Biotechnology* 7, 1. https://doi.org/10.1186/s40104-015-0057-5

Majewski, M., 2014. Allium sativum: Facts and myths regarding human health. *Roczniki Państwowego Zakładu Higieny* 65, 1–8.

McCormick, R.K., 2007. Osteoporosis: Integrating biomarkers and other diagnostic correlates into the management of bone fragility. *Alternative Medicine Review* 12, 113–145.

McDonald, D., Hyde, E., Debelius, J.W., Morton, J.T. *et al.*, 2018. American Gut: An open platform for citizen science microbiome research. *mSystems* 3. https://doi.org/10.1128/mSystems.00031-18

McMullin, M.F., Young, P.B., Bailie, K.E., Savage, G.A., Lappin, T.R., White, R., 2001. Homocysteine and methylmalonic acid as indicators of folate and vitamin B12 deficiency in pregnancy. *Clinical and Laboratory Haematology* 23, 161–165.

Micali, S., Isgro, G., Bianchi, G., Miceli, N., Calapai, G., Navarra, M., 2014. Cranberry and recurrent cystitis: More than marketing? *Critical Reviews in Food Science and Nutrition* 54, 1063–1075. https://doi.org/10.1080/10408398.2011.625574

Mikkelsen, K., Stojanovska, L., Apostolopoulos, V., 2016. The effects of vitamin B in depression. *Current Medical Chemistry* 23, 38. http://www.eurekaselect.com/145648/article

Mouraviev, V., McDonald, M., 2018. An implementation of next generation sequencing for prevention and diagnosis of urinary tract infection in urology. *Canadian Journal of Urology* 25, 9349–9356.

Naito, Y., Uchiyama, K., Takagi, T., 2018. A next-generation beneficial microbe: *Akkermansia muciniphila*. *Journal of Clinical Biochemistry and Nutrition* 63, 33–35. https://doi.org/10.3164/jcbn.18-57

Nanayakkara, W.S., Skidmore, P.M., O'Brien, L., Wilkinson, T.J., Gearry, R.B., 2016. Efficacy of the low FODMAP diet for treating irritable bowel syndrome: The evidence to date. *Clinical and Experimental Gastroenterology* 9, 131–142. https://doi.org/10.2147/CEG.S86798

Nayan, S., Maby, A., Endam, L.M., Desrosiers, M., 2015. Dietary modifications for refractory chronic rhinosinusitis? Manipulating diet for the modulation of inflammation. *American Journal of Rhinology and Allergy* 29, e170–174. https://doi.org/10.2500/ajra.2015.29.4220

NHS, 2017. Urinary tract infections (UTIs). Accessed on 14/06/2019 at www.nhs.uk/conditions/urinary-tract-infections-utis

Patterson, R.E., Laughlin, G.A., Sears, D.D., LaCroix, A.Z. *et al.*, 2015. Intermittent fasting and human metabolic health. *Journal of the Academy of Nutrition and Dietetics* 115, 1203–1212. https://doi.org/10.1016/j.jand.2015.02.018

Pound, M.W., May, D.B., 2005. Proposed mechanisms and preventative options of Jarisch–Herxheimer reactions. *Journal of Clinical Pharmacy and Therapeutics* 30, 291–295. https://doi.org/10.1111/j.1365-2710.2005.00631.x

Powell, B.S., Dhaher, Y.Y., Szleifer, I.G., 2015. Review of the multiscale effects of female sex hormones on matrix metalloproteinase-mediated collagen degradation. *Critical Reviews in Biomedical Engineering* 43, 401–428. https://doi.org/10.1615/CritRevBiomedEng.2016016590

Rao, S.S.C., Rehman, A., Yu, S., Andino, N.M. de, 2018. Brain fogginess, gas and bloating: A link between SIBO, probiotics and metabolic acidosis. *Clinical and Translational Gastroenterology* 9, 162. https://doi.org/10.1038/s41424-018-0030-7

Ryan, J., Ancelin, M.-L., 2012. Polymorphisms of estrogen receptors and risk of depression: Therapeutic implications. *Drugs* 72, 1725–1738. https://doi.org/10.2165/11635960-000000000-00000

Siebecker, A., n.d. SIBO – Small Intestine Bacterial Overgrowth. Accessed on 26/05/2019 at www.siboinfo.com

Thevaranjan, N., Puchta, A., Schulz, C., Naidoo, A. *et al.*, 2017. Age-associated microbial dysbiosis promotes intestinal permeability, systemic inflammation, and macrophage dysfunction. *Cell Host and Microbe* 21, 455–466.e4. https://doi.org/10.1016/j.chom.2017.03.002

Thornton, M.J., 2013. Estrogens and aging skin. *Dermato-Endocrinology* 5, 264–270. https://doi.org/10.4161/derm.23872

Vostalova, J., Vidlar, A., Simanek, V., Galandakova, A. *et al.*, 2015. Are high proanthocyanidins key to cranberry efficacy in the prevention of recurrent urinary tract infection? *Phytotherapy Research* 29, 1559–1567. https://doi.org/10.1002/ptr.5427

Wang, H., Braun, C., Enck, P., 2018. Effects of rifaximin on central responses to social stress – a pilot experiment. *Neurotherapeutics* 15, 807–818. https://doi.org/10.1007/s13311-018-0627-2

Wang, W.-M., Jin, H.-Z., 2017. Homocysteine: A potential common route for cardiovascular risk and DNA methylation in psoriasis. *Chinese Medical Journal* 130, 1980–1986. https://doi.org/10.4103/0366-6999.211895

Wienecke, E., Nolden, C., 2016. [Long-term HRV analysis shows stress reduction by magnesium intake]. *MMW Fortschritte der Medizin* 158, 12–16. https://doi.org/10.1007/s15006-016-9054-7

World Health Organization, 2011. Waist circumference and waist–hip ratio: Report of a WHO expert consultation, Geneva, 8–11 December 2008. World Health Organization, Geneva.

Zhu, L., Zhang, D., Zhu, H., Zhu, J. *et al.*, 2018. Berberine treatment increases *Akkermansia* in the gut and improves high-fat diet-induced atherosclerosis in Apoe$^{-/-}$ mice. *Atherosclerosis* 268, 117–126. https://doi.org/10.1016/j.atherosclerosis.2017.11.023

5

Chronic Fatigue Syndrome

Practitioner: Helen Lynam

Additional contribution to case write-up: Angela Walker

Setting the scene

Chronic fatigue syndrome (CFS) or myalgic encephalomyelitis (ME) is a multifactorial chronic illness, normally diagnosed by the exclusion of other more specific disorders. It is characterized by long-term fatigue that interferes with normal life, which is unexplained, persistent or recurrent and lasts for at least four months (NICE, 2007). The severity varies considerably from one person to another. One person may be able to work full-time if they manage the rest of their life to minimize any further activity; some can be bed-bound.

The average length of the illness is around six years, although some people live with CFS/ME for decades (Nisenbaum *et al.*, 2000). Many people adopt coping mechanisms over time to accept a reduced level of life that helps to manage their symptoms and this often includes a withdrawal from work (Brown, Brown and Jason, 2010). Research published in 2017 estimated the cost of CFS/ME to the UK economy at £3.3bn (2020 Health, 2017).

The causes of CFS/ME are unknown and it is generally accepted now that there is unlikely to be a single cause. The U.S Centers for Disease

Control and Prevention (CDC) state the possibility for two or more triggers to act as causes for the illness. Such triggers include infections, immune function changes, stress, changes in energy production and genetics (CDC, 2017a).

There is no diagnostic test and therefore clinical or symptomatic diagnostic criteria are used, of which there are several. The primary diagnostic criteria are: the CDC 1994 criteria often referred to as the Fukuda definition (Fukuda *et al.*, 1995), the International Consensus Criteria, also known as the Canadian criteria (Carruthers *et al.*, 2003), and, more recently, the Institute of Medicine (2015) which renamed the condition systemic exertion intolerance disease. A description of the diagnostic criteria can be found in Appendix 5.1.

According to NICE (2007), the symptoms that can lead to a CFS/ME diagnosis include: sleep problems; headaches; pain in the muscles or joints; sore throat or sore glands that aren't swollen; problems thinking, remembering, concentrating or planning; flu-like symptoms; feeling dizzy or sick or having palpitations; exercising or concentrating on something which makes the symptoms worse. An adult will have a diagnosis if these symptoms have persisted for at least four months.

Conventional treatment is limited. The NICE (2007) guidelines list symptom management such as sleep, rest and relaxation, pacing, diet and equipment to maintain independence. The only interventions that are sometimes offered are cognitive behavioural therapy (CBT); graded exercise therapy (GET); painkillers; antidepressants at normal dose for depression, or at low dose for muscle pain relief.

Initial case presentation

MA was 32 years old when she presented with overwhelming fatigue which onset a year earlier following a viral infection. Her main symptoms were fatigue and low weight, with a body mass index (BMI) of 17.3.

MA was frustrated with her current situation. All blood tests taken by her general practitioner (GP) were within ranges from conventional pathology laboratories, and she was told there was no treatment and that her health would eventually improve 'in its own time'. She thought her diet had room for improvement and had started to make changes, but she was confused by the many different dietary suggestions in the public domain. She wanted to be able work full-time and socialize with her friends again.

At the onset of her illness, MA had the following symptoms: unable to stand or walk, feeling 'shaky', a tingling sensation throughout her entire body, unable to think or concentrate, difficulty holding a conversation, sore throat, sensitivity to noise, feelings of depression.

Over the following 11 months her symptoms had improved a little to the extent that her mood had lifted and she was feeling more positive. The progress had been very slow and she experienced frequent dips. She was not working but had a job offer for three afternoons a week from home.

MA went to bed at 10pm but took over an hour to fall asleep. She would wake up at 7am to her husband's alarm. Without the alarm, she would sleep until 9am. Sleep was unrefreshing and she often had nightmares. On waking, MA felt fatigued and often nauseous, she frequently stayed in bed during the morning. Her menstrual cycle, once regular, was now infrequent and she experienced premenstrual pain and cramping.

During subsequent consultations, it became clear that MA envisaged her future as a mother and was concerned that this might not be possible or that she would be too unwell to cope with motherhood. Later in MA's recovery, this became a focus of attention.

Timeline of health

- Childhood:
  - Upper respiratory tract infection most years, without complications. No other childhood illnesses.
  - Prescribed vaccinations in accordance with the National Health Service (NHS) policy at the time, which included polio, diphtheria, whooping cough and tetanus as an infant; measles, rubella and tuberculosis while at school.

- A happy childhood, described as loving, secure and supportive.
  - Childhood diet was 'meat and two vegetables', with most food cooked from scratch. Lunch was taken at school.
  - Desserts or puddings were eaten with lunch and evening meal, but sweets and chocolate were only consumed on special occasions (birthdays, Easter and Christmas).
- Teens and early 20s:
  - Healthy with no memorable illnesses causing her to miss school, university or work.
  - MA was active, playing badminton at least weekly and going for long bike rides and walks as part of her social life.
  - At university, MA had what she described as a typical student experience – reliant on takeaways and 'junk' food as well as late nights.
- Age 28:
  - MA got married and her diet improved a little, eating regular meals (three per day and no snacks), although they were often processed/prepared meals in the evening and sandwiches at lunchtime.
- Age 29:
  - While travelling in Asia she experienced several suspected gastrointestinal infections. Suspected because no infection was ever identified, although she was given unspecified antibiotics. At this point, MA lost around 5 kg (10 lb) in weight, which she had not regained.
  - On return to the UK, gastrointestinal pain and diarrhoea continued for a total of nine months before clearing up. No further treatment was taken.
- Age 30:
  - MA took redundancy and started a new job, which came with high stress levels.
  - MA socialized in the evenings and at weekends and described her lifestyle as 'hectic'.
  - Two upper respiratory infections that seemed to clear, so did not cause concern at the time.
  - Declining libido.

- Age 31:
  - Close relative died.
  - Contracted a non-specified virus from which she did not recover and as a result she had to stop work.

Supplements and medications
MA took no prescription medication. She had taken antibiotics for gastrointestinal infections she had experienced two years previously while travelling, but did not recall details. She had started to take a supermarket brand of multivitamin and minerals daily three months into her fatigue and had always taken vitamin C if she felt a cold coming on, although in the previous six months she took this daily.

Diet
MA had cravings for and ate sugary foods, chocolate and a high-carbohydrate diet. In the previous months she had increased her fruit and vegetable intake and switched her grain-containing foods to higher-fibre versions (e.g. white bread switched to seeded bread or oatcakes).

- Breakfast: a high-fibre cereal which came with dried fruit and she added semi-skimmed milk, or a sweetened muesli with a high dried fruit content with Greek yogurt and orange juice or a vitamin C tablet dissolved in water.
- Lunch: oatcakes or seeded bread with cheese or ham and tomatoes and sometimes cucumber and lettuce.
- Dinner: meat or fish (often prepacked in a sauce), with rice and two portions of vegetables (often pre-cut and packaged), with a packaged sweet desert such as a crème caramel.
- Snacks: including chocolate and chocolate biscuits.
- Drinks: tea, coffee, unfiltered water and occasional alcohol.

MA had never drunk excessive amounts of alcohol. At the time of the initial consultation, she would have a glass of white wine or a Pimm's cocktail only once or twice a week.

Environment and lifestyle

MA lived in the centre of a city and her previous job had required her to commute using public transport. She took great pride in doing a good job and work could be a cause of stress. She typically puts others before herself. Her husband and family were very supportive during her illness.

Initial investigations

Blood chemistry re-evaluation

Table 5.1 summarizes the out-of-range results taken over the previous 11 months. Although they had been noted by her medical practitioner as being in range, where unexplained symptoms exist, it is proposed that targeting an optimal reference range, which is a subset of normal ranges, may help identify an individual's underlying root causes of symptoms (see Chapter 3). Weatherby and Ferguson (2002) have documented optimal reference ranges for these situations which are used in Table 5.1.

Table 5.1 Summary of blood chemistry out-of-range results over past 11 months*

Test	Result (H or L based on optimal reference range)	Lower optimum	Upper optimum
Glucose mmol/L	4.4 L	4.44	5.55
Urea (BUN) mmol/L	3.5 L	3.57	5.71
Total Protein g/L	68 L	69	74
Creatinine umol/L	63 L	70.7	97.2
Monocytes % WBC and other fractions normal	10% H	0	7%
MCV	98 H	82	89.9
MCH pg/cell	33.5 H	28	31.9

* Only out-of-range results (compared with optimal ranges) are shown.

Source: Lower and upper optimal reference ranges taken from Blood Chemistry and CBC Analysis (Weatherby and Ferguson, 2002)

Simple home tests for the evaluation of stomach acidity and changes in the pH of saliva in response to a lemon (acidic) challenge were used (Weatherby and Ferguson, 2005). The evidence to support use of these tests is only anecdotal. In this practitioner's experience, they are reflective of improvements in symptoms and can be helpful in engaging and motivating the client. The results are summarized in Table 5.2.

Table 5.2 Summary of results from home tests

Test	Expected result	MA result
Stomach acid bicarbonate challenge test	Significant belch within 10–20 minutes	No belch of any kind, at any point
Lemon challenge test for electrolyte response (patient drinks lemon juice and salivary pH is measured over 5 minutes)	pH at start of 7 pH after lemon juice of 4.5 Then slow return back to 7 over 5 minutes	pH of 6 pH of 5 pH of 5.5 pH of 6 pH of 6.25 pH of 6.25

Four-point salivary cortisol test plus DHEA

Given MA's poor sleep and episodes of high stress in her timeline, the practitioner wanted to explore functional imbalance in the hypothalamus–pituitary–adrenal (HPA) axis. This test was discussed further in Chapter 3. Although some studies have found hypocortisolaemia to be more common in those with CFS compared with controls (Jerjes et al., 2005; Nater et al., 2008; Strickland et al., 1998), it is unclear whether HPA imbalance is a contributing factor in CFS. In a review, Cleare (2004) concluded HPA axis disturbance is less likely to be present at the onset of CFS but can evolve during the course of the condition. Furthermore, HPA disturbances can prolong CFS, but can be reversed by addressing contributing factors such as unresolved stress and sleep disturbance. The results are shown in Figure 5.1.

Cortisol levels	Inside range	Outside range	
Sample 1 (post awakening)	16.9		
Sample 2 (+4–5 hours)	5.6		
Sample 3 (+4–5 hours)	5.0		
Sample 4 (prior to sleep)		0.7	L
Total daily cortisol	28.2		
	Range 21–41nmol/L		
DHEA levels			
Sample 2 (am)		0.28	L
Sample 3 (pm)		0.30	L
DHEA:Cortisol ratio		1.03	L

Figure 5.1 Four-point salivary cortisol and DHEA results (see online colour plate)

Case interpretation and analysis

It became clear that several functional systems were compromised, which is a 'typical' finding when working with a CFS/ME case. These were as follows.

Defence and repair/immune system

MA had regular upper respiratory tract infections as a child and had two further upper respiratory tract infections at age 30. She had an ongoing sore throat, and a non-specified viral infection had been the final trigger for her fatigue.

MA had antibiotic treatment while travelling in Asia. Certain antibiotics can change the microbiome composition and diversity for up to 12 months (Zaura *et al.*, 2015). There is thought to be an interaction between the microbiome and the immune system whereby the microbiome 'entrains' the immune system (see Box 5.1). The antibiotic treatments could potentially have impacted on MA's immune system function.

The full blood count revealed a small imbalance in her white blood cells: monocytes accounted for over 10% of her total white blood cells. Although this is considered normal by conventional pathology laboratories, the rationale for applying a tighter reference range in cases of unexplained symptoms was outlined in Chapter 3. The optimal reference range used by this practitioner is 0–7% (Weatherby and Ferguson, 2002). This tighter reference range seemed particularly relevant given that the final trigger for MA's fatigue had been a viral infection: monocytes are the second line of defence against infection, producing the antiviral agent interferon. The practitioner hypothesized that the continued elevation could indicate unresolved antiviral activity.

BOX 5.1 MICROBIOME IMMUNE SYSTEM INTERACTION

The microbiome is thought to play a key role in the induction, training and function of the immune system. This is still an emerging understanding of the potential mechanisms involved, but examples that have been described include:

- Commensal bacteria promote the induction of regulatory T-cells and Th17 cells.
- Short-chain fatty acids (SCFAs) such as butyrate, metabolites of commensal bacteria, can inhibit expression of pro-inflammatory cytokines.
- Quorum sensing (QS) signals are part of the bacterial regulation mechanisms to perceive and promote synchronized behaviours. Depending on the bacteria, QS signals can trigger an inflammatory or anti-inflammatory gene expression at target cells within the gastrointestinal tract.
- *Commensal* is a term used to represent bacteria that can derive benefit from and do not inflict harm on the host. A given bacterium may have the capacity to shift from a mutualistic (both host and bacterium benefit) to a commensal or parasitic (harm to host) position depending on the environment and activation of the host.

Adapted from Belkaid and Hand (2014);
Lin and Zhang (2017) by Angela Walker

Communication/hormones

MA's sleep was unrefreshing, her menstrual cycle was irregular, she had lost her libido and she was experiencing cognitive issues. The incidence of CFS/ME is higher in the female population, and although the mechanism is not fully understood, oestrogen metabolism is suspected to be involved (Soyupek *et al.*, 2017). MA had experienced several incidents of acute and chronic stress exposure, which is perhaps reflected in the results for the four-point salivary cortisol and DHEA tests; these are interpreted and discussed below. Thyroid-stimulating hormone was within the conventional reference range and only 0.1 mIU/L outside an optimal reference range and so further thyroid investigation were not prioritized at that stage.

Assimilation

This practitioner looks at trends in blood chemistry results and correlates this to the patient's symptom pattern. MA had low total protein, low urea, low creatinine and raised MCV and MCH, all of which can be due to hypochlorhydria and reduced digestive enzymes when overall dietary protein intake is sufficient, as was the case for MA (Weatherby and Ferguson, 2002). In addition, MA had halitosis, nausea and gastrointestinal bloating. The lack of belch following the bicarbonate challenge is also thought to be due to low stomach acidity (Weatherby and Ferguson, 2005). These symptom and test result analysis, coupled with unintended weight loss, led the practitioner to query whether assimilation of nutrients from her diet was optimal. Optimal digestion and assimilation involves integration of gut peptide, enzyme and bile acid secretion, all of which may be disturbed by stress and or microbiome imbalance (Ojeda *et al.*, 2016), irrespective of regular bowel movements.

Fluid and electrolyte balance

Electrolytes (minerals with an electric charge) are important for maintaining optimal pH levels and ionic equilibrium in the body. Electrolytes help regulate water in the body fluids and are involved in some of the transport routes across the cell membrane and in nerve impulse transmission.

MA had an excessive thirst, tingling of the skin and low blood pressure, combined with occasional rapid heartbeat and cold hands and feet. While there is a paucity of published data to support this, in this practitioner's clinical experience these symptoms can be related to an electrolyte imbalance (i.e. lack of alkalizing minerals), often triggered when the body is under stress (Heintze and Dymling, 1985). This was highlighted by the results of the lemon challenge test which looks to see whether the body has the alkaline reserves necessary to respond to the acidity of lemon juice by using the buffering effects of electrolytes.

Lifestyle factors
While time in bed appeared sufficient, MA found it difficult to fall asleep (taking over one hour) and was unrefreshed on waking, which led the practitioner to suspect suboptimal sleep quality. Stage 3 of non-REM sleep is thought to be necessary for an individual to feel refreshed the next day (NIH, 2018); perhaps MA was not achieving all stages of the sleep cycle, which are required for optimal sleep quality (Walker, 2018). In CFS, pacing refers to a balance between energy availability and expenditure. The practitioner suspected that MA frequently expended too much energy, contributing to a later dip in energy levels.

Areas to focus on in the future

- **Energy:** MA's primary symptom and reason for seeking help was fatigue. The practitioner's approach was to focus on the foundations of her diet, digestion, immune and adrenal function first, before investigating mitochondria function. The progress and development section below covers investigations into mitochondria function and production of energy adenosine triphosphate (ATP).
- **Biotransformation and elimination/detoxification:** While digestive symptoms were not a priority from MA's perspective, she had experienced a series of gastrointestinal infections while travelling in Asia which had continued for some months after her return. There is some evidence to link CFS with gastrointestinal infections (Donnachie *et al.*, 2018). In addition, there were

signs that digestion was suboptimal, as discussed above under 'Assimilation'.

Initial recommendations

Dietary guidance

MA felt confused about the components of an optimal diet, so the practitioner's approach was to build awareness and confidence over food choices. Given the unintended weight loss, the practitioner did not want to introduce strict dietary restrictions, but rather to support MA in gradual changes that would be simple, given her current limited available energy. The clinic this practitioner works from publishes a Healthy Eating Guide booklet to help clients make those initial diet changes. The booklet provides top-level guidelines on how to make dietary changes. For each food group it gives healthy versus less healthy examples – under the category 'fish', for example, processed fish or seafood products such as fish fingers are listed as least helpful, tinned or smoked fish is listed as helpful, and wild, line-caught, fresh fish is listed as 'fantastic'. A 14-day plan and practical suggestions on where to source foods is included. The 14-day plan is not intended to be prescriptive, rather to provide 14 examples of breakfast, lunch and dinner to inspire and motivate individuals to find meals they can enjoy.

MA's dietary guidance can be summarized as follows:

- Reduce gluten – not to eliminate it but to reduce reliance on gluten-containing foods.
- Increase vegetables for fibre and phytonutrients.
- Increase variety and regularity of protein.
- Reduce simple sugars relative to carbohydrates and protein.
- Eliminate caffeine.

Making dietary changes when energy is low can be quite difficult, so these were specifically called 'guidelines' and MA was coached over time to do what she was able. As her energy increased, she was encouraged to invest that energy in her meal preparations.

Dietary rationale

Sensitivities to foods such as wheat and gluten are now recognized as contributing to a variety of symptoms, including digestive issues, weight loss and immune activation (Catassi *et al.*, 2013). Non-coeliac gluten sensitivity is now a recognized condition with a self-reported prevalence in the UK of around 13% (Silvester *et al.*, 2016). More recently, it was shown that a subgroup of ME/CFS patients have a sensitivity to wheat which is related to their symptoms (Uhde *et al.*, 2018).

When reducing foods, it is vital that these are replaced to ensure that calorie and nutrient intake is maintained, which was especially important for MA, given her unintended weight loss. MA was given simple suggestions for gluten-free grains such as brown, wild and red rice, quinoa and buckwheat, as well as starchy vegetables such as swede, carrot, turnip and sweet potato. These suggestions would add variety to MA's diet in the form of additional fibre and flavonoids which may improve the microbiota composition (Klinder *et al.*, 2016) and therefore should positively impact on assimilation and immune function (see Box 5.1).

The practitioner worked with MA to identify simple changes. For example, MA was eating 3–4 portions of vegetables and drinking orange juice each day. MA was encouraged to increase her vegetable intake to seven portions a day (a portion equals 80 g). These changes alone would increase her antioxidant availability, vitamin and mineral status, fibre and electrolytes from their water content (Klinder *et al.*, 2016; Oyebode *et al.*, 2014). In addition, replacing orange juice for a piece for fruit would reduce simple sugar intake and increase fibre (Bazzano *et al.*, 2008).

Although there may be some loss of micronutrient levels in pre-chopped vegetables (Hodges and Toivonen, 2008) the practitioner decided that, given current energy levels, these should be continued as they helped to simplify meal preparation.

An increase in the amount and quality of MA's protein intake was recommended, particularly at breakfast. Ham, which she was having around 3–4 times a week, was replaced with a less processed and sodium-rich protein. Simple, quick protein sources such as eggs, tinned mackerel, sardine or salmon and goats' cheese were recommended, with specific portion sizes given for guidance: two eggs, a small tin of fish or 80 g goats' cheese.

Larger salads were recommended for lunches, containing green leaves, a mix of other vegetables, seeds, beans, and dressings. The seeds and beans were suggested to help provide additional protein, fats and fibre, while also introducing new foods to her diet to increase diversity. These were also easy for her to add when her energy was low.

Her high-fibre cereal and milk was switched to a nutty granola with a protein-to-carbohydrate ratio of 1:4 (SACN, 2015) and full-fat organic yogurt. This simple swap reduced the sugar and increased the total amount of protein in her diet (her previous muesli had a protein-to-carbohydrate ratio of 1:12).

Stress response and nervous system

MA's adrenal test results showed that her cortisol levels were all in normal range; however, she had low DHEA, indicating that cortisol production may have been prioritized, and it was possible that in time cortisol levels might drop without further action. DHEA production was supported with 7-hydroxydehydroepiandrosterone. Despite there being limited published studies to support this supplement (Hampl *et al.*, 2000), anecdotal clinical evidence is supportive. Caffeine can cause hyper-stimulation of cortisol secretion (Lovallo *et al.*, 2005); therefore, to support adrenal function and stabilize the stress response, caffeine was eliminated. Given that she only had one or two cups of coffee a day, this was eliminated immediately rather than gradually reduced.

Techniques to manage stress levels were discussed. As a practising Christian, prayer was recommended over meditation, as this has been found to help with cognitive and emotional wellbeing (Jarvis, 2017) and to have a positive impact on cortisol output (Hulett *et al.*, 2018).

Sleep and pacing

Sleep hygiene was discussed and new habits were recommended with a view to helping MA get to sleep quicker and improve sleep quality. Use of lavender essential oil, either as drops on the pillow or via a diffuser, may help sleep quality (Lewith, Godfrey and Prescott, 2005). Having at least 30 minutes of natural daylight each day can aid the pineal gland to regulate sleep (Sloane, Figueiro and Cohen, 2008). MA was advised to avoid blue light from screens (TV and computer) and devices (mobile phone and tablets) for at least an hour before bed as this light may suppress melatonin production (Wood *et al.*, 2013). Switching off her mobile phone at least 30 minutes before bedtime also enabled her to 'unplug' from social media which has also been found to disturb sleep (Hysing *et al.*, 2015). She was also advised to switch off the internet router at night, based on emerging evidence that electromagnetic fields may disrupt sleep (Lewczuk *et al.*, 2014).

MA was coached on how to listen to her body with regard to available energy and adjust her activity accordingly. This approach is thought to be suitable for most people with CFS to make steady process (NICE, 2007). Initially, MA was advised to rest more than she had been doing in order to find her baseline. In time, she was encouraged to explore how her energy was increasing by doing a little more activity. She was only encouraged to continue this new level of activity if there were no repercussions and she was able to sustain it over consecutive days. This approach is designed to ensure available energy is maintained for repair and restoration and not all 'spent' on activity.

Immune system

An extract of coriolus mushroom was recommended which has been shown to activate natural killer (NK) cells (Jiménez *et al.*, 2005), in one study doubling NK cells in eight weeks (Monro, 2003). NK cells are part of the innate immune system response to viral infections; this intervention was therefore intended to help resolve any viral response that was perhaps persisting, given the high monocyte count.

Assimilation

An extract of papaya and pineapple was recommended, which studies have shown may support digestion and assimilation (Abdelkafi *et al.*, 2009; Pavan *et al.*, 2012).

Maric and colleagues (2014) showed that a multivitamin and mineral can lead to quantitative improvements (in SODase levels, as an assessment of antioxidant status) as well as qualitative improvements (reduced fatigue levels, improved symptoms and sleep quality) in chronic fatigue sufferers. A multivitamin and mineral was added to support the work described above on assimilation and immune function.

Cognition

Dietary intake of long-chain omega 3 fatty acids had been low. Long-chain fatty acids are essential for neurodevelopment and cognitive maintenance (Karr, Alexander and Winningham, 2011); this is thought to be related to their role in cell membrane structures (McCann and Ames, 2005) and endothelial vasodilation function (Kuszewski, Wong and Howe, 2017). While meta-analysis on omega 3 fatty acid supplementation and cognitive function has not demonstrated a significant benefit (Cooper *et al.*, 2015), this may be due to individual variability in essential fatty acid status. Furthermore, it has been hypothesized that in CFS cases, persistent viral infections may impair the delta-6-desaturase enzyme responsible for elongation of the omega 3 and 6 fatty acids chains, which may further inhibit the optimal functional status of essential fatty acids in this group (Puri, 2007).

Essential fatty acids status had not been tested. Under these circumstances, the practitioner always chooses a blend of omega 3 and 6 fatty acids, and a supplement containing omega 3 fatty acids in the form of eicosapentaenoic acid (EPA) and docosahexaenoic acid (DHA) as well as omega 6 fatty acids as gamma-linolenic acid (GLA) was recommended.

Summary of initial supplement recommendations

- Papaya and pineapple enzyme (see Appendix 5.2 for formula and dose).
- Multivitamin and mineral (see Appendix 5.2 for formula and dose).
- 5 mg of 7-hydroxydehydroepiandrosterone blended with 30 mcg of superoxide dismutase and 30 mcg of catalase, twice a day.
- *Coriolus versicolour* 3 g per day for two weeks then 1.5 g for six weeks.
- Essential fats: 270 mg EPA, 180 mg DHA, 160 mg GLA per day.

Progress and development

Within six months of implementing the above programme, MA had made progress, reporting that over the winter months she had not had any viral infections, despite those around her having colds and flu. Her menstrual cycle became more regular, although she was experiencing premenstrual syndrome (PMS) symptoms of abdominal bloating and tearfulness, which were now more apparent due to her more regular cycles.

To support PMS symptoms, one portion of brassica vegetables every day was added. The mechanisms by which the phytonutrients within brassica vegetables may support oestrogen metabolism are described in a review paper on the detoxification functions of food components and their clinical application (Hodges and Minich, 2015). In addition, one dessertspoon of flax seeds every day and two bean-based meals a week were recommended to increase her intake of phytoestrogens (Sirotkin and Harrath, 2014). Phytoestrogens are plant-based oestrogens that compete with endogenous oestrogen to bind to oestrogen receptors in the body. The reader will find a more thorough discussion on the use of foods and supplements to support oestrogen metabolism in Chapter 11.

After ten months, MA's energy levels had improved to the extent that she could typically work every day (and was travelling to the office every day) and socialize once a week. There were, however, still times where she needed to work from home or use a taxi rather than public transport. The practitioner now turned attention to mitochondria function and production of ATP.

Testing mitochondria function

The practitioner used an ATP profile test for over ten years to assess mitochondria function, but this test is no longer available to practitioners. This section will therefore include the main findings from the tests undertaken on MA and how they could be assessed using alternative and currently available functional tests. Table 5.3 describes MA's test results for the ATP profile as well as alternative and currently available ways to test these functions.

Oxidation of carbohydrates or fatty acids takes place in the mitochondria and is the energy system which produces the most significant quantity of ATP molecules per substrate. Box 5.2 describes this in more detail alongside the other two main energy systems by which ATP can be produced. Mitochondria production of ATP can be impaired by cofactor deficiency or inhibition due to toxicity (Myhill, Booth and McLaren-Howard, 2013).

BOX 5.2 ENERGY SYSTEMS PRODUCING ATP

ATP-PCr: Takes place in the muscle cells. Typically used by explosive sporting activity. An individual will use their supply of ATP-PCr resource within 30 seconds of intensive activity.

Glycolysis: Takes place in the cytosol. Anaerobic. Glucose or glycogen is reduced anaerobically producing lactate. Two to three molecules of ATP produced by each molecule of glucose or glycogen which makes it much less efficient than oxidative phosphorylation

Oxidative phosphorylation: Occurs in the mitochondria. Requires oxygen. The tricarboxylic acid (TCA) cycle oxidizes acetyl CoA, derived from carbohydrates, proteins, ketone bodies and fatty acids to produce NADH and FADH2 which are used in the respiratory chain to synthesize ATP. Theoretically, 32 or 33 molecules of ATP can be produced from each substrate molecule, making this the most efficient method for producing ATP.

Adapted from Bralley and Lord (2008); Galloway (2011); Mathieu and Ruohola-Baker (2017); McArdle (2010); Salway (2004), by Angela Walker

---

MA's mitochondria function test showed a low normal output of ATP as shown in Table 5.3.

An alternative testing option is the use of urinary organic acids which can provide insight on central energy systems in the following ways:

- Elevated lactate with concurrent low pyruvate can be caused by lack of sufficient mitochondrial ATP (Bralley and Lord, 2008; Lord and Bralley, 2008).
- Elevations of intermediaries of the Krebs cycle – succinate, fumarate, malate and citrate – may indicate a functional insufficiency of the immune mitochondria membrane coenzyme Q_{10} (CoQ$_{10}$) to maintain a flow of electrons, and hence are proposed as a functional marker for low mitochondria ATP.
- See Chapter 3 for a fuller discussion on the use of the organic acids test.

Magnesium is a key cofactor for ATPase (Barbagallo *et al.*, 1999; Gröber, Schmidt and Kisters, 2015). MA's ratio of ATP to magnesium-ATP was low, as shown in Table 5.3, which suggests the available magnesium inside the mitochondria was low (Booth *et al.*, 2012; Myhill, Booth and McLaren-Howard, 2013).

Magnesium can be measured in serum or plasma, although red blood cell magnesium has been found empirically to be a more reliable marker of magnesium status (Biolab, 2018) as the magnesium pool in red blood cells is higher than in serum (Alfrey, Miller and Butkus, 1974; Bralley and Lord, 2008; Simşek, Karabay and Kocabay, 2005).

The active coenzyme forms of B3 (Niacin) are nicotinamide adenine dinucleotide (NAD) and nicotinamide adenine dinucleotide phosphate (NADH). In these forms they function as coenzymes in oxidation and reduction reactions. NAD and NADH cycle between their reduced states NADH + H$^+$ and NADHP + H$^+$. In the central energy pathways this oxidation/reduction reaction is essential for the lactate-to-pyruvate pathway. As outlined in Box 5.2, these are also key substrates in oxidative phosphorylation.

MA's NAD was low, as shown in Table 5.3, which would potentially inhibit mitochondria production of ATP. Niacin red blood cell NAD activation is an equivalent marker which continues to be an available test.

Table 5.3 Results from mitochondria function (out-of-range results) and comparable tests

Mitochondria Function Test Component	MA result (reference range) and comment	Comparable, available test
ATP produced by whole cells	1.68 nmol/10^6 cells (1.6–2.9) Low normal	Urinary organic acids: serum CoQ_{10}
Ratio of ATP to Magnesium-ATP	0.58 (> 0.65) Magnesium-related ATP is low	Red blood cell magnesium
Red cell NAD	12.8 mcg/ml (14–30) Low NAD activity	Niacin red blood cell NAD activation
DNA adducts (chemicals bound to DNA)	Phenoxyethanol, phloroglucinol, resorcinol	Toxicity screen

CoQ_{10} has two key roles in mitochondria function. It is a mobile electron carrier, transferring electrons through the various complexes (1–3) in the electron transport chain. In its reduced form it acts as an antioxidant and is the only lipophilic endogenously produced antioxidant (Molyneux *et al.*, 2008). Since the practitioner was able to measure ATP output using the mitochondria function test, MA's CoQ_{10} level was not measured. Serum CoQ_{10} continues to be an available test and may be helpful for practitioners assessing mitochondria function.

DNA adducts are a form of DNA damage, where a chemical is covalently bound to the DNA, and it causes a mutation of that DNA so that it cannot replicate normally. The chemical can potentially come from any substance the body is exposed to. Examples include a metal such as nickel, a plastic such as bisphenol A (BPA) or a chemical found in hair dye or body products. While most research on DNA adducts is in relation to carcinogenesis, that process involves a mutation which can influence enzymes functioning within the mitochondria (Van Houten, Hunter and Meyer, 2016), which is why testing these can be useful for mitochondria function.

MA's test reported presence of phenoxyethanol on the SOD2 gene, phloroglucinol on the adenylate cyclase gene and resorcinol on a non-gene area. The alternative way to explore toxicant impact on mitochondria function is to use toxicant profile for the presence of toxicants (metals as well as non-metals), usually via urine. Although these will identify the *presence* of a toxicant, that doesn't automatically mean it is disturbing mitochondria function. Some profiles include a marker called tiglyglycine, which is elevated due to mitochondria disorders of fatty acid metabolism. Tiglyglycine can therefore be used as a marker for toxicant impact on mitochondria function (Shaw, 2017).

Mitochondria function support

The first action was to address exposure to these exogenous toxicants. MA was given a referenced data sheet on how to reduce toxicant exposure in general. Phenoxyethanol is used as a preservative in cosmetics and so she was asked to reduce usage of these products to minimize ongoing exposure.

Updated supplementation after mitochondrial testing:

- 400 mg of glutathione a day, for three months
- 500 mg of calcium d-glucarate a day, for three months.

These supplements support specific detoxification pathways relevant to the three chemicals: in particular calcium-d-glucarate for phenoxyethanol (Scientific Committee on Consumer Safety, 2016) and resorcinol (Kim and Matthews, 1987) and glutathione for phloroglucinol (Antoce, Badea and Cojocaru, 2016).

- 200 mg of magnesium, in the form of magnesium glycinate as this appears to be well absorbed and can help improve the quality of sleep (Bannai and Kawai, 2012).
- Multinutrient formula designed to support mitochondrial ATP production. The full formula is shown in Appendix 5.2. In summary, it includes a multivitamin and mineral in low doses plus 500 mg curcuma and 25 mg carnitine. In cell studies, curcumin has been shown to reverse mitochondrial damage

(Daverey and Agrawal, 2016), and in animal studies to stimulate mitochondria biogenesis (Hamidie *et al.*, 2015). Carnitine is essential for the transport of long-chain fatty acids across the mitochondrial membrane for beta oxidation (Longo, Frigeni and Pasquali, 2016).

- Digestive enzyme and essential fats continued.

Supplements stopped:

- Previous multivitamin and mineral.
- 7-Hydroxydehydroepiandrosterone and superoxide dismutase.
- *Coriolus versicolour* (this was only taken for eight weeks).

Progress

As is often the case, life stressors intervened and probably slowed the healing process. Individuals are rarely able to heal in an inert environment (and even if they are able to stay at a retreat or ashram, they still have to reintegrate into 'real life' at some point). For MA there was a death of someone she was close to, stressors at work, a change of job, a house sale, purchase and move. The mitochondria function was repeated two years after the first test, showing significant improvements. These are summarized in Table 5.4.

Table 5.4 Compared results from initial and follow-up mitochondria function tests

Mitochondria function test	Initial result (reference range) and comment	Follow-up results (reference range) and comment
ATP produced by whole cells	1.68 nmol/10^6 cells (1.6–2.9) Low normal	2.55 nmol/10^6 cells (1.6–2.9) Normal
Ratio of ATP to magnesium-ATP	0.58 (> 0.65) Low	0.65 (> 0.65) Borderline normal

Red cell NAD	12.8 mcg/ml (14–30) Low	16.8 mcg/ml (14–30) Normal
DNA adducts	Phenoxyethanol, phloroglucinol, resorcinol	None Normal

These results were particularly encouraging for MA to see in black and white; they gave her confidence to gradually increase her activity and it was at this point she turned her attention more towards her fertility. The previous supplements were stopped and MA was recommended to take the following supplements:

- A multivitamin and mineral designed for use in conception. The formula is provided in Appendix 5.2.
- 1000 mg fish oil per day containing 500 mg DHA and 100 mg EPA. Sufficient maternal DHA status has been shown in an observational study to improve infant cognitive function (Braarud *et al.*, 2018).
- A formula containing nutrients which have an antioxidant function – the full formula is shown in Appendix 5.2. Reactive oxygen species have been linked to egg damage that can increase with ageing (Agarwal, Saleh and Bedaiwy, 2003). In addition, vitamin E (total combined with the multivitamin and mineral of 12 mg) may help oocyte maturation and higher-quality embryo maturation (Bahadori *et al.*, 2017).

At year four, as part of fertility investigations, MA was told she had an enlarged bowel. MA's digestive and elimination function had varied throughout the previous years; however, even at their worst they had been quite minor compared with her other symptoms. That said, as the rest of MA's health improved, her gastrointestinal symptoms came to have greater significance. There had been hesitation to order a comprehensive stool test as, depending on the findings, any antimicrobial herbs that we might use would be incompatible with pregnancy. It was now agreed to complete a comprehensive stool test (using PCR methodology, see Chapter 3). The results showed the following:

- raised levels of microsporidia (intracellular parasitic fungi (CDC, 2017b))
- modest levels of *Candida* species
- low secretory IgA (sIgA)
- high beta-glucuronidase (see Box 5.3)
- elevated antigliadin IgA.

Following the digestive function testing, the following supplements were added:

- Calcium-d-glucarate (500 mg TID) for two months. Calcium-D-glucarate is used to reduce beta-glucuronidase activity based on clinical observation and animal studies ('Calcium-D-glucarate', 2002; Dwivedi *et al.*, 1990).
- *Saccharomyces boulardii* (3 billion CFUs (colony forming units)) and proteolytic enzyme, taken on an empty stomach for three months to allow the proteolytic enzyme to break down the cell walls of the microsporidium. Cell wall proteins on yeasts and fungi are thought to be involved in their adhesion to host tissues (Chaffin *et al.*, 1998). *S. boulardii* may interfere with intestinal pathogens and could increase sIgA levels in the intestine (McFarland, 2010).
- Pregnancy preparation supplementation was continued.

Elevated faecal IgA antibodies to gluten indicated an immune response to gluten (Halblaub *et al.*, 2004); MA was now advised to strictly eliminate all gluten. MA agreed to use protection during sex and put any attempts to conceive on hold for three months so that she could undergo a supplementation programme to address the findings. This was ultra-cautious, but there is no research to show that calcium-d-glucarate and proteolytic enzymes are safe during pregnancy.

This appeared to be the final step in MA's recovery. By her final appointment (which occurred 12 months following the digestive function test), she was living life to the full, working as much as she wanted and had conceived and had a successful full-term pregnancy.

> **BOX 5.3 BETA-GLUCURONIDASE**
> Beta-glucuronidase is an enzyme produced by bacteria in the large intestine. The enzyme has a number of functions including the breakdown of complex carbohydrates and the deconjugation of glucuronide molecules. Glucuronide molecules are produced as part of the detoxification and metabolism of a variety of endogenous substances such as hormones and exogenous toxicants. Beta-glucuronidase activity must be sufficient for deconjugation of desirable molecules yet low enough to prevent deconjugation and reabsorption of toxicants and other undesirable substances.

Discussion and conclusion

As much as any case can be, MA's case is typical. It was complex, involving at least four different functions in the body – defence and repair, endocrine, energy and absorption – and it took time. CFS/ME cases can often take time to resolve for many different reasons: time for the client to implement the changes, time for the body to heal, financial pacing of the cost of tests and supplements, and fitting in the rest of life. For instance, in this time MA moved house, changed jobs and had to cope with a family bereavement.

Also, although it seemed initially in her eyes that the fatigue was sudden onset, on reflection, going through her history, the previous two years had probably laid the foundations for the final trigger of the viral infection.

It was interesting to observe that as some symptoms are resolved, other symptoms can arise. For MA, as her menstrual cycle became regular, she then started to get regular PMS symptoms, in particular menstrual cramps and tearfulness. As is often the case for females, her CFS/ME symptoms also got worse in the last few days of her cycle. Based on the frequency with it is raised on CFS/ME forums, PMS is a major concern to those who experience it and it is certainly something frequently seen by this practitioner, although the mechanism for this is poorly understood. Research has found a higher rate of autoimmune, endocrine disorders, fibromyalgia and CFS in women with endometriosis (Sinaii *et al.*, 2002); however, there is little information beyond that. This is hardly surprising, given that both hormone imbalance and CFS/ME are very individual, with a multitude of triggers. Although MA did not have endometriosis, it is a condition like PMS involving hormone imbalance. For MA, it is possible that the raised levels of beta-glucuronidase may have increased unconjugated levels of oestrogen, contributing to a hormonal imbalance. Raised beta-glucuronidation is associated with an increase in oestrogen-receptor positive breast cancer (Kwa *et al.*, 2016) and colon cancer (Waszkiewicz *et al.*, 2015). Some gut bacteria produce the enzyme beta-glucuronidase, which deconjugates glucuronic acid from oestrogen in the gut. This reverses the normal detoxification process and so the now free oestrogen is available to be reabsorbed, thereby increasing the total oestrogen in circulation and possible oestrogen dominance.

This demonstrates the effect of using a root-cause approach to CFS/ME. In the case of MA, the additional benefit of addressing all the factors involved in her fatigue, such as the raised beta-glucuronidase and the full 'jigsaw puzzle' of her health, enabled her to achieve full health.

In working with CFS/ME, the support network can be very important. MA had a loving childhood, with healthy parents who would come and stay to care for her if her husband was away. She had a loving husband who was considerate of her needs. She was believed at all times by those around her and given the space to heal at her own pace. This can actually be quite rare, and although there are few statistics on it, clinical experience has shown that clients may have children, partners or older parents that they feel they need to care for before their own health. They may feel the pressure to work to earn money not just for therapy but also for day-to-day living, although over 50% of people with CFS/ME are unable to work (Collin *et al.*, 2011) and they may not be believed. Some lay people (often of an older generation) continue to label CFS/ME as 'Yuppie flu' and do not take it seriously, and newspaper articles continue to cite examples of the scepticism of medical professionals towards the reality of CFS/ME (Chainey, 2017).

As people recover from CFS/ME, reintegration into 'normal' life can prove to be the next challenge, with some people wanting to pick up life where they left off, risking a relapse. Others can be over-cautious, having lost trust in their bodies, whereas others get it just right. When CFS/ME is at its worse, people do not have to make any decisions about whether they do something or not – their body makes the decision for them; as they recover and they have more energy, they have to give careful consideration to assess if there would be delayed fatigue, also known as post-exertional fatigue. Follow-up testing can play an important role here. Sometimes finances mean that retesting is not an option and we can only work on symptoms. Sometimes retesting is used to assess progress and whether the therapeutic actions are having an effect or need to be changed. Follow-up testing can also inform parents and family that the client is still recovering and they should not be pushed to do more. For MA, the results from follow-up testing gave her confidence in her body and improved health capabilities.

Q&A

AW: MA hadn't seen lots of practitioners, which is unusual for a CFS client. How did this help you? Were there any ways this was a challenge?

HL: You are correct: it is rare that someone finds a specialist clinic such as ours at the start of their illness. It is more normal to find that people have seen many different practitioners including doctors, consultants, alternative and complementary therapists. This can mean that clients have often spent a lot of money on their recovery, meaning they are left on a very tight budget or they are very reluctant to spend any more. They have often been made false promises, and so, while they have not given up hope, they can be understandably very sceptical or desperate. Clients can have a lot of test results and obviously feel that they are a long way through their journey and can therefore be impatient, expecting the latest practitioner to be able to start where any previous practitioner left off. Although it's important to prepare and go over recent and historical health records, it is a new relationship, which is going to take time to establish. For instance, different clients respond to dietary changes in different ways; some may need to be taken through stages of dietary changes and can take a couple of years to be able to prepare themselves mentally and practically to start something like an autoimmune Palaeo diet, whereas others can make that change within just a week or two.

MA was right at the start of her recovery journey, having only seen her medical practitioner beforehand. I would say that this was an advantage on the whole. It did mean that she had little understanding of what to expect, and simple dietary changes took time. A lot of the biology was new, but MA was inquisitive and keen to have things explained.

AW: Reflecting on the case, is there anything you would you have done differently?

HL: It seems quite obvious on reflection now that a stool test earlier on could have been helpful and potentially may have sped up the recovery process. Although overt symptoms such as IBS were lacking, there were constant hints that the health of her GI tract was not optimal (inability to gain weight, nausea and bloating) and, of course, she had the gut infections whilst travelling in Asia two years before she started with CFS. I also see more and more how there can be problems with gut health that are expressed in ways other than the blatant IBS-type symptoms. I now consider stool or breath testing for large or small intestine health when perhaps there are signs of poor nutrient absorption issues through weight or appetite and, of course, when finances allow it.

AW: Is it unusual for a client with CFS to have had a seemingly 'normal' childhood and upbringing – i.e. good health, no stressful episodes?

HL: I would say there are no usual or unusual circumstances for CFS based on my years of working with it to date. Although there may be some 'rules of thumb' with regard to precursors to CFS/ME, I find every single case to be unique. For instance, while many people with CFS/ME may have had the Epstein Barr virus (EBV) many years or even just months before their diagnosis, there are also many people who have never had such an infection, and, of course, those who have had EBV and never developed CFS/ME. Some people can have traumatic childhoods and have a healthy adulthood, while, as in MA's case, others can have a wonderful childhood and early adulthood, but a buildup of several health issues in a relatively short period of time can be overwhelming to their body. That is really why we need to take a person-centred approach to addressing the condition and why that approach can be so constructive, compared with an allopathic or 'treat the symptoms' approach.

Appendix 5.1 Summary of diagnostic criteria for CFS/ME

NICE (2007)	CDC/Fukuda (1994)	Canadian Criteria (Carruthers *et al.* 2003)	Institute of Medicine (2015)
4 months for an adult 3 months for a minor	6 months for an adult	6 months for an adult	6 months
Has fatigue with all of the following features: • new or had a specific onset (that is, it is not lifelong) • persistent and/or recurrent • unexplained by other conditions • has resulted in a substantial reduction in activity level • characterized by post-exertional malaise and/or fatigue (typically delayed, for example, by at least 24 hours, with slow recovery over several days)	Has four or more of these symptoms concurrently present for ≥6 months: • impaired memory or concentration • sore throat • tender cervical or axillary lymph nodes • muscle pain • multi-joint pain • new headaches • unrefreshing sleep • post-exertion malaise	Has all of these symptoms: • fatigue • post-exertional malaise and/or fatigue • sleep dysfunction • pain • two or more neurological/ cognitive manifestations	Has all of these symptoms: • impaired day-to-day functioning due to fatigue • malaise after exertion (physical, cognitive or emotional) • unrefreshing sleep

cont.

NICE (2007)	CDC/Fukuda (1994)	Canadian Criteria (Carruthers *et al.* 2003)	Institute of Medicine (2015)
Has one or more of the following symptoms: • difficulty with sleeping, such as insomnia, hypersomnia, unrefreshing sleep, a disturbed sleep–wake cycle • muscle and/or joint pain that is multi-site and without evidence of inflammation • headaches • painful lymph nodes without pathological enlargement • sore throat • cognitive dysfunction, such as difficulty thinking, inability to concentrate, impairment of short-term memory, and difficulties with word-finding, planning/organizing thoughts and information processing • physical or mental exertion makes symptoms worse • general malaise or 'flu-like' symptoms • dizziness and/or nausea • palpitations in the absence of identified cardiac pathology		At least one symptom from two of the following categories: • autonomic • neuroendocrine • immune	At least of one of these two symptoms: • cognitive impairment • orthostatic intolerance

Appendix 5.2 Supplement formulas used

Multivitamin and mineral (used initially)	Daily dose
Vitamin A (as beta-carotene with mixed carotenoids)	5000 IU
Vitamin C (as calcium ascorbate)	200 mg
Vitamin D (as cholecalciferol)	2000 IU
Vitamin E (contains tocopherols d-alpha, d-beta, d-gamma, d-delta and tocotrienols)	30 IU
Vitamin K1 (as FoodState)	50 mcg
Vitamin B1 (as thiamine HCl)	5 mg
Vitamin B2 (as riboflavin 5-phosphate)	5 mg
Niacin (as niacinamide)	20 mg
Vitamin B6 (as pyridoxal-5-phosphate)	6 mg
Folate (as FoodState)	400 mcg
Vitamin B12 (as methycobalamin)	1000 mcg
Biotin (as FoodState)	300 mcg
Pantothenic acid (as d-calcium pantothenate)	10 mg
Calcium (as Albioncalcium citrate malate)	300 mg
Iodine (as kelp)	150 mcg
Magnesium (as magnesium glycinate complex)	300 mg
Zinc (as zinc bisglycinate complex)	15 mg
Selenium (as Albionselenium glycinate complex)	25 mcg
Copper (as TRAACScopper glycinate chelate)	500 mcg
Manganese (as TRAACSmanganese glycinate chelate)	1 mg
Chromium (as chromium glycinate complex)	50 mcg
Molybdenum (as TRAACSmolybdenum glycinate chelate)	20 mcg
Potassium	10 mg
Boron (as boron glycinate complex)	200 mcg
Vanadium (as vanadium glycinate complex)	25 mcg
Choline (as choline bitartrate)	25 mg
Coenzyme Q_{10} (ubiquinone)	50 mg
Arabinogalactan	200 mg
Citrus Bioflavonoid Peel	50 mg

cont.

Papaya and pineapple enzyme (used initially)	Daily dose
Pineapple concentrate (Ananas comosus fruit)	325 mg
Papaya concentrate	270 mg
Gamma oryzanol	300 mg
Lactobacillus acidophilus, Bifidobacterium bifidum, Bifidobacterium lactis	3 billion viable cells
Multinutrient formula designed for mitochondrial support (used after mitochondria testing)	**Daily dose**
α-Lipoic acid	9.00 mg
Agaricus blazei Murill (almond fungus)	450.00 mg
Biotin	135.00 mcg
Bromelain (enzyme)	9.00 mg
Chromium	60.50 mcg
Coenzyme Q_{10}	2.70 mg
Curcuma powder	599.40 mg
Folic acid/folate ((6S)-5-methyltetrahydrofolic acid, glucosamine salt)	495.00 mcg
Pomegranate extract	90.00 mg
L-carnitine	30.60 mg
Lecithin from sunflowers	40.50 mg
L-glutathione	135.00 mg
Ling Zhi (Glossy Lackporling)	13.50 mg
Lutein	900.00 mcg
Manganese	1.00 mg
Orotic	22.50 mg
Rice bran	450.00 mg
Rice protein	1350.00 mg
Selenium	33.30 mcg
Shiitake (Pasani mushroom)	450.00 mg
Taurine	60.00 mg
Grape seed extract (OPC)	450.00 mg
Vitamin B1 (thiamine hydrochloride)	2.13 mg
Vitamin B2 (riboflavin)	3.15 mg

Vitamin B3 (nicotinamide)	27.00 mg
Vitamin B5 (calcium pantothenate)	12.42 mg
Vitamin B6 (pyridoxal 5'-phosphate)	3.15 mg
Vitamin B12 (methylcobalamin)	67.50 mcg
Vitamin C (L-ascorbic acid)	225.00 mg
Vitamin D3 (cholecalciferol)	11.25 mcg
Vitamin E (mixture of tocopherols and tocotrienols)	7.80 mg (α-tocopherol equivalents)
Yam	450.00 mg
Zinc	11.84 mg
Includes 1350 mg rice protein providing: L-alanine 57.38 mg L-arginine 88.52 mg L-aspartic acid 96.73 mg L-cysteine 18.66 mg L-glutamic acid 190.48 mg glycine 45.43 mg L-histidine 25.28 mg L-isoleucine 45.97 mg L-leucine 90.55 mg L-lysine 38.39 mg L-methionine 39.46 mg L-phenylalanine 58.34 mg L-proline 47.14 mg L-serine 52.47 mg L-threonine 39.46 mg L-tryptophan 9.81 mg L-tyrosine 35.73 mg L-valine 65.48 mg	

Multivitamin and mineral (suitable for pregnancy, used later in programme)	Daily dose
Vitamin D 3	1000 IU 25 mcg
Vitamin E	9 IU 6 mg TE
Vitamin C	180 mg

cont.

Multivitamin and mineral (suitable for pregnancy, used later in programme)	Daily dose
Riboflavin (vitamin B2)	40 mg
Niacin (vitamin B3)	20 mg NE
Vitamin B6	10 mg
Folate (as 5-MTHF)	400 mcg
Vitamin B12	20 mcg
Biotin	200 mcg
Pantothenic acid (vitamin B5)	50 mg
Calcium	120 mg
Magnesium	150 mg
Iron	15 mg
Zinc	15 mg
Iodine	150 mcg
Manganese	1 mg
Copper	1000 mcg
Selenium	150 mcg
Chromium	20 mcg
Alpha lipoic acid	50 mg
N-acetyl-L-cysteine	75 mg
Inositol	2 mg
Beta-carotene	5 mg
Lycopene	2 mg
Lutein	2 mg
Coenzyme Q_{10}	40 mg
Bilberry	12.5 mg
Blackberry	12.5 mg
Blackcurrant	12.5 mg
Blueberry	12.5 mg
Pomegranate extract	50 mg
Grapeskin extract	25 mg
Prune juice extract	10 mg

Antioxidant formula (suitable for pregnancy, used later in programme)	Daily dose
Vitamin E	8.9 IU 6 mg TE
Vitamin B12	100 mcg
Vitamin C	170 mg
Magnesium	150 mg
Iodine	150 mcg
Manganese	2 mg
Selenium	50 mcg
Beta-carotene	4 mg
N-acetyl-L-cysteine	80 mg
Alpha lipoic acid	70 mg
Quercetin	50 mg
Coenzyme Q_{10}	10 mg
Mixed berry extract	20 mg
Pomegranate extract	10 mg
Resveratrol	10 mg
Pine bark extract	10 mg
Spirulina	10 mg
Chlorella	10 mg
Bilberry fruit extract	10 mg
Watercress extract	5 mg

References

2020 Health, 2017. *Counting the Cost: Chronic Fatigue Syndrome/Myalgic Encephalomyelitis.* Accessed on 26/05/2019 at www. meassociation.org.uk/wp-content/ uploads/2020Health-Counting-the-Cost-Sept-2017.pdf

Abdelkafi, S., Fouquet, B., Barouh, N., Durner, S. et al., 2009. *In vitro* comparisons between *Carica papaya* and pancreatic lipases during test meal lipolysis: Potential use of CPL in enzyme replacement therapy. *Food Chemistry* 115, 488–494. https://doi. org/10.1016/j.foodchem.2008.12.043

Agarwal, A., Saleh, R.A., Bedaiwy, M.A., 2003. Role of reactive oxygen species in the pathophysiology of human reproduction. *Fertility and Sterility* 79, 829–843. https://doi. org/10.1016/S0015-0282(02)04948-8

Alfrey, A.C., Miller, N.L., Butkus, D., 1974. Evaluation of body magnesium stores. *Journal of Laboratory and Clinical Medicine* 84, 153–162.

Antoce, A.O., Badea, G.A., Cojocaru, G.A., 2016. Effects of glutathione and ascorbic acid addition on the CIE*Lab* chromatic characteristics of Muscat Ottonel wines. *Agriculture and Agricultural Science Procedia* 10, 206–214. https://doi.org/10.1016/j. aaspro.2016.09.054

Bahadori, M.H., Sharami, S.H., Fakor, F., Milani, F., Pourmarzi, D., Dalil-Heirati, S.F., 2017. Level of vitamin E in follicular fluid and serum and oocyte morphology and embryo quality in patients undergoing IVF treatment. *Journal of Family Planning and Reproductive Health* 11, 74–81.

Bannai, M., Kawai, N., 2012. New therapeutic strategy for amino acid medicine: Glycine improves the quality of sleep. *Journal of Pharmacological Sciences* 118, 145–148. https://doi.org/10.1254/jphs.11R04FM

Barbagallo, M., Dominguez, L.J., Tagliamonte, M.R., Resnick, L.M., Paolisso, G., 1999. Effects of glutathione on red blood cell intracellular magnesium: Relation to glucose metabolism. *Hypertension* 1979, 34, 76–82.

Bazzano, L.A., Li, T.Y., Joshipura, K.J., Hu, F.B., 2008. Intake of fruit, vegetables, and fruit juices and risk of diabetes in women. *Diabetes Care* 31, 1311–1317. https://doi. org/10.2337/dc08-0080

Belkaid, Y., Hand, T., 2014. Role of the microbiota in immunity and inflammation. *Cell* 157, 121–141. https://doi.org/10.1016/j. cell.2014.03.011

Biolab, 2018. Magnesium Data Sheet. Accessed on 18/05/2019 at www.biolab.co.uk/docs/ magnesium.pdf

Booth, N.E., Myhill, S., McLaren-Howard, J., 2012. Mitochondrial dysfunction and the pathophysiology of myalgic encephalomyelitis/chronic fatigue syndrome (ME/CFS). *Int. Journal of Clinical and Experimental Medicine* 5, 208–220.

Braarud, H.C., Markhus, M.W., Skotheim, S., Stormark, K.M. *et al.*, 2018. Maternal DHA status during pregnancy has a positive impact on infant problem solving: A Norwegian prospective observation study. *Nutrients* 10. https://doi.org/10.3390/ nu10050529

Bralley, J.A., Lord, R.S., 2008. *Laboratory Evaluations for Integrative and Functional Medicine*, 2nd ed. Metametrix Institute.

Brown, M.M., Brown, A.A., Jason, L.A., 2010. Illness duration and coping style in chronic fatigue syndrome. *Psychological Reports* 106, 383–393. https://doi.org/10.2466/ PR0.106.2.383-393

Calcium-D-glucarate, 2002. *Alternative Medicine Review* 7, 336–339.

Carruthers, B.M., Jain, A.K., De Meirleir, K.L., Peterson, D.L. *et al.*, 2003. Myalgic encephalomyelitis/chronic fatigue syndrome: Clinical working case definition, diagnostic and treatment protocols. *Journal of Chronic Fatigue Syndrome* 11, 7–115. https://doi.org/10.1300/J092v11n01_02

Catassi, C., Bai, J.C., Bonaz, B., Bouma, G. *et al.*, 2013. Non-celiac gluten sensitivity: The new frontier of gluten related disorders. *Nutrients* 5, 3839–3853. https://doi. org/10.3390/nu5103839

CDC, 2017a. Myalgic Encephalomyelitis/ Chronic Fatigue Syndrome: Possible Causes. Accessed on 26/05/2019 at www.cdc.gov/ me-cfs/about/possible-causes.html

CDC, 2017b. Microsporidiosis. Accessed on 26/05/2019 at www.cdc.gov/dpdx/microsporidiosis/index.html

Chaffin, W.L., López-Ribot, J.L., Casanova, M., Gozalbo, D., Martínez, J.P., 1998. Cell wall and secreted proteins of *Candida albicans*: Identification, function, and expression. *Microbiology and Molecular Biology Reviews* 62, 130–180.

Chainey, N., 2017. Yet more research shows chronic fatigue syndrome is real. When will health services catch up? *The Guardian*, 21 March. Accessed on 26/5/2019 at www.theguardian.com/commentisfree/2017/mar/21/yet-more-research-shows-chronic-fatigue-syndrome-is-real-when-will-health-services-catch-up

Cleare, A.J., 2004. The HPA axis and the genesis of chronic fatigue syndrome. *Trends in Endocrinology and Metabolism* 15, 55–59. https://doi.org/10.1016/j.tem.2003.12.002

Collin, S.M., Crawley, E., May, M.T., Sterne, J.A.C., Hollingworth, W., 2011. The impact of CFS/ME on employment and productivity in the UK: A cross-sectional study based on the CFS/ME national outcomes database. *BMC Health Services Research* 11, 217. https://doi.org/10.1186/1472-6963-11-217

Cooper, R.E., Tye, C., Kuntsi, J., Vassos, E., Asherson, P., 2015. Omega-3 polyunsaturated fatty acid supplementation and cognition: A systematic review and meta-analysis. *Journal of Psychopharmacology* 29, 753–763. https://doi.org/10.1177/0269881115587958

Daverey, A., Agrawal, S.K., 2016. Curcumin alleviates oxidative stress and mitochondrial dysfunction in astrocytes. *Neuroscience* 333, 92–103. https://doi.org/10.1016/j.neuroscience.2016.07.012

Donnachie, E., Schneider, A., Mehring, M., Enck, P., 2018. Incidence of irritable bowel syndrome and chronic fatigue following GI infection: A population-level study using routinely collected claims data. *Gut* 67, 1078–1086. https://doi.org/10.1136/gutjnl-2017-313713

Dwivedi, C., Heck, W.J., Downie, A.A., Larroya, S., Webb, T.E., 1990. Effect of calcium glucarate on beta-glucuronidase activity and glucarate content of certain vegetables and fruits. *Biochemical Medicine and Metabolic Biology* 43, 83–92.

Fukuda, K., Straus, S.E., Hickie, I., Sharpe, M., Dobbins, J.G., Komaroff, A., 1995. The chronic fatigue syndrome: A comprehensive approach to its definition and study. *Annals of Internal Medicine* 121, 953–959. https://doi.org/10.7326/0003-4819-121-12-199412150-00009

Galloway, 2011. Exercise Physiology. In S.J. Lanham-New, S.J. Steer, S.M. Sherrifs, A.L. Collins (eds) *Sports and Exercise Metabolism*. Wiley-Blackwell.

Gröber, U., Schmidt, J., Kisters, K., 2015. Magnesium in prevention and therapy. *Nutrients* 7, 8199–8226. https://doi.org/10.3390/nu7095388

Halblaub, J.M.L., Renno, J., Kempf, A., Bartel, J., Schmidt-Gayk, H., 2004. Comparison of different salivary and fecal antibodies for the diagnosis of celiac disease. *Clinical Laboratory* 50, 551–557.

Hamidie, R.D.R., Yamada, T., Ishizawa, R., Saito, Y., Masuda, K., 2015. Curcumin treatment enhances the effect of exercise on mitochondrial biogenesis in skeletal muscle by increasing cAMP levels. *Metabolism* 64, 1334–1347. https://doi.org/10.1016/j.metabol.2015.07.010

Hampl, R., Lapcík, O., Hill, M., Klak, J. *et al.*, 2000. 7-Hydroxydehydroepiandrosterone – a natural antiglucocorticoid and a candidate for steroid replacement therapy? *Physiological Research* 49, Suppl 1, S107–112.

Heintze, U., Dymling, J.F., 1985. Buffer effect, secretion rate, pH and electrolytes of stimulated whole saliva in relation to the renin-aldosterone system. *Swedish Dental Journal* 9, 249–254.

Hodges, D.M., Toivonen, P.M.A., 2008. Quality of fresh-cut fruits and vegetables as affected by exposure to abiotic stress. *Postharvest Biology and Technology* 48, 155–162. https://doi.org/10.1016/j.postharvbio.2007.10.016

Hodges, R.E., Minich, D.M., 2015. Modulation of metabolic detoxification pathways using foods and food-derived components: A scientific review with clinical application. *Journal of Nutrition and Metabolism* 2015. https://doi.org/10.1155/2015/760689

Hulett, J.M., Armer, J.M., Leary, E., Stewart, B.R., McDaniel, R., Smith, K., Millspaugh, R., Millspaugh, J., 2018. Religiousness, spirituality, and salivary cortisol in breast cancer survivorship: A pilot study. *Cancer Nursing* 41.

Hysing, M., Pallesen, S., Stormark, K.M., Jakobsen, R., Lundervold, A.J., Sivertsen, B., 2015. Sleep and use of electronic devices in adolescence: Results from a large population-based study. *BMJ Open* 5, e006748. https://doi.org/10.1136/bmjopen-2014-006748

Institute of Medicine, Committee on the Diagnostic Criteria for Myalgic Encephalomyelitis/Chronic Fatigue Syndrome, Board on the Health of Select Populations, 2015. *Beyond Myalgic Encephalomyelitis/Chronic Fatigue Syndrome: Redefining an Illness, The National Academies Collection: Reports funded by National Institutes of Health*. National Academies Press (US), Washington, DC.

Jarvis, M., 2017. Meditation and yoga associated with changes in brain. *Science* 358, 461–461. https://doi.org/10.1126/science.358.6362.461

Jerjes, W.K., Cleare, A.J., Wessely, S., Wood, P.J., Taylor, N.F., 2005. Diurnal patterns of salivary cortisol and cortisone output in chronic fatigue syndrome. *Journal of Affective Disorders* 87, 299–304. https://doi.org/10.1016/j.jad.2005.03.013

Jiménez, E., Garcia-Lora, A., Martinez, M., Garrido, F., 2005. Identification of the protein components of protein-bound polysaccharide (PSK) that interact with NKL cells. *Cancer Immunology, Immunotherapy* CII 54, 395–399. https://doi.org/10.1007/s00262-004-0601-1

Karr, J.E., Alexander, J.E., Winningham, R.G., 2011. Omega-3 polyunsaturated fatty acids and cognition throughout the lifespan: A review. *Nutritional Neuroscience* 14, 216–225. https://doi.org/10.1179/1476830511Y.0000000012

Kim, Y.C., Matthews, H.B., 1987. Comparative metabolism and excretion of resorcinol in male and female F344 rats. *Fundamental and Applied Toxicology* 9, 409–414. https://doi.org/10.1016/0272-0590(87)90023-6

Klinder, A., Shen, Q., Heppel, S., Lovegrove, J.A., Rowland, I., Tuohy, K.M., 2016. Impact of increasing fruit and vegetables and flavonoid intake on the human gut microbiota. *Food and Function* 7, 1788–1796. https://doi.org/10.1039/c5fo01096a

Kuszewski, J.C., Wong, R.H.X., Howe, P.R.C., 2017. Effects of long-chain omega-3 polyunsaturated fatty acids on endothelial vasodilator function and cognition – are they interrelated? *Nutrients* 9. https://doi.org/10.3390/nu9050487

Kwa, M., Plottel, C.S., Blaser, M.J., Adams, S., 2016. The intestinal microbiome and estrogen receptor-positive female breast cancer. *JNCI: Journal of the National Cancer Institute* 108, djw029. https://doi.org/10.1093/jnci/djw029

Lewczuk, B., Redlarski, G., Zak, A., Ziółkowska, N., Przybylska-Gornowicz, B., Krawczuk, M., 2014. Influence of electric, magnetic, and electromagnetic fields on the circadian system: Current stage of knowledge. *BioMed Research International* 2014, 169459. https://doi.org/10.1155/2014/169459

Lewith, G.T., Godfrey, A.D., Prescott, P., 2005. A single-blinded, randomized pilot study evaluating the aroma of *Lavandula augustifolia* as a treatment for mild insomnia. *Journal of Alternative and Complementary Medicine* 11, 631–637. https://doi.org/10.1089/acm.2005.11.631

Lin, L., Zhang, J., 2017. Role of intestinal microbiota and metabolites on gut homeostasis and human diseases. *BMC Immunology* 18. https://doi.org/10.1186/s12865-016-0187-3

Longo, N., Frigeni, M., Pasquali, M., 2016. Carnitine transport and fatty acid oxidation. *Biochimica et Biophysica Acta* 1863, 2422–2435. https://doi.org/10.1016/j.bbamcr.2016.01.023

Lord, R.S., Bralley, J.A., 2008. Clinical applications of urinary organic acids. Part I: Detoxification markers. *Alternative Medicine Review* 13, 205–215.

Lovallo, W.R., Whitsett, T.L., al'Absi, M., Sung, B.H., Vincent, A.S., Wilson, M.F., 2005. Caffeine stimulation of cortisol secretion across the waking hours in relation to caffeine intake levels. *Psychosomatic Medicine* 67, 734–739. https://doi.org/10.1097/01.psy.0000181270.20036.06

Maric, D., Brkic, S., Tomic, S., Novakov Mikic, A., Cebovic, T., Turkulov, V., 2014. Multivitamin mineral supplementation in patients with chronic fatigue syndrome. *Medical Science Monitor* 20, 47–53. https://doi.org/10.12659/MSM.889333

Mathieu, J., Ruohola-Baker, H., 2017. Metabolic remodeling during the loss and acquisition of pluripotency. *Development* 144, 541–551. https://doi.org/10.1242/dev.128389

McArdle, W.D., 2010. *Exercise Physiology: Nutrition, Energy and Human Performance*. Lippincott Williams & Wilkins.

McCann, J.C., Ames, B.N., 2005. Is docosahexaenoic acid, an n-3 long-chain polyunsaturated fatty acid, required for development of normal brain function? An overview of evidence from cognitive and behavioral tests in humans and animals. *American Journal of Clinical Nutrition* 82, 281–295. https://doi.org/10.1093/ajcn.82.2.281

McFarland, L.V., 2010. Systematic review and meta-analysis of *Saccharomyces boulardii* in adult patients. *World Journal of Gastroenterology* 16, 2202–2222. https://doi.org/10.3748/wjg.v16.i18.2202

Molyneux, S.L., Young, J.M., Florkowski, C.M., Lever, M., George, P.M., 2008. Coenzyme Q$_{10}$: Is there a clinical role and a case for measurement? *Clinical Biochemist Reviews* 29, 71–82.

Monro, J.A., 2003. Treatment of cancer with mushroom products. *Archives of Environmental Health* 58, 533–537. https://doi.org/10.3200/AEOH.58.8.533-537

Myhill, S., Booth, N., McLaren-Howard, J., 2013. Targeting mitochondrial dysfunction in the treatment of myalgic encephalomyelitis/chronic fatigue syndrome (ME/CFS) – a clinical audit. *International Journal of Clinical and Experimental Medicine* 6, 1–15.

Nater, U.M., Maloney, E., Boneva, R.S., Gurbaxani, B.M. *et al.*, 2008. Attenuated morning salivary cortisol concentrations in a population-based study of persons with chronic fatigue syndrome and well controls. *Journal of Clinical Endocrinology and Metabolism* 93, 703–709. https://doi.org/10.1210/jc.2007-1747

NICE, 2007. Chronic fatigue syndrome/myalgic encephalomyelitis (or encephalopathy): diagnosis and management. Accessed on 26/05/2019 at www.nice.org.uk/guidance/cg53/chapter/1-Guidance#diagnosis

NIH, 2018. Brain Basics: Understanding Sleep. Accessed on 26/05/2019 at www.ninds.nih.gov/Disorders/Patient-Caregiver-Education/Understanding-Sleep

Nisenbaum, R., Jones, A., Jones, J., Reeves, W., 2000. Longitudinal analysis of symptoms reported by patients with chronic fatigue syndrome. *Annals of Epidemiology* 10, 458.

Ojeda, P., Bobe, A., Dolan, K., Leone, V., Martinez, K., 2016. Nutritional modulation of gut microbiota – the impact on metabolic disease pathophysiology. *Journal of Nutritional Biochemistry* 28, 191–200. https://doi.org/10.1016/j.jnutbio.2015.08.013

Oyebode, O., Gordon-Dseagu, V., Walker, A., Mindell, J.S., 2014. Fruit and vegetable consumption and all-cause, cancer and CVD mortality: Analysis of Health Survey for England data. *Journal of Epidemiology and Community Health* 68, 856–862. https://doi.org/10.1136/jech-2013-203500

Pavan, R., Jain, S., Shraddha, Kumar, A., 2012. Properties and therapeutic application of bromelain: A review. *Biotechnology Research International* 2012, 976203. https://doi.org/10.1155/2012/976203

Puri, B.K., 2007. Long-chain polyunsaturated fatty acids and the pathophysiology of myalgic encephalomyelitis (chronic fatigue syndrome). *Journal of Clinical Pathology* 60, 122–124. https://doi.org/10.1136/jcp.2006.042424

Salway, J., 2004. *Metabolism at a Glance*, 3rd ed. Blackwell.

Scientific Advisory Committee on Nutrition (SACN), 2015. SACN Carbohydrates and Health Report. Accessed on 26/05/2019 at www.gov.uk/government/publications/sacn-carbohydrates-and-health-report

Scientific Committee on Consumer Safety, 2016. Scientific Committee on Consumer Safety (SCCS): Opinion on Phenoxyethanol. Accessed on 18/06/2019 at https://ec.europa.eu/health/scientific_committees/consumer_safety/docs/sccs_o_195.pdf

Shaw, W., 2017. Elevated urinary glyphosate and clostridia metabolites with altered dopamine metabolism in triplets with autistic spectrum disorder or suspected seizure disorder: A case study. *Integrative Medicine* 16, 50–57.

Silvester, J.A., Weiten, D., Graff, L.A., Walker, J.R., Duerksen, D.R., 2016. Living gluten-free: Adherence, knowledge, lifestyle adaptations and feelings towards a gluten-free diet. *Journal of Human Nutrition and Dietetics* 29, 374–382. https://doi.org/10.1111/jhn.12316

Simşek, E., Karabay, M., Kocabay, K., 2005. Assessment of magnesium status in newly diagnosed diabetic children: Measurement of erythrocyte magnesium level and magnesium tolerance testing. *Turkish Journal of Pediatrics* 47, 132–137.

Sinaii, N., Cleary, S.D., Ballweg, M.L., Nieman, L.K., Stratton, P., 2002. High rates of autoimmune and endocrine disorders, fibromyalgia, chronic fatigue syndrome and atopic diseases among women with endometriosis: A survey analysis. *Human Reproduction* 17, 2715–2724.

Sirotkin, A.V., Harrath, A.H., 2014. Phytoestrogens and their effects. *European Journal of Pharmacology* 741, 230–236. https://doi.org/10.1016/j.ejphar.2014.07.057

Sloane, P.D., Figueiro, M., Cohen, L., 2008. Light as therapy for sleep disorders and depression in older adults. *Clinics in Geriatric Medicine* 16, 25–31.

Soyupek, F., Aydogan, C., Guney, M., Kose, S.A., 2017. Premenstrual syndrome and fibromyalgia: The frequency of the coexistence and their effects on quality of life. *Gynecological Endocrinology* 33, 577–582. https://doi.org/10.1080/09513590.2017.12 96126

Strickland, P., Morriss, R., Wearden, A., Deakin, B., 1998. A comparison of salivary cortisol in chronic fatigue syndrome, community depression and healthy controls. *Journal of Affective Disorders* 47, 191–194. https://doi.org/10.1016/S0165-0327(97)00134-1

Uhde, M., Indart, A.C., Yu, X.B., Jang, S.S. *et al.*, 2018. Markers of non-coeliac wheat sensitivity in patients with myalgic encephalomyelitis/chronic fatigue syndrome. *Gut* gutjnl-2018-316133. https://doi.org/10.1136/gutjnl-2018-316133

Van Houten, B., Hunter, S.E., Meyer, J.N., 2016. Mitochondrial DNA damage induced autophagy, cell death, and disease. *Frontiers in Bioscience – Landmark Ed.* 21, 42–54.

Walker, M., 2018. Why We Sleep. Penguin.

Waszkiewicz, N., Szajda, S.D., Konarzewska-Duchnowska, E., Zalewska-Szajda, B. *et al.*, 2015. Serum β-glucuronidase as a potential colon cancer marker: A preliminary study. *Advances in Hygiene and Experimental Medicine* 69, 436–439. https://doi.org/10.5604/17322693.1148704

Weatherby, D., Ferguson, S., 2002. *Blood Chemistry and CBC Analysis: Clinical Laboratory Testing from a Functional Perspective*. Bear Mountain Publishing.

Weatherby, D., Ferguson, S., 2005. *The Complete Practitioner's Guide to Take-Home Testing, Tools for Gathering More Valuable Patient Data*, 1st ed. Emperors Group LLC.

Wood, B., Rea, M.S., Plitnick, B., Figueiro, M.G., 2013. Light level and duration of exposure determine the impact of self-luminous tablets on melatonin suppression. *Applied Ergonomics* 44, 237–240. https://doi.org/10.1016/j.apergo.2012.07.008

Zaura, E., Brandt, B.W., Teixeira de Mattos, M.J., Buijs, M.J. *et al.*, 2015. Same exposure but two radically different responses to antibiotics: Resilience of the salivary microbiome versus long-term microbial shifts in feces. *mBio* 6. https://doi.org/10.1128/mBio.01693-15

6

Morbid Obesity and Weight Loss Resistance

Nutrition Practitioner: Romilly Hodges

Case Physician: Kara Fitzgerald

Introduction

Overweight and obesity affect over one-third of the world's population and continue to trend upwards (Hruby and Hu, 2015). Obesity, and especially morbid obesity, is associated with extremely high risk of weight-related comorbidities including type 2 diabetes, hypertension, dyslipidaemia, infertility, certain cancers, depression and more. Morbid obesity, defined as body mass index (BMI) 40.0–59.9 kg/m^2, also known as obese class III, is associated with substantially increased rates of total mortality, averaging 6.5–13.7 years of life lost, with most deaths relating to the comorbidities of cardiovascular disease, cancer and diabetes (Kitahara *et al.*, 2014).

Calorie restriction alone isn't often effective for sustained weight loss. Personalized nutrition provides a much more comprehensive view of the underlying aetiological factors and contributors to undesired weight gain, and therefore presents an opportunity to address weight loss with greater success, as this case will show.

Initial case presentation

This case involved a number of medications. Potential drug–nutrient interactions were all reviewed and overseen by the case physician.

AR was 43 years old when she presented with primary concerns of morbid obesity and weight-loss resistance. At six feet tall and 365 lbs (165.5 kg), her BMI of 49.5 put her at extremely high risk for weight-related comorbidities and mortality.

History of weight gain

Starting in her 20s, AR had experienced binge-eating patterns, cyclical weight fluctuations and an overall trend of weight gain. AR had tried dieting in the past, including restricting energy intake to 800 kcal per day for 12 weeks. This had resulted in a 45 lbs (20.4 kg) weight loss but she found that after the 12 weeks her weight-loss resistance had worsened. Her current diet typically consisted of cereal and milk for breakfast, a sandwich with meat and cheese plus a Caesar salad for lunch, and a dinner of pasta or rice with chicken or red meat. She chose organic produce most of the time and avoided artificial sweeteners and high-fructose corn syrup. She experienced significant cravings for cheese, chocolate, pizza and other sugar/carbohydrates. She noted that she felt worse after eating high-carbohydrate foods and that high-protein foods made her feel better. Her eating patterns were 'sporadic', ranging from just one meal per day in the late afternoon to grazing on 'junk' food all day long.

History of comorbidities

AR had hypertension, which had reached a high of 198 systolic, 98 diastolic one year prior to initial consultation. At time of presentation, she was on blood-pressure-lowering medication. AR also had hot flushes, severe abdominal premenstrual pain, irritability and cravings, and painful periods. She had dry skin and significant hair loss, and reported that she would get seasonal allergies in the springtime, often resulting in asthma symptoms and sinusitis that were treated with steroids and antibiotics. Perfume smells made her feel nauseous and gave her a headache. AR had a resting tremor that had started about six months prior. She had depression and anxiety, which worsened during menstruation, insomnia (with nocturia), and low energy, which made exercising difficult. AR also felt very self-conscious about exercising.

During her early childhood years AR had recurrent strep throat (streptococcal pharyngitis) and took several rounds of antibiotics. She had a history of depression and anxiety starting in her teens. She had seen several psychiatrists and therapists, tried many antidepressant medications, but found that they were never helpful and made her feel 'disconnected from herself'. She self-prescribed 5-hydroxytryptophan and St John's Wort, finding them somewhat helpful.

At 38 years old, AR was diagnosed with an endometrioma on one of her ovaries and Hashimoto's thyroiditis. She had been started on levothyroxine thyroid hormone (T4) replacement with no impact on weight symptoms. Two years ago (age 41), she was switched to levothyroxine and liothyronine (T3) replacement medication, which she reported helpful; it appeared to have prompted some quick and easy weight loss of about 35 lbs (15.8 kg), but since then weight loss has plateaued.

AR quit smoking seven years ago, having smoked 20 cigarettes per day for 20 years.

AR reported regular bowel movements, one or two times per day, with some constipation around the time of menses.

Family medical history

Both AR's parents were living, and both had suffered ischaemic heart disease. Between them they also had osteoarthritis, type 2 diabetes and kidney disease. Her brothers had hypertension and hyperlipidaemia. On her mother's side of the family there was one incidence of Parkinson's disease. There was no family history of obesity.

Readiness to change

Despite being highly motivated to change and wanting to prevent the need for surgical intervention, AR was struggling with feelings of hopelessness. In her words, 'I know my eating is bad now, but I don't even bother because I can't lose weight when I try! It gets very frustrating to be continuously told it is all my fault. It's difficult not to lose hope for help.'

Current medications and supplements

Table 6.1 shows the supplements and medications AR was taking on presentation. Supplements were self-prescribed; medications were physician prescribed.

Table 6.1 Supplements and medications taken on presentation

Medication or supplement	Daily dose	Duration
Losartan potassium (antihypertensive angiotensin-receptor blocker)	50 mg	3 years
Levothyroxine and liothyronine (T3 and T4)	120 mg AM, 60 mg PM	15 years
St John's Wort	300 mg	4 months
EPA/DHA	EPA 110 mg DHA 500 mg	4 months
Zinc with copper	25 mg zinc 2.5 mg copper	4 months
5-hydroxytryptophan	100 mg	4 months
Probiotic (unspecified)	3 capsules	4 months
Melatonin	3–5 mg at night	2+ years
Vitamin D	10,000 IU	2 years

Investigations

Physical examination

A physical examination revealed the following notable findings:

- **Skin:** Excess hair growth on the upper lip (AR confirmed she regularly shaved her facial hair) as well as several skin tags. Both findings have been associated with sex hormone imbalances, in particular oestrogen dominance, and insulin resistance (Crespo et al., 2018).

- **Nails:** Her fingernails showed signs of brittleness, deep vertical ridging and Beau's lines (transverse ridging), suggesting multiple potential nutrient deficiencies. Both nail findings can associate with general maldigestion, malabsorption or poor circulation (Seshadri and De, 2012).
- **Oral cavity:** Oral examination revealed a thick white tongue coating, indicative of oropharyngeal candidiasis (thrush) (Pankhurst, 2013).

Subjective questionnaires

Table 6.2 shows the summary results of AR's subjective questionnaire (MSQ) at the initial consultation. The client is asked to score symptoms in each, based on the last 14 days (for initial intake) and past 30 days for follow-up questionnaires. Clients score ranges from 0 for never have the symptom to 4 for frequently have it, effect is severe. Scores are added to give a total for each body system listed in each column of Table 6.2. The number of individual symptoms vary by body system. The resources section of this book provides a link to find a copy of the questionnaire.

Table 6.2 Results of subjective questionnaire: Medical Symptom/Toxicity Questionnaire (MSQ) – baseline results

Symptom area	Score
Gastrointestinal	5
Ears	10
Emotions	14
Energy	8
Eyes	2
Head	7
Heart	0
Joints/muscles	8
Lungs	1
Mind	0

cont.

Symptom area	Score
Mouth/throat	1
Nose	1
Skin	15
Weight	20
Other	4
Total	96

Laboratory tests ordered and rationale (only significant findings are presented)

Further information about advanced lipid testing, IgG food sensitivity, urinary organic acids, stress response testing and comprehensive stool testing is found in Chapter 3.

1. **Anaemia/iron investigation:** Complete blood count, chemistry screen and iron panel ruled out the presence of frank anaemia (red blood cell count, haemoglobin and haematocrit were within normal limits). However, iron saturation fell just under the reference range at 19% (range 20–50%) and ferritin was 38 mcg/L (low normal), compared with an ideal range of 50–75 mcg/L. Increasing a ferritin level of below 50 mcg/L, even when haemoglobin is normal, has been shown to improve fatigue levels in women (Vaucher *et al.*, 2012).

2. **Thyroid investigations:** It was important to establish a baseline assessment of her thyroid autoimmunity (Hashimoto's thyroiditis) while on the current medication.
   - **Thyroid hormone pathways:** Thyroid stimulating hormone (TSH) <0.01 mIU/L (low), free T3 10.18 pmol/L (high), reverse T3 35 ng/dL (high) (NB free T4 normal at 16.34 pmol/L)
   - **Antibodies:** Anti-thyroperoxidase (anti-TPO) antibodies 367 IU/mL (high).

3. **Sex hormone investigations:**
   - **Oestrogen/progesterone (luteal phase):** Serum total oestrogen, oestrone, oestradiol, oestriol, progesterone, follicle-stimulating hormone (FSH) and luteinizing hormone (LH) were all within normal limits. However, oestradiol was high normal, and progesterone was low normal, creating a relative imbalance of higher oestrogen to progesterone.
   - **Androgens:** Serum total testosterone, free testosterone and DHEAS were within normal limits.

4. **Cardiometabolic investigations:**
   - **Basic cardiovascular:** Fasting triglycerides 2.37 mmol/L (high), LDL cholesterol 2.79 mmol/L (normal), HDL cholesterol 1.22 mmol/L (normal), total cholesterol 5.76 mmol/L (high normal)
   - **Advanced cardiovascular lipids:** LDL particle number 1350 nmol/L (moderate risk), Apo B 92 mg/dL (moderate risk), Lp(a) 12 nmol/L (normal), LDL Pattern A (optimal)
   - **Metabolic:** HbA1c 33.3 mmol/mol (normal), fasting insulin 34.5 uIU/mL (high), fasting glucose 97 mg/dL (high normal)
   - **Inflammation:** hs-CRP 5.0 mg/L (high), fibrinogen 544 mg/dL (high), ferritin 38 mcg/L (normal).

5. **Immunological investigations:**
   - **Food-specific IgG antibodies:** IgG antibodies to all tested foods came back above the reference range. These are shown in Table 6.3

Table 6.3 IgG food sensitivity results

	Result (mcg/mL)	Reference range
Soybean	4.9	<2
Casein/cow milk	29.6	<2
Wheat	28.0	<2
Maize/corn	9.9	<2
Gluten	22.0	<2

cont.

	Result (mcg/mL)	Reference range
Yeast	2.8	<2
Almond	5.9	<2
Egg (yolk and white)	14.4	<2
Rye	16.6	<2
Oat	12.8	<2

- **Coeliac predisposition:** HLA DQ2 and HLA DQ8 were negative
- **Thyroid antibodies:** As above.

6. **Urinary organic acids plus blood multi-panel test:**
   - **Plasma amino acids:** Arginine, glycine, serine, histidine, threonine, asparagine were all below reference range. Ratio of glutamate to glutamine was high.
   - **Methylation:** Plasma homocysteine was elevated (10.1 nmol/mL), an indicator of methylation deficiency (King *et al.*, 2012) (potentially as a result of her methylene tetrahydrofolate reductase (MTHFR) gene variants as well as nutrient deficiencies). Formiminoglutamate (FIGLU), a marker of functional levels of folate, was 1.1 (high normal).
   - **Toxic elements:** High blood aluminium and cadmium.
   - **Oxidative stress:** Serum lipid peroxides were on the high end of normal range.
   - **Nutrient status:** Low serum beta-carotene. 25-hydroxyvitamin D, a biomarker for vitamin D status, was 202.5 nmol/L (high), urinary alpha-keto acids were below detectable limits (suggestive of functional deficiency of B1, B2, B3, B5 and/or lipoate).
   - **Fatty acid metabolism:** High urinary ethylmalonate indicated some difficulty with oxidation of fatty acids for energy.
   - **Carbohydrate metabolism and central energy pathways:** Urinary pyruvate levels were below detectable limits, yet L-lactate was within range without deficiency. Several urinary

citric acid cycle markers were overall on the low end of normal or below detectable limits.

- **Neurotransmitters metabolites:** High urinary 5-hydro-xyindoleacetic acid (5-HIAA, likely due to 5-HTP supplementation), high urinary kynurenate and quinolinate suggesting imbalanced excitatory signalling in the central nervous system.
- **Dysbiosis:** AR had very high urinary D-lactate, which is specific to bacterial origin (rather than metabolic) and can cause neurological symptoms including depression (Kang, Lee and Kang, 2006).

7. **Methylation:** AR was heterozygous for the MTHFR polymorphisms C677T and A1298C. (AR's genetic testing was ordered through conventional laboratories and, at that point in time, this was the only methylation-related single nucleotide polymorphism (SNP) tested for.)

8. **Stress response:**
   - Four-point cortisol: AR's first morning cortisol was significantly depressed. At the three other times measured throughout the day, cortisol was on the low end of normal. This is shown in Figure 6.1.

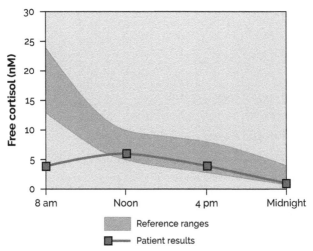

Figure 6.1 Four-point cortisol result (see online colour plate)

9. **Comprehensive stool test:**
   - **Faecal bacteria:** Low levels of beneficial bacteria were present. *Escherichia coli* species were in the top quintile (see Figure 6.2). Strains were not specified in this test.
   - **Faecal immunological markers:** High faecal secretory IgA, which results from active immunological stress in the digestive tract (see Figure 6.2).

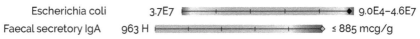

Escherichia coli   3.7E7   9.0E4–4.6E7
Faecal secretory IgA   963 H   ≤ 885 mcg/g

Figure 6.2 Excerpts from the comprehensive stool test (see online colour plate)

Case interpretation and analysis

A summary of the clinical diagnosis (made by the overseeing physician) and symptoms:

- morbid obesity (BMI 49.5)
- weight-loss resistance
- hypertension (controlled with medication)
- severe premenstrual syndrome (PMS)
- xeroderma (dry skin)
- hair loss
- seasonal allergies
- asthma
- chemical sensitivity (perfumes)
- resting tremor
- depression and anxiety
- insomnia
- fatigue
- Hashimoto's thyroiditis
- insulin resistance
- hypertriglyceridemia
- gut dysbiosis
- oropharyngeal candidiasis

- past medical history: endometrioma, sinusitis, smoking, traumatic childhood.

Mechanisms at work that underpin the above diagnosis, signs and symptoms

- **Insulin dysregulation:** Even though AR's HbA1c and fasting glucose were within normal range, measuring fasting insulin was extremely revealing in her case. Insulin is an anabolic hormone, promoting weight gain and stalling weight loss. Insulin also upregulates aromatase activity, promoting oestrogen imbalance that can lead to PMS symptoms (DiSilvestro *et al.*, 2014).
- **GI dysfunction:** Intestinal dysbiosis is indicated in AR's case by the elevated D-lactate organic acid marker and low beneficial flora reported on the stool test. (See Box 9.2 in Chapter 9 for a definition of dysbiosis.) Dysbiosis and intestinal hyperpermeability is also strongly suggested by her history of multiple instances of antibiotic use, and the presence of multiple IgG food sensitivities – in fact, to every food that was tested – as well as her autoimmune and allergic conditions (Sturgeon and Fasano, 2016). Observed oral thrush provides additional evidence of dysbiosis and potential sources of inflammation (Feller *et al.*, 2014). Although AR reported regularity of bowel movements, her low-fibre diet (which would otherwise normally promote constipation) suggests that she may rather be experiencing mild diarrhoea.
- **Immune dysregulation:** AR's presentation included several aspects of immune dysregulation including autoimmune thyroiditis, seasonal allergies, delayed (IgG) food sensitivities, high faecal sIgA, inflammation (high hs-CRP and fibrinogen) and oxidative stress (high lipid peroxides). These active immune processes all perpetuate ongoing inflammation. Inflammation is a core driver of cardiometabolic disturbance. Inflammation also plays a significant role in central nervous system (CNS) dysfunction including depression (Kiecolt-Glaser, Derry and Fagundes, 2015; Strawbridge *et al.*, 2015). A history of frequent

antibiotic use and poor diet is suggestive of altered microbiome and increased intestinal permeability, both of which predispose to dysregulated immune activity (Belkaid and Hand, 2014).

- **Methylation imbalance:** AR's homocysteine, at 10.1 nmol/mL, was elevated. FIGLU seen in her urinary multi-panel was high normal, indicating a functional deficiency of folate, a critical cofactor in methylation pathways (Shojania, 1982). Lastly, AR was heterozygous for the MTHFR C677T single nucleotide polymorphism, indicating a lower level of enzyme activity. Impairments in methylation activity have been linked with depression and other mood disorders (in AR's case, compounded with childhood trauma), as well as insomnia (Gilbody, Lewis and Lightfoot, 2007). Methylation via catechol-O-methyltransferase (COMT) is a critical step in catecholamine metabolism, and so deficiencies can impair clearance of adrenaline and noradrenaline, worsening anxiety (Ursini *et al.*, 2011). COMT also functions to metabolize oestrogen metabolites and so deficiency can lead to hormone imbalance (Männistö and Kaakkola, 1999). Elevated homocysteine is a positive predictive risk factor for cardiovascular disease and may play a role in the pathophysiology of neurodegenerative disease including Parkinson's disease, in part due to its potential to increase oxidative stress (Saadat *et al.*, 2018; Sławek *et al.*, 2013). Homocysteine also relates to hypertension with a U-shaped curve relationship (Wang *et al.*,2014).

- **Low cortisol output:** Low or low normal cortisol output across all four time points, and especially upon rising, strongly correlate with fatigue symptoms and indicate a later stage of adrenal dysfunction (Hall *et al.*, 2014). Including movement in AR's therapeutic plan was going to be difficult until her fatigue from hypo-adrenal function and insomnia could be addressed effectively. Adrenal, thyroid and sex hormones are also closely interrelated, and should be addressed in that order.

- **Overwhelmed biotransformation and elimination:** AR's elevated cadmium and aluminium, along with a high MSQ (questionnaire) score of 96, chemical sensitivity to perfumes and recent-onset resting tremor (with family history of Parkinson's disease) indicate or strongly suggest ongoing toxin exposure and/or an inability of her detoxification and elimination pathways to match the toxin load she is carrying (Ahmed and Santosh, 2010). Weight-loss resistance alone can be perpetuated by excess environmental toxins that interfere with normal hormonal signalling (see below for further discussion on this). Toxicants have also been linked with hypertension, neurological symptoms and hormone disruption (Rancière *et al.*, 2015; Vandenberg *et al.*, 2012).

Additional notes
While laboratory investigations indicated that sex hormone levels were within normal limits, AR's PMS symptoms and history of endometrioma are suggestive of sex hormone imbalances. Her high normal oestradiol compared with a low normal progesterone presented a relative deficiency of progesterone to oestrogen. Insulin is a potent stimulator of aromatase, which is expressed in adipose tissue, further adding to a potential picture of oestrogen dominance. Addressing AR's clear sign of insulin resistance would also address hormonal imbalances. The intention with AR was to follow up with more detailed investigations of sex hormone metabolites, if needed, although this proved not to be necessary.

Apparent primary underlying factors contributing to the above

- **Poor diet:** AR's diet continued to be high in processed foods and refined carbohydrates, both having a pro-inflammatory impact in the body. Processed foods also carry a higher toxin burden, including a class of endocrine-disrupting chemicals (primarily pesticides, herbicides and plastics) called 'obesogens' within the scientific community for their ability to promote weight gain (Baillie-Hamilton, 2002; Heindel, Newbold and Schug, 2015; Janesick and Blumberg, 2016; Yang *et al.*, 2015). Refined carbohydrates are also the most direct stimulator of insulin signalling, and with increasing insulin resistance at the cellular level, circulating levels of insulin build up significantly. AR also consumed very little phytonutrient content since her diet was lacking in varied plant foods such as vegetables, fruits, nuts and seeds, which act as antioxidants and epigenetic regulators (see Box 6.1) in their own right. Low levels of beneficial fibres from plant foods starve beneficial bacteria in the gut.

BOX 6.1 EPIGENETIC REGULATORS DEFINITION

Epigenetics refers to the study of heritable yet potentially reversible changes to our gene expressions that occur without alterations in DNA sequence. Epigenetic processes are part of normal cellular regulation and control. The three most common epigenetic mechanisms are DNA methylation, histone modifications and non-coding RNAs. Dietary phenolic compounds, such as curcumin, resveratrol, flavonoids and proanthocyanidins, have been shown (in animal and cell studies) to interact with epigenetic mechanisms. Luteolin, for example, is a flavonoid with DNA-methylation-inhibiting properties. It is found in thyme, Brussels sprouts, cabbage, onion and many other plant foods. Quercetin, another flavonoid, has been shown to inhibit histone-deacetylase enzymes and DNA methylation enzymes. Quercetin is present in many plant foods, especially onions, broccoli and leafy green vegetables. These dietary phenols can be referred to therefore as epigenetic regulators.

Sources: Jiang et al. (2018); Nian et al. (2009);
Pan et al. (2013); Thakur et al. (2013)

- **Nutrient deficiencies:** AR's laboratory investigations indicated nutrient deficiencies in several areas. Folate is one identified deficiency, indicated by high normal levels of FIGLU. Several essential amino acids were all below reference range, including arginine which is a key amino acid for regulating blood pressure. Deficiencies of citric acid cycle intermediates suggest either insufficient anaplerotic reactions (see Box 6.2), which can be due to insufficient amino acid substrate, and/or impaired entry to the citric acid cycle. The combined deficiency of pyruvate, normal

L-lactate, low citric cycle intermediates, all in the context of a high-carbohydrate diet, indicate inhibition of carbohydrate metabolism and cellular energy production. Excess conversion of pyruvate to L-lactate and alpha-keto acids below detectable limits indicate likely functional deficiencies of B1, B2, B3, B5 and/or lipoate, since all those reactions require dehydrogenase activity which uses these micronutrients as cofactor.

BOX 6.2 ANAPLEROSIS

Anaplerosis is the act of replenishing tricarboxylic acid (TCA) cycle intermediates that have been extracted for biosynthesis (in what are called anaplerotic reactions). The TCA cycle is a hub of metabolism, with central importance in both energy production and biosynthesis. The TCA cycle is discussed further in Chapter 5 in relation to mitochondria function.

- **Environmental toxins:** AR had raised blood levels of cadmium and aluminium. Cadmium levels in urine, serum, plasma and blood are significantly correlated with exposure to tobacco products (Richter, Faroon and Pappas, 2017). AR was no longer smoking, but was still exposed to second-hand smoke. Cadmium can also bioaccumulate in food and water. Common sources of aluminium exposure include deodorants, aluminium foil and aluminium baking pans.

Initial management plan

Dietary intervention

- Paleo elimination diet (removes grains/gluten, legumes, dairy, egg, soy, peanut, shellfish) including identified IgG food sensitivities > 5.0 mcg/mL.

- Foods that contain abundant levels of substrates and cofactors that feed or support the formation of the universal methyl donor S-adenosylmethionine (SAMe) (e.g. folate, methionine, betaine, zinc). Such foods include dark leafy greens, liver, seeds and beetroot.
- Foods that contain epigenetic regulators to support DNA methylation and histone modification such as garlic (Xu et al., 2018), rosemary (Jang, Hwang and Choi, 2018), shiitake mushrooms (Yang et al., 2013).
- Total carbohydrates 70 g per day or less; no added sugars, grains, legumes, starchy vegetables; low-glycaemic-load fruits only from the following list: wild berries, lemon, lime, avocado and olives.
- Increase phytonutrient and fibre intake. AR was advised to eat at least seven portions of vegetables, in a variety of colours (one portion equals 80 g per day).
- Beta-carotene sources (e.g. dark leafy greens, red/yellow peppers, broccoli).
- Vitamin E food sources (e.g. avocado, nuts, seeds).
- No processed foods.
- No aluminium pans, canned food or aluminium foil.

Lifestyle

- Swimming, try for 2–3 times per week, gentle exercise.
- Meditation/quiet time, start with 2–3 minutes daily.
- Sleep hygiene.
- Household water analysis for toxic elements.

Supplements

- Berberine 1000 mg BID.
- Oil of oregano 150 mg QD.
- Botanical antimicrobial formula including bilberry, milk thistle, echinacea, goldenseal, white willow bark, garlic, grapeseed extract, black walnut, tea tree and oregano, 10 drops BID (swish in mouth then swallow).

- B complex with 25 mg thiamine, 25 mg riboflavin, 150 mg niacin, 55 mg B6, 800 mcg L-methylfolate, 1000 mcg methylcobalamin QD (for additional methylation support).
- Bovine adrenal glandular, 320 mg QD.
- Omega-3 fatty acids providing 2000 mg EPA and 1000 mg DHA QD.
- Rhubarb extract (ERr731) 4 mg QD.
- Chelated iron (bisglycinate) 30 mg QD.
- Continue 5HTP, St John's Wort, multivitamin/mineral, melatonin.
- Stop zinc/copper, probiotic.
- Reduce vitamin D to 2000 IU QD.

Rationale

Diet is a powerful leverage point to turn around insulin-driven weight-loss resistance. Removing grains, legumes and dairy, as outlined in the Palaeo diet (see Box 9.1 in Chapter 9) is a convenient structure in which to reduce carbohydrates and remove the most problematic food sensitivities that can get in the way of sensitive insulin signalling and weight loss due to the low-grade inflammation they can induce. A meta-analysis of four trials involving 159 subjects supported the use of a Palaeolithic diet for short-term improvements in metabolic syndrome compared with guideline-based control diets (Manheimer *et al.*, 2015).

It was important that reduced carbohydrate intake would not be at the expense of fibre and phytonutrients, which were considered essential for gut restoration, antioxidant and detoxification support, as well as improved endothelial function (for blood pressure). What to exclude in the diet is as important as what to include, and cutting out immune-provoking and processed foods that come with higher levels of pesticides, sugars, trans fats and other toxins was essential in AR's case. Methylation-supportive foods were added to reduce homocysteine, balance mood and support epigenetic regulation of favourable gene expression (Shankar, Kumar and Srivastava, 2013; vel Szic *et al.*, 2015).

To address dysbiosis, AR's initial management plan leaned heavily on botanical antimicrobials including berberine, oil of oregano and a combination drop formula that could be swished in the oral cavity before swallowing to improve oral thrush (Bassolé and Juliani, 2012;

Hammer, Carson and Riley, 1999). AR tolerated this combination well, although some individuals may find they experience symptoms related to toxicant load from microbe lysis. Berberine has the added benefit of improving insulin sensitivity (Zhang *et al.*, 2008).

Energy and mood were critical components to give AR enough resilience to be able to enact her weight-loss protocol – challenging dietary changes as well as beginning to incorporate regular gentle movement. Several angles were pursued to assist with this:

- **Central energy and methylation:** Supplemental B vitamins were added to directly support AR's deficient central energy and methylation pathways, a need indicated by her laboratory workup. A highly absorbable form of iron was recommended based on low percentage iron saturation to assist with oxygen transport and energy (Milman *et al.*, 2014). Iron supplementation should only be initiated based on laboratory testing indicating a need and should be tracked closely to avoid excess iron.
- **Adrenal:** This clinic uses reputably sourced glandular extracts based on their long traditional use in medicine systems and the concept of food as medicine. While studies are dated, evidence exists to support the use to adrenal extracts to support adrenal function (Hartman *et al.*, 1932).
- **Hormone balance:** Long-chain omega-3 fatty acids, especially EPA, help to reduce inflammation, including reducing the pro-inflammatory prostaglandin PGE2 which directly stimulates aromatase (in conjunction with insulin) to create an oestrogen-dominant pattern, with corresponding PMS symptoms, mood swings and cravings (Ferrero *et al.*, 2014; Trebble *et al.*, 2003). Rhubarb extract was also added to balance those same symptoms (Hajirahimkhan, Dietz and Bolton, 2013).
- **Sleep:** Sleep hygiene recommendations were provided that included reduced blue-light exposure in evenings, dark and cool sleeping environment, avoiding brain-stimulating reading or activities in the evening, early-morning sun exposure. Avoid fluids within two hours of going to bed to minimize nocturia.

- **Meditation:** Meditation can help improve adrenal output, balance hormones and improve sleep (Nagendra, Maruthai and Kutty, 2012). A causal connection between stress and autoimmune thyroiditis is thought to exist (Damian *et al.*, 2016).
- Continue St John's Wort (SJW) and 5HTP. The mechanism by which SJW supports mood is not fully understood but is thought to involve neurotransmitter modulation and anti-inflammatory effect (Schmidt and Butterweck, 2015). AR felt SJW and 5HTP helped her and in order to sustain motivation for the dietary and lifestyle changes it was decided to continue with these.
- As AR's vitamin D result was high, her supplement dose was reduced from 10,000 IU to 2000 IU QD. Vitamin D status would be monitored during the following months and indeed, as expected, the level dropped to optimal ranges. There is some indication from the published literature that requirements for vitamin D are increased in obesity (Vanlint, 2013).

Physician-only prescriptions

The case was overseen by a physician who prescribed the following (as these are outside the personalized nutrition remit, they will not be discussed further):

- melatonin
- topical progesterone
- continue other medications as prescribed by external physicians (losartan and levothyroxine).

Drug–nutrient interactions

Drug–nutrient interactions were checked using the Natural Medicines Comprehensive Database (see Appendix A). SJW can induce cytochrome P450 3A4 and may induce cytochrome P450 2C9 which are two of the metabolic pathways used by losartan ('Natural Medicines Interaction Checker', n.d.; Sica, Gehr and Ghosh, 2005). It is possible that the half-life of losartan could be reduced by the concomitant use of SJW, thus reducing the medication effect. Given that the diet and lifestyle programme was designed to support weight loss and that AR had already self-prescribed the combination for four months, the case physician was satisfied that AR could continue with SJW.

Topical delivery of progesterone eliminates first-pass metabolism, and therefore interactions with substances (food or supplement) that inhibit or induce drug metabolism in liver and small intestine will be avoided.

Case management

Months 0–3

Monthly follow-ups for the first three months were planned to quickly address any factors that might derail compliance. Cravings were initially challenging, but lessened significantly after two weeks of following the lower-carbohydrate intake level. By three months there were no more cravings. She was able to swim three days a week and added weight training three days each week.

Over the first three months, AR lost 32 lbs (14.5 kg). A number of symptoms completely resolved including menstrual symptoms, hot flushes, insomnia, nasal congestion, constipation and abdominal cramping. Her hair loss lessened. AR reported that her energy was overall 'great', although she still felt some sluggishness in the mornings. Her blood pressure was much improved, such that her cardiologist reduced her losartan dose by half. Oregano oil was stopped.

Table 6.4 describes the adjustments to plan after three months and rationale.

Table 6.4 Adjustments made after three months

Adjustment	Clinical rationale
Increase adrenal glandular to 1200 mg in morning	Persistent morning fatigue
Omega-3-rich fish (low-mercury species) three times per week	Support reduction in inflammation Goal was to encourage dietary sources in order to reduced reliance on supplementation in the future

Reduce fruit consumption, to maintain total carbohydrate intake below 70 g per day	Ongoing weight loss
Initiate food challenges	Minimize effect of restricted diet and identify delayed food sensitivities
Nutrient intake analysis following food challenges	Support optimal dietary nutrient intakes

Nutrient intake analysis and food challenges at four months

AR's detailed diet diary and computerized nutrient intake analysis most notably indicated a need for additional calcium, since her average daily consumption averaged only 306 mg (compared with a recommended daily intake of 700 mg per day in the UK, or 1000 mg per day in the US). Her main calcium-contributing foods were almonds, kale and the brand of mineral water she used. Magnesium consumption was also slightly low at 238 mg average daily intake. Her dietary folate intake only provided half of her recommended intake levels, although the shortfall was currently being covered in her supplement plan.

AR experienced some difficulty going through the carefully planned food challenge process. She successfully tested and reintroduced egg, almond and soy. Her dairy challenge initially did not seem to indicate a problem; however, she did subsequently notice a worsening of her PMS symptoms and the return of seasonal allergy and asthma symptoms. These issues resolved on removal of dairy again.

The most difficult experience was challenging grains. She experienced mood swings, a return of thrush and severe fatigue that made it hard for her to get out of bed before 10 am. Challenging gluten-containing grains added symptoms of swollen joints and bloating. Weight loss stalled immediately during these grain/gluten challenges and cravings returned with a vengeance, which were hard to bring back under control.

Adjustments to plan after four months:

- Calcium/magnesium combination providing 500 mg QD calcium, 200 mg magnesium.
- Continue to avoid dairy and grains/gluten based on food challenges.

- Temporary use of mild ketogenic diet, with nutritionist support, to bring cravings back under control and restart weight loss (see Q&A section).
- Oregano oil reintroduced. It was suspected that the intense cravings experienced during grain challenges indicated negative changes in her microbiome. To help rebalance her microbiome as quickly as possible (and help her with cravings), the oregano oil was added back.

Six-month follow-up

At six months, AR weighed 295 lbs (133 kg) (having lost 79 lbs/35.8 kg) and was delighted with her progress. Her waist measurement had reduced to 46 inches (116.8 cm) (from 55 inches/139.7 cm at baseline) and her hip measurement to 48 inches (121.9 cm) (from 60 inches/152.4 cm at baseline). She had no symptoms of depression and her energy remained good overall, despite ongoing sluggishness in the morning.

AR was now up to moderate exercising six days per week. Her cardiologist was 'very impressed', and under close supervision ceased her blood pressure medication and reduced her thyroid medication by half. Discussions about proceeding with bariatric surgery were postponed as long as she could maintain her weight-loss trajectory for at least another 40 lbs (18 kg) (bringing her BMI under 35).

Table 6.5 shows the follow-up laboratory assessment at five months.

Table 6.5 Selection of laboratory results at five months (all results within range unless indicated otherwise)

Test	Result
Fasting blood glucose	4.773 mmol/L
Triglycerides	1.3 mmol/L
HDL cholesterol	1.23 mmol/L
LDL cholesterol	4.27 mmol/L (high)

Total cholesterol	6.2 mmol/L (high)
LDL pattern	A (optimal)
Apolipoprotein B	128 mg/dL (high)
Insulin	8.1 uIU/mL
Vitamin D	112.5 nmol/L
Anti-TPO antibodies	346 IU/mL (high)
Ferritin	56 ng/L

Table 6.6 shows the summary results of the follow-up subjective questionnaires.

Table 6.6 Results of subjective questionnaire: Medical Symptoms/Toxicity Questionnaire (MSQ) – six-month results

Symptom area	Score
Gastrointestinal	1
Ears	3
Emotions	0
Energy	1
Eyes	0
Head	0
Heart	0
Joints/muscles	0
Lungs	0
Mind	0
Mouth/throat	0
Nose	0

cont.

Symptom area	Score
Skin	3
Weight	0
Other	0
Total	8

Overall, AR was on a good trajectory with significant symptom improvement and steady ongoing weight loss. Adjustments to plan after six months:

- Adaptogenic botanicals added: ashwagandha 300 mg, rhodiola 400 mg, eleuthero 300 mg, holy basil 200 mg, Maca 150 mg per day.
- Iron (bisglycinate) reduced to 15 mg QOD.
- Dietary:
  - Relax ketogenic macronutrient targets.
  - Continue to focus on high phytonutrient, high fibre.
  - Foods to prioritize: green or oolong tea, capers, sesame seeds.
  - Reduce egg consumption to 2–3 times per week.
  - Reduce saturated fat intake to 10% calories, replace with unheated polyunsaturated fats.

AR had experienced improvement in her overall energy, but she continued to experience low morning energy. The adaptogen botanicals listed in her adjusted plan above are also known to assist in adrenal recovery and were therefore added at this stage (Bhattacharya, Bhattacharya and Chakrabarti, 2000; White *et al.*, 2016).

Follow-up lab screening showed that while AR's triglycerides had normalized, her LDL cholesterol, total cholesterol and apolipoprotein B had risen. In the clinic's experience, some (but not all) individuals on a ketogenic diet do experience a temporary increase in LDL and total cholesterol levels, and biomarkers are therefore tracked closely; in most cases, the overall pattern A vs B remains favourable, and triglycerides, insulin and glucose levels are dramatically improved.

To err on the side of caution, the ketogenic macronutrient targets were relaxed after weight loss had been reinitiated, and foods to support cholesterol elimination and apolipoprotein B balance were added. High-fibre and high-plant-sterol intake, as well as sesame intake, all increase bile acid (and therefore cholesterol) excretion (Visavadiya and Narasimhacharya, 2008); fibre also reduces cholesterol enterohepatic recirculation. Epigallocatechin gallate (EGCG) from green and oolong teas lowers apolipoprotein B (Kohlstadt, 2012) and is an epigenetic regulator. AR enjoyed capers, which are an excellent source of quercetin, as well as an epigenetic regulator and immune balancer (Hodges and Minich, 2015). Quercetin may also help resolve intestinal hyperpermeability and is a source of sterols to reduce cholesterol and apolipoprotein B (Kohlstadt, 2012). Sesame seeds may also reduce blood pressure, inhibit HMG CoA reductase, inhibit LDL oxidation and reduce intestinal cholesterol absorption (Kohlstadt, 2012).

Since AR was consuming about 600 mg cholesterol daily and 15% calories from saturated fats, her consumption of eggs and saturated fatty acids was reduced.

Months 9–12

AR continued to do well at staying true to her protocol supported with monthly meetings with the nutritionist. At nine months, AR had lost a total of 95 lbs (43 kg) and by 12 months 122 lbs (55 kg). Her weight after one year was 243 lbs (110 kg), giving her a BMI of 32.5. While this still falls within the BMI category obese class 1, it also meant that she was no longer a candidate for surgical intervention.

AR reported that her morning energy was now much improved. All her other symptoms remained absent or minimal. She continued to keep her blood pressure within target ranges without medication. She continued to do well at half her original dose of thyroid hormone replacement (T3/T4 combination). The adrenal glandular and oregano oil were stopped. A probiotic was introduced at nine months to support the microbiome following use of antimicrobials. A fuller discussion on the use of probiotics with a microbiome support programme can be found in Chapter 9.

Table 6.7 shows follow-up laboratory assessment at 11 months.

Table 6.7 Follow-up laboratory assessments at 11 months (all results within range unless indicated otherwise)

Test	Result
Fasting blood glucose	4.7 mmol/L
Triglycerides	1.2 mmol/L
HDL cholesterol	1.3 mmol/L
LDL cholesterol	3.16 mmol/L
Total cholesterol	5.1 mmol/L
LDL pattern	A (optimal)
Apolipoprotein B	117 mg/dL
Insulin	5.2 uIU/mL
Anti-TPO antibodies	94 IU/mL (high)

These results show a great improvement in AR's insulin resistance, with her insulin nearly below 5 uIU/mL which was associated with the lowest risk of cardiovascular disease in the San Antonio Heart Study (Hanley *et al.*, 2002). Cholesterol was now normal and thyroid antibodies significantly reduced.

Over the course of the second year she found that if she deviated from her list of 'avoid' foods, she would notice a return of symptoms, stalled weight loss and cravings, and her anti-TPO antibodies would rise.

Discussion

AR's case illustrates the multifactorial contributions to weight gain and weight-loss resistance. While many cases of overweight and obesity may not be as complex, this case shows how effective a broad, comprehensive approach can be.

A central driver of AR's unwanted weight gain was insulin resistance. While visceral adiposity is known to correlate with peripheral insulin resistance (Preis *et al.*, 2010), if the practitioner had relied on fasting glucose or HbA1c as indicators of dysglycemia alone, they would have missed the significant elevation of fasting insulin. Insulin is potently anabolic, and rises are known to precede glycaemic elevations by several years. Pennings, Jaber and Ahiawodzi (2018) recently showed that subjects with elevated insulin and insulin resistance have higher weight gain than those with normal insulin levels over a ten-year period, with gains in weight realized before glycaemic levels started to elevate (Pennings *et al.*, 2018).

Also important to address were AR's dysbiosis and yeast overgrowth, likely long-standing issues for AR due to multiple rounds of antibiotics, other medications, and high consumption of sugar and processed food. The microbiome can be a central factor in addressing the underlying drivers of several chronic conditions, many of which AR had, including weight gain, insulin resistance, depression, fatigue, hormone imbalance and immune activation (Belkaid and Hand, 2014; Sekirov *et al.*, 2010). Choosing a fairly aggressive botanical antimicrobial (active against both bacteria and fungi) was instrumental in helping reduce presumed lipopolysaccharide circulation that can often drive CNS dysfunction, low energy/insomnia and significant cravings (Xiao *et al.*, 2014). In the experience of this clinic, cravings are often driven by an overgrowth of pathogenic species in the gut microbiome. Providing methylation support through dietary and supplemental nutrients likely also helped her depression and anxiety (Gilbody *et al.*, 2007; Shankar *et al.*, 2013). Nutrient support for central energy pathways helped to restore mitochondrial energy output (Ames, 2010). Without supporting these aspects, it would have been likely impossible for AR to enact the dietary and exercise changes she would need to address the insulin imbalance and initiate weight loss.

Avoiding specific food triggers also proved to be a key factor in AR's case, most clearly indicated by the observation that during her food challenge period she experienced a return of symptoms, stalled weight loss and intense cravings. Delayed immunological reactions (Type IV hypersensitivity) may also have been playing a role in her thyroid autoimmunity, given that she was able to reduce her thyroid medication by half when the avoided her known trigger foods. Non-coeliac gluten sensitivity is associated with thyroid autoimmunity (Losurdo *et al.*, 2018).

Reducing her exposure to toxins and supporting gentle detoxification through fibre, adequate protein and phytonutrients may help her immune system regain improved balance over time (Martucci *et al.*, 2017; Xiao *et al.*, 2014). It is also important to think about detoxification support during any period of weight loss since fat-soluble toxins will be released from adipose stores into circulation.

Finally, AR's plan provided palliative support for her symptoms of oestrogen imbalance, low cortisol output, and mood. These extra components helped AR experience more rapid symptom reduction, supporting her motivation and ability to enact some of the more challenging aspects of her protocol. Over time, AR's need for these aids lessened, as the underlying work she put in on her diet and lifestyle would serve to correct dysfunction in those areas.

Conclusion

Overweight and obesity are common complaints and are significant drivers of the top causes of morbidity and mortality. Some cases of weight loss can be resolved simply by cleaning up the diet, limiting refined carbohydrates and adding regular exercise. However, an increasing number of cases are proving more complex and difficult to address due to the multifactorial aetiologies of weight gain and challenges with adhering to weight-loss protocols.

To that end, the case of AR illustrates how a comprehensive personalized nutrition and functional medicine approach can provide the keys that unlock all the pieces of the weight-loss puzzle simultaneously, enabling AR to successfully lose a dramatic 122 lbs (55 kg) as well as her insulin resistance, hypertension, depression, anxiety, PMS, seasonal allergies and more.

Q&A

AW: Many practitioners have first-hand experience of the power of elimination diets, but we are always concerned about the long-term impact of these, so I love how you used the food challenge to help re-expand the AR's diet after the initial phase. Can you tell us more about how you did the food challenge?

RH: I ask clients to try the least likely problem foods first, leaving more common problem foods such as dairy and gluten as late in the process as possible. I like to have individuals also consume the challenge food up until mid-afternoon only, to give the remainder of the day to observe symptoms and to minimize any potential sleep disruption.

I tell them to choose simple or single-ingredient foods – for example, when challenging egg, they use boiled egg rather than a cake containing egg. I tell them to eat the food for one day, with three servings each day (e.g. a quarter boiled egg in the morning, half at mid-morning and a whole boiled egg mid-afternoon) and then continue to observe two further full days for reactions.

I ask them to fill in a sheet to track any symptoms or reactions. We use a template for this which includes the main reactions and symptoms, but ask them also to fill in any of their own. The main symptoms are: digestion/bowel function; joint/muscle aches/neuropathic pain; headache/pressure; nasal or chest congestion; skin changes; energy level; sleep; mood/wellbeing; blood pressure or heart rate. Examples of the other symptoms a client may track depending on their case include urination and weight gain.

If they notice a reaction, I tell them to stop eating that food, to monitor symptoms and not to start on the next test food until the symptoms have stopped and they have had a bowel movement. If they have had no reaction, then start on the next food challenge on day 4 and after having a complete bowel movement. I tell them not to reintroduce any of the test foods into the normal diet until the entire challenge process has been completed. We have these instructions set up as a handout for clients and then I guide them through how to personalize it and choose the test foods.

While the process is very helpful to follow, it doesn't always catch *all* reactions. Some can take even longer than the three-day challenge period to materialize, as was the case with dairy for AR, especially since its effects were associated with symptoms that were cyclical.

AW: You used a ketogenic diet for a short period of time with AR to great effect, to restart weight loss and eliminate cravings. Can you give us a bit more information on how you guided her on this diet?

RH: I gave her calorie and macronutrient targets to get her started and talked through how she would like to monitor these. She was already using an app for tracking her diet, so she knew her macronutrient levels. I am flexible with tracking tools as long as they work for the individual and provide the information that she and I need.

These were her targets: Daily target: 1600 calories, > 120 g fat, < 50 g total carbohydrate, 80–100 g protein.

For weight loss, we sometimes find it necessary to adjust the daily targets at follow-up sessions to either dial down carbohydrate intake further if needed to prompt weight loss, or to relax them if weight loss is proceeding too rapidly and high levels of ketosis are recorded. I use total carbohydrates rather than net (see Box 6.3) as I find it's a simpler starting point for patients to implement and it results in a stricter implementation, at least initially; for that reason we had given AR a pretty liberal carbohydrate target < 50 g/d for ketosis). As we work with individuals over time, we will educate them about total and net carbs when appropriate, and have them experiment with adjusting their goals to net carbs – responses vary here and for some this will thwart ketosis. This mechanism is not fully known, but I suspect, based on my clinical experience, that it has to do with variability of the microbiome and how that acts on dietary fibre. It can be an iterative process of refinement to reach personalized macro goals that are the most liberal but still deliver the end results we're after.

> **BOX 6.3 NET CARBOHYDRATES**
>
> The distinction between net and total carbohydrates is sometimes used in the context of ketogenic diets. Net carbohydrate refers to the total amount of carbohydrate in a food or meal minus the fibrous or non-digestible carbohydrates. As non-digestible fibre is not absorbed, only the net carbohydrates will influence metabolism in respect of insulin response and maintaining ketosis. In practice, metabolic responses to fibre vary by individual, possibly due to differences in microbial activity on fibre components, and so effects should be closely monitored.

AR was especially unsure about what she could eat for breakfast and snacks, so I sent her compatible breakfast/snack recipes, ideas and some store-bought snack options. We discussed how to include compatible foods that were also high in phytonutrients and fibre, such as non-starchy vegetables, avocados, herbs/spices, nuts/seeds. I recommended adequate hydration and had her drink the following electrolyte formula twice a day over the first week, then as needed thereafter, to help reduce the symptoms that can occur during transition into ketosis (sometimes called 'keto flu'):

- 8 oz water
- ¼ tsp baking soda
- ¼ tsp high potassium salt
- juice of ½ lemon/lime.

After two days of hitting these macro targets, she was to start monitoring urinary ketones using over-the-counter test strips. Her target was mild-to-moderate urinary ketones. We did not use blood monitoring since we do not usually use that for weight-loss situations, only for cancer. In cancer cases we are looking to meet specific blood glucose and ketone targets that have been shown to be most favourable for cancer outcomes according to the research of Thomas Seyfried at Boston College. However, for weight loss, we can measure the desired response by measuring weight changes. The urinary keto strips are helpful for the client to know that they are on the right track, and many find them motivating.

We met weekly for two weeks during this time, then every other week until her next physician follow-up appointment (two months total on the ketogenic diet was sufficient to restart weight loss and eliminate cravings).

AW: I was interested to see you used a detailed nutrient analysis to help monitor micronutrient intake levels. Is that something you use with all cases or only when you are using an elimination-style diet?

RH: We do regularly use intermittent nutrient analyses to help monitor micronutrient intake levels, and especially on any kind of restricted diet. This serves several purposes. First, it allows us to ensure that we are doing what we can to avoid nutrient shortfalls when we remove major food groups (such as calcium when dairy foods are removed). Second, it allows us to optimize nutrient intake through food, which we consider to be a better choice than supplements where possible. Third, it helps to educate our clinic patients about their food choices and how they impact nutrient intake.

AW: Did you have any concerns about switching from a keto-style diet to one much higher in fibre and lower in fats – more of a Mediterranean-style diet? Were you concerned that it might stall her weight loss (even though you did it because of the tracked advanced lipid markers)?

RH: We see in clinic that not everyone responds in the same way to dietary macronutrient shifts. While our implementation of a ketogenic diet is also high in plant fibre, certainly as she moved off that diet to a more Mediterranean-style one, she would still have increased her fibre intake from moderate amounts of additional vegetable choices such as sweet potato and squashes, legumes and other fruits.

Tracking the effect on weight loss was key during this stage to ensure that the dietary transition did not adversely affect weight loss. Fortunately, this was not the case, as long as AR did not deviate from her avoided food sensitivities. It is always a case of monitoring the individual.

AW: Barriers to change can be a big issue in eight loss. What did you implement to overcome AR's key barriers to change?

RH: You're absolutely right that change can be difficult and that many factors can stand in its way. Depression, anxiety and fatigue were present in AR's case, and so we were deliberate in our interventions to give her some relief early on. Getting some 'quick wins' in the early stages also helped strengthen AR's trust in our approach – improving her blood pressure, menstrual, gastrointestinal, insomnia and energy symptoms were compelling steps forward. Frank conversations about the role of dysbiosis in driving food cravings, how dietary choices can exacerbate microbially driven hunger signals and how herbal antimicrobials can initially worsen but then improve symptoms of cravings where dysbiosis exists helped prepare AR mentally for the inevitable bumps in the journey.

References

Ahmed, S.S.S.J., Santosh, W., 2010. Metallomic profiling and linkage map analysis of early Parkinson's disease: A new insight to aluminum marker for the possible diagnosis. *PLoS ONE* 5. https://doi.org/10.1371/journal.pone.0011252

Ames, B.N., 2010. Optimal micronutrients delay mitochondrial decay and age-associated diseases. *Mechanisms of Ageing and Development* 131, 473–479. https://doi.org/10.1016/j.mad.2010.04.005

Baillie-Hamilton, P.F., 2002. Chemical toxins: a hypothesis to explain the global obesity epidemic. *Journal of Alternative and Complementary Medicine* N 8, 185–192. https://doi.org/10.1089/107555302317371479

Bassolé, I.H.N., Juliani, H.R., 2012. Essential oils in combination and their antimicrobial properties. *Molecules* 17, 3989–4006. https://doi.org/10.3390/molecules17043989

Belkaid, Y., Hand, T., 2014. Role of the microbiota in immunity and inflammation. *Cell* 157, 121–141. https://doi.org/10.1016/j.cell.2014.03.011

Bhattacharya, S.K., Bhattacharya, A., Chakrabarti, A., 2000. Adaptogenic activity of Siotone, a polyherbal formulation of Ayurvedic rasayanas. *Indian Journal of Experimental Biology* 38, 119–128.

Crespo, R.P., Bachega, T.A.S.S., Mendonça, B.B., Gomes, L.G., 2018. An update of genetic basis of PCOS pathogenesis. *Archives of Endocrinology and Metabolism* 62, 352–361. https://doi.org/10.20945/2359-3997000000049

Damian, L., Ghiciuc, C.M., Dima-Cozma, L.C., Ungureanu, M.C., Cozma, S., Patacchioli, F.R., Lupusoru, C.E., 2016. No definitive evidence for a connection between autoimmune thyroid diseases and stress in women. *Neuro Endocrinology Letters* 37, 155–162.

DiSilvestro, D., Petrosino, J., Aldoori, A., Melgar-Bermudez, E., Wells, A., Ziouzenkova, O., 2014. Enzymatic intracrine regulation of white adipose tissue. *Hormone Molecular Biology and Clinical Investigation* 19, 39–55. https://doi.org/10.1515/hmbci-2014-0019

Feller, L., Khammissa, R.A.G., Chandran, R., Altini, M., Lemmer, J., 2014. Oral candidosis in relation to oral immunity. *Journal of Oral Pathology and Medicine* 43, 563–569. https://doi.org/10.1111/jop.12120

Ferrero, S., Remorgida, V., Maganza, C., Venturini, P.L. *et al.*, 2014. Aromatase and endometriosis: Estrogens play a role. *Annals of the New York Academy of Sciences* 1317, 17–23. https://doi.org/10.1111/nyas.12411

Gilbody, S., Lewis, S., Lightfoot, T., 2007. Methylenetetrahydrofolate reductase (MTHFR) genetic polymorphisms and psychiatric disorders: A HuGE review. *American Journal of Epidemiology* 165, 1–13. https://doi.org/10.1093/aje/kwj347

Hajirahimkhan, A., Dietz, B.M., Bolton, J.L., 2013. Botanical modulation of menopausal symptoms: Mechanisms of action? *Planta Medica* 79, 538–553. https://doi.org/10.1055/s-0032-1328187

Hall, D.L., Lattie, E.G., Antoni, M.H., Fletcher, M.A. *et al.*, 2014. Stress management skills, cortisol awakening response, and post-exertional malaise in chronic fatigue syndrome. *Psychoneuroendocrinology* 49, 26–31. https://doi.org/10.1016/j.psyneuen.2014.06.021

Hammer, K.A., Carson, C.F., Riley, T.V., 1999. Antimicrobial activity of essential oils and other plant extracts. *Journal of Applied Microbiology* 86, 985–990.

Hanley, A.J.G., Williams, K., Stern, M.P., Haffner, S.M., 2002. Homeostasis model assessment of insulin resistance in relation to the incidence of cardiovascular disease: The San Antonio Heart Study. *Diabetes Care* 25, 1177–1184.

Hartman, F.A., Thorn, G.W., Lockie, L.M., Greene, C.W., Bowen, B.D., 1932. Treatment of Addison's disease with an extract of supra-renal cortex (cortin). *JAMA* 98, 788–793. https://doi.org/10.1001/jama.1932.02730360010003

Heindel, J.J., Newbold, R., Schug, T.T., 2015. Endocrine disruptors and obesity. *Nature Reviews Endocrinology* 11, 653–661. https://doi.org/10.1038/nrendo.2015.163

Hodges, R.E., Minich, D.M., 2015. Modulation of metabolic detoxification pathways using foods and food-derived components: A scientific review with clinical application. *Journal of Nutrition and Metabolism* 2015. https://doi.org/10.1155/2015/760689

Hruby, A., Hu, F.B., 2015. The epidemiology of obesity: A big picture. *PharmacoEconomics* 33, 673–689. https://doi.org/10.1007/s40273-014-0243-x

Janesick, A.S., Blumberg, B., 2016. Obesogens: An emerging threat to public health. *American Journal of Obstetrics and Gynecology* 214, 559–565. https://doi.org/10.1016/j.ajog.2016.01.182

Jang, Y.-G., Hwang, K.-A., Choi, K.-C., 2018. Rosmarinic acid, a component of rosemary tea, induced the cell cycle arrest and apoptosis through modulation of HDAC2 expression in prostate cancer cell lines. *Nutrients* 10. https://doi.org/10.3390/nu10111784

Jiang, X., Liu, Y., Ma, L., Ji, R. *et al.*, 2018. Chemopreventive activity of sulforaphane. Drug Design, *Development and Therapy* 12, 2905–2913. https://doi.org/10.2147/DDDT.S100534

Kang, K.P., Lee, S., Kang, S.K., 2006. D-lactic acidosis in humans: Review of update. *Electrolyte and Blood Pressure* E & BP 4, 53–56. https://doi.org/10.5049/EBP.2006.4.1.53

Kiecolt-Glaser, J.K., Derry, H.M., Fagundes, C.P., 2015. Inflammation: Depression fans the flames and feasts on the heat. *American Journal of Psychiatry* 172, 1075–1091. https://doi.org/10.1176/appi.ajp.2015.15020152

King, W.D., Ho, V., Dodds, L., Perkins, S.L., Casson, R.I., Massey, T.E., 2012. Relationships among biomarkers of one-carbon metabolism. *Molecular Biology Reports* 39, 7805–7812. https://doi.org/10.1007/s11033-012-1623-y

Kitahara, C.M., Flint, A.J., Berrington de Gonzalez, A., Bernstein, L., Brotzman, M. *et al.*, 2014. Association between class III obesity (BMI of 40–59 kg/m^2) and mortality: A pooled analysis of 20 prospective studies. *PLoS Medicine* 11, e1001673. https://doi.org/10.1371/journal.pmed.1001673

Kohlstadt, I., 2012. *Advancing Medicine with Food and Nutrients*, 2nd ed. CRC Press.

Losurdo, G., Principi, M., Iannone, A., Amoruso, A. *et al.*, 2018. Extra-intestinal manifestations of non-celiac gluten sensitivity: An expanding paradigm. *World Journal of Gastroenterology* 24, 1521–1530. https://doi.org/10.3748/wjg.v24.i14.1521

Manheimer, E.W., van Zuuren, E.J., Fedorowicz, Z., Pijl, H., 2015. Paleolithic nutrition for metabolic syndrome: Systematic review and meta-analysis. *American Journal of Clinical Nutrition* 102, 922–932. https://doi.org/10.3945/ajcn.115.113613

Männistö, P.T., Kaakkola, S., 1999. Catechol-O-methyltransferase (COMT): Biochemistry, molecular biology, pharmacology, and clinical efficacy of the new selective COMT inhibitors. *Pharmacological Reviews* 51, 593–628.

Martucci, M., Ostan, R., Biondi, F., Bellavista, E. *et al.*, 2017. Mediterranean diet and inflammaging within the hormesis paradigm. *Nutrition Reviews* 75, 442–455. https://doi.org/10.1093/nutrit/nux013

Milman, N., Jønsson, L., Dyre, P., Pedersen, P.L., Larsen, L.G., 2014. Ferrous bisglycinate 25 mg iron is as effective as ferrous sulfate 50 mg iron in the prophylaxis of iron deficiency and anemia during pregnancy in a randomized trial. *Journal of Perinatal Medicine* 42, 197–206. https://doi.org/10.1515/jpm-2013-0153

Nagendra, R.P., Maruthai, N., Kutty, B.M., 2012. Meditation and its regulatory role on sleep. *Frontiers in Neurology* 3. https://doi.org/10.3389/fneur.2012.00054

Natural Medicines Interaction Checker n.d. Natural Medicines. Accessed on 26/05/2019 at https://naturalmedicines.therapeuticresearch.com

Nian, H., Delage, B., Ho, E., Dashwood, R.H., 2009. Modulation of histone deacetylase activity by dietary isothiocyanates and allyl sulfides: Studies with sulforaphane and garlic organosulfur compounds. *Environmental and Molecular Mutagenesis* 50, 213–221. https://doi.org/10.1002/em.20454

Pan, M.-H., Lai, C.S., Wu, J.-C., Ho, C.-T., 2013. Epigenetic and disease targets by polyphenols. *Current Pharmaceutical Design* 19, 34. https://doi.org/10.2174/1381612811319340010

Pankhurst, C.L., 2013. Candidiasis (oropharyngeal). *BMJ Clinical Evidence* 2013.

Pennings, N., Jaber, J., Ahiawodzi, P., 2018. Ten-year weight gain is associated with elevated fasting insulin levels and precedes glucose elevation. *Diabetes Metabolism Research and Reviews* 34, e2986. https://doi.org/10.1002/dmrr.2986

Preis, S.R., Massaro, J.M., Robins, S.J., Hoffmann, U. *et al.*, 2010. Abdominal subcutaneous and visceral adipose tissue and insulin resistance in the Framingham heart study. *Obesity* 18, 2191–2198. https://doi.org/10.1038/oby.2010.59

Rancière, F., Lyons, J.G., Loh, V.H.Y., Botton, J. *et al.*, 2015. Bisphenol A and the risk of cardiometabolic disorders: A systematic review with meta-analysis of the epidemiological evidence. *Environmental Health* 14. https://doi.org/10.1186/s12940-015-0036-5

Richter, P., Faroon, O., Pappas, R.S., 2017. Cadmium and cadmium/zinc ratios and tobacco-related morbidities. *International Journal of Environmental Research and Public Health* 14. https://doi.org/10.3390/ijerph14101154

Saadat, P., Ahmadi Ahangar, A., Samaei, S.E., Firozjaie, A. *et al.*, 2018. Serum homocysteine level in Parkinson's Disease and its association with duration, cardinal manifestation, and severity of disease. *Parkinson's Disease* 2018, 5813084. https://doi.org/10.1155/2018/5813084

Schmidt, M., Butterweck, V., 2015. The mechanisms of action of St. John's wort: An update. *Wiener Medizinische Wochenschrift* 1946 165, 229–235. https://doi.org/10.1007/s10354-015-0372-7

Sekirov, I., Russell, S.L., Antunes, L.C.M., Finlay, B.B., 2010. Gut microbiota in health and disease. *Physiological Reviews* 90, 859–904. https://doi.org/10.1152/physrev.00045.2009

Seshadri, D., De, D., 2012. Nails in nutritional deficiencies. *Indian Journal of Dermatology, Venereology and Leprology* 78, 237. https://doi.org/10.4103/0378-6323.95437

Shankar, S., Kumar, D., Srivastava, R.K., 2013. Epigenetic modifications by dietary phytochemicals: implications for personalized nutrition. *Pharmacology and Therapeutics* 138, 1–17. https://doi.org/10.1016/j.pharmthera.2012.11.002

Shojania, A.M., 1982. Oral contraceptives: Effect of folate and vitamin B12 metabolism. *Canadian Medical Association Journal* 126, 244–247.

Sica, D.A., Gehr, T.W.B., Ghosh, S., 2005. Clinical pharmacokinetics of losartan. *Clinical Pharmacokinetics* 44, 797–814. https://doi.org/10.2165/00003088-200544080-00003

Sławek, J., Roszmann, A., Robowski, P., Dubaniewicz, M. *et al.*, 2013. The impact of MRI white matter hyperintensities on dementia in Parkinson's disease in relation to the homocysteine level and other vascular risk factors. *Neurodegenerative Diseases* 12, 1–12. https://doi.org/10.1159/000338610

Strawbridge, R., Arnone, D., Danese, A., Papadopoulos, A., Herane Vives, A., Cleare, A.J., 2015. Inflammation and clinical response to treatment in depression: A meta-analysis. *European Neuropsychopharmacology* 25, 1532–1543. https://doi.org/10.1016/j.euroneuro.2015.06.007

Sturgeon, C., Fasano, A., 2016. Zonulin, a regulator of epithelial and endothelial barrier functions, and its involvement in chronic inflammatory diseases. *Tissue Barriers* 4, e1251384. https://doi.org/10.1080/21688370.2016.1251384

Thakur, V.S., Deb, G., Babcook, M.A., Gupta, S., 2013. Plant phytochemicals as epigenetic modulators: Role in cancer chemoprevention. *AAPS Journal* 16, 151–163. https://doi.org/10.1208/s12248-013-9548-5

Trebble, T.M., Wootton, S.A., Miles, E.A., Mullee, M. *et al.*, 2003. Prostaglandin E2 production and T cell function after fish-oil supplementation: Response to antioxidant cosupplementation. *American Journal of Clinical Nutrition* 78, 376–382. https://doi.org/10.1093/ajcn/78.3.376

Ursini, G., Bollati, V., Fazio, L., Porcelli, A. *et al.*, 2011. Stress-related methylation of the catechol-O-methyltransferase Val 158 allele predicts human prefrontal cognition and activity. *Journal of Neuroscience* 31, 6692–6698. https://doi.org/10.1523/JNEUROSCI.6631-10.2011

Vandenberg, L.N., Colborn, T., Hayes, T.B., Heindel, J.J. *et al.*, 2012. Hormones and endocrine-disrupting chemicals: Low-dose effects and nonmonotonic dose responses. *Endocrine Reviews* 33, 378–455. https://doi.org/10.1210/er.2011-1050

Vanlint, S., 2013. Vitamin D and obesity. *Nutrients* 5, 949–956. https://doi.org/10.3390/nu5030949

Vaucher, P., Druais, P.-L., Waldvogel, S., Favrat, B., 2012. Effect of iron supplementation on fatigue in nonanemic menstruating women with low ferritin: A randomized controlled trial. *CMAJ* 184, 1247–1254. https://doi.org/10.1503/cmaj.110950

vel Szic, K.S., Declerck, K., Vidaković, M., Vanden Berghe, W., 2015. From inflammaging to healthy aging by dietary lifestyle choices: Is epigenetics the key to personalized nutrition? *Clinical Epigenetics* 7. https://doi.org/10.1186/s13148-015-0068-2

Visavadiya, N.P., Narasimhacharya, A.V.R.L., 2008. Sesame as a hypocholesteraemic and antioxidant dietary component. *Food and Chemical Toxicology* 46, 1889–1895. https://doi.org/10.1016/j.fct.2008.01.012

Wang, Y., Chen, S., Yao, T., Li, D. *et al.*, 2014. Homocysteine as a risk factor for hypertension: A 2-year follow-up study. *PloS ONE* 9, e108223. https://doi.org/10.1371/journal.pone.0108223

White, P.T., Subramanian, C., Motiwala, H.F., Cohen, M.S., 2016. Natural withanolides in the treatment of chronic diseases. *Anti-inflammatory Nutraceuticals and Chronic Diseases* 928, 329–373. https://doi.org/10.1007/978-3-319-41334-1_14

Xiao, S., Fei, N., Pang, X., Shen, J. *et al.*, 2014. A gut microbiota-targeted dietary intervention for amelioration of chronic inflammation underlying metabolic syndrome. *FEMS Microbiology Ecology* 87, 357–367. https://doi.org/10.1111/1574-6941.12228

Xu, Y., Su, D., Zhu, L., Zhang, S. *et al.*, 2018. S-allylcysteine suppresses ovarian cancer cell proliferation by DNA methylation through DNMT1. *Journal of Ovarian Research* 11, 39. https://doi.org/10.1186/s13048-018-0412-1

Yang, H., Hwang, I., Kim, S., Ahn, C., Hong, E.-J., Jeung, E.-B., 2013. Preventive effects of Lentinus edodes on homocysteinemia in mice. *Experimental and Therapeutic Medicine* 6, 465–468. https://doi.org/10.3892/etm.2013.1130

Yang, O., Kim, H.L., Weon, J.-I., Seo, Y.R., 2015. Endocrine-disrupting chemicals: Review of toxicological mechanisms using molecular pathway analysis. *Journal of Cancer Prevention* 20, 12–24. https://doi.org/10.15430/JCP.2015.20.1.12

Zhang, Y., Li, X., Zou, D., Liu, W. *et al.*, 2008. Treatment of type 2 diabetes and dyslipidemia with the natural plant alkaloid berberine. *Journal of Clinical Endocrinology and Metabolism* 93, 2559–2565. https://doi.org/10.1210/jc.2007-2404

7

Cognitive Health through Gut–Brain Communication

Practitioner: Miguel Toribio-Mateas

Introduction

This chapter documents the case report of GA, a female client seeking nutrition and lifestyle advice for the management of insomnia, anxiety and low energy with borderline depressive mood, accompanied by bloating and gastrointestinal discomfort. The case aims to illustrate how neurological and cognitive symptoms can be related to the gastrointestinal system and why working upstream from the gut should be considered as a potential clinical strategy for improving cognitive health.

Initial case presentation

GA is a 72-year-old female who has been under the care of a nutrition practitioner for more than seven years, initially seeking support for the dietary management of ulcerative colitis (UC), loss of bone density as a result of steroid treatment for UC, and borderline hypothyroidism. Although these issues will be referred to as we navigate through our client's individual health trajectory, the focus of this chapter is on cognitive health and on the translatability of various pieces of evidence to the case in a way that practitioners are able to apply in clinical practice. The case study focuses on a six-month period when cognitive health became the focus for the practitioner and client.

The gut microbiome is of particular interest for this case because of GA's history of UC. The microbe population living in the gastrointestinal (GI) tract, traditionally referred to as 'gut flora', and collectively known as 'gut microbiota' or 'gut microbiome' if including the microbes' genes (Marchesi and Ravel, 2015), interacts with GA as a host through a number of pathways, including neural, immune and neuroendocrine. These act as communication channels through which gut microbes cast local as well as systemic effects on the host biology, both in health and disease (Toribio-Mateas, 2018). Inflammatory bowel diseases (IBDs) such as UC and Crohn's disease (CD) are characterized by alterations in normal composition of commensal gut microbiota or dysbiosis, seen as a key contributory factor to the inflammation underlying these conditions (Basso, Câmara and Sales-Campos, 2018; Knox *et al.*, 2019; Qiao, Cai and Ran, 2016; Sartor and Wu, 2017). Calprotectin is used as a routine biomarker to assess the extent to which the gut is compromised by inflammatory processes (Hold *et al.*, 2014; Nissilä *et al.*, 2017; Zhou *et al.* 2018). Dysbiosis is also seen in functional gastrointestinal disorders (FGIDs) such as irritable bowel syndrome (IBS), constipation, dyspepsia and oesophageal disorders, which the new Rome IV criterion defines as disorders of gut–brain interaction (Drossman, 2016; Drossman and Hasler, 2016; Tack and Drossman, 2017). Last but not least, dysbiosis is widely seen as a mediator in the pathogenesis of a number of other conditions. Particularly relevant to this case are metabolic (Buford, 2017; Lau *et al.*, 2017; Ma and Li, 2018; Nagpal, Yadav and Marotta, 2014) and cardiovascular diseases (Battson *et al.*, 2018a, 2018b).

The client had been working with this practitioner since 2011. In her late 30s and early 40s GA had experienced what she describes as 'gut issues', featuring ongoing loose, watery and frequent bowel movements. She was tested for common causes of her symptoms, such as the presence of *Escherichia coli*, *Campylobacter*, *Shigella* or *Salmonella* (Lääveri *et al.*, 2016; Porter *et al.*, 2017). Parasitology was negative, so no treatment was issued at the time – it was very much a case of 'we cannot find anything wrong with you'. For more than ten years she tried to 'manage her gut' by avoiding ultra-processed foods and alcohol, as these would trigger undesirable symptoms that could last for days. In 2011, at age 65, she was finally diagnosed with UC after a severe episode of blood in the stool and being hospitalized for ten days. She was prescribed prednisolone (40 mg/day) as an anti-inflammatory agent and the aminosalicylate mesalamine as suppositories and orally for the management of the rectal bleeding and diarrhoea. Six months after being discharged, she decided she wanted to manage her condition by means of diet and lifestyle. This is when she had her first nutrition appointment with the personalized nutrition practitioner.

The practitioner used the Measure Yourself Medical Outcome Profile (MYMOP) tool to assess GA's primary symptoms. This is shown in Table 7.1. Note that while the concerns rated in the MYMOP are long-standing, the scoring was taken at a consultation six months prior to the recommendations covered below.

Table 7.1 Pre-intervention MYMOP questionnaire for GA

Concern	Rating	Makes difficult or prevents
Anxiety	0 1 2 3 4 5 ⑥	Makes day-to-day life difficult
Fatigue	0 1 2 3 4 5 ⑥	Shopping, house chores
Sleep	0 1 2 3 4 5 ⑥	Makes day-to-day life difficult
General feeling of wellbeing	0 1 2 3 4 ⑤ 6	

The MYMOP questionnaire was created by general practitioner Dr Charlotte Paterson in the mid-1990s (Paterson, 1996) and was then developed and validated by a research team at the University of Bristol (UK) to be used in any clinical settings where a client presents with symptoms, which can be physical, emotional or social (Paterson, 2004; Paterson and Britten, 2000). It allows the client to rate their own choice of symptoms using a seven-point scale where 0 is 'as good as it could be' and 6 is 'as bad as it could be'. Clients can also rate their general feeling of wellbeing, and any activities that the symptoms prevent the client from doing.

Looking at the body through a wide-angle lens

While GA has a generally positive outlook on life, she is prone to worry. In recent years this trait has been intensified by having to deal with a difficult personal situation. Her long-term partner – 79 years old – has metastasized prostate cancer affecting several organs and is also affected by cardiovascular disease. Moreover, she is very close to an older family friend who is terminally ill in a nursing home. Additionally, a few months ago, she was physically attacked while taking money out of an ATM, which severely affected her confidence. All of these situations are seen to have contributed to a great degree of the anxiety and borderline depression experienced by the client.

Diet and nutraceutical history

Shortly after the UC diagnosis, GA had started following the specific carbohydrate diet (SCD), and she had adhered strictly to the principles of no grains, sugars (except for honey), processed foods or milk. The SCD purports decreased intestinal inflammation by restoring the balance of bacteria within the bowels and resolving the associated dysbiosis found in IBD (Suskind *et al.*, 2016). Because of her fear of food triggering UC symptoms, her diet had become restrictive and repetitive and mostly based on the following:

- Vegetables: Onions, butternut squash, broccoli, cabbage, spinach, frozen peas, watercress, tomatoes, mushrooms, peppers.
- Fruit: Blueberries, raspberries, bananas, apple, apricot puree, grapes.
- Meat and fish: chicken, tuna.
- Fats: olive oil.
- Nuts: Walnuts.

The client was aware of this and, in order to mitigate potential nutrient deficiencies, she had experimented with a variety of supplements. In the following summary, 'current' corresponds to the time the MYMOP in Table 7.1 was completed.

- A range of practitioner-grade multivitamin-type products. Currently taking a good-quality multivitamin and mineral complex with added botanicals including green tea extract, curcumin and other nutrients such as lutein and resveratrol.
- Iron, various forms including ferrous bisglycinate, from 5 mg to 50 mg a day. Currently taking 7.5 mg/day food-state iron in addition to 4 mg ferrous bisglycinate in the multivitamin.
- Zinc, also various forms, from citrate to bisglycinate, from 10 mg to 30 mg/day. Currently taking 20 mg zinc as bisglycinate as part of the multivitamin complex.
- A range of probiotic products, from single strain to multi-strain. Currently not taking any.
- Pepsin, betaine and digestive enzymes. Currently not taking any.

Antecedents, triggers and mediators

GA had presented with high levels of low-density lipoprotein cholesterol (LDL-C) for some time before the UC diagnosis. By itself this would normally not be a red flag, but she also had a family history of cardiovascular and neurodegenerative disease. The client's mother had hypertension and her maternal grandmother had developed late-onset Alzheimer's disease (LOAD) in her 80s and she herself carries one copy of the apolipoprotein E (APOE) ε4 allele (see Table 7.2). A practitioner with a good all-round view of a client's condition would look through a wide-angle lens and see her gastrointestinal issues in context, taking into account that dysbiosis of gut microbiota is seen not only in gastrointestinal disorders, as discussed previously, but also in clients with stroke and transient ischaemic attack (TIA). Pre-clinical evidence documenting this relationship has been available for some time (Bu and Wang, 2018; Richards et al., 2017), and recent clinical data confirms it (Awoyemi et al., 2018; Yin et al., 2015).

Additionally, focusing on the client's family history of neurode-generative disease, a systems-oriented practitioner would also wonder about chronically raised calprotectin and its links with cognitive impairment. Calprotectin is a heterodimer formed by pro-inflammatory proteins S100A8 and S100A9. Both neutrophils and monocytes are first-line immune defence cells and contain huge amounts of the S100A8/A9 in their cytoplasm. They are recruited to sites of inflammation during infection or sterile injury. Besides its role as a clinically relevant biomarker to monitor disease activity in chronic inflammatory disorders including IBDs and rheumatoid arthritis, extracellular calprotectin interacts with the pattern recognition receptors toll-like receptor 4 (TLR4) and receptor for advanced glycation end products (RAGE) promoting cell activation and recruitment (Pruenster *et al.*, 2016). Most relevantly for GA's case, it has been established as a biomarker for the diagnosis and progression of Alzheimer's disease (AD) and dementia (Horvath *et al.*, 2016; Wang *et al.*, 2018).

The client also reports having had cellulitis of the legs at age 72, having had antibiotics for this condition also at 65 and 66 years of age. The antibiotic prescribed was amoxicillin, 200 mg TID. Pre-clinical data suggests that antibiotic-induced dysbiosis may lead to severe damage of the enteric nervous system (ENS) and how, in animal models, this is coupled with potential long-lasting dysregulation of the microbiota–gut–brain axis, the main line of communication between the gut and the brain (Caputi *et al.*, 2017; Stefano, Samuel and Kream, 2017). The additional potential disruption to the gut ecosystem following the antibiotic treatment, alongside existing disruptions characteristic of UC, should be taken into account when evaluating this case through a wide-angle lens.

Investigations

During the seven years the practitioner had worked with GA, a number of tests had been ordered by the practitioner or her medical practitioner. The most relevant investigations are summarized in Tables 7.2, 7.3 and 7.4, with some context. Tables 7.3 and 7.4 include results from as early as 2011 and up to as recently as six months before the case study was written. The aim is to provide an overview of the markers assessed as part of the management of the long-standing issues affecting the patient.

Table 7.2 Genetic testing/genotyping

Gene	Rationale	Result	Significance
APOE	Family history of cardiovascular disease (CVD) and neurodegenerative disease	APOE3/4 genotype, i.e. carries one copy of the APOE-ε4 allele	Increased risk of CVD and Alzheimer's disease (AD)/ dementia
FTO	Family history of neurodegenerative disease	AA genotype for rs6499640, a set of variants for the FTO gene including gene variations in FTO rs6499640, FTO rs8044769 and FTO rs9939609	Increased risk of AD/ dementia
MTHFR	Family history of CVD and neurodegenerative disease, in addition to clinical presentation with anxiety and low mood	GT genotype for rs1801131 (MTHFR A1298C) and AG genotype for rs1801133 (MTHFR C677T)	Reduced MTHFR enzyme activity, compared with people with other genotypes
Cat-echol-O-meth-yltransferase (COMT)	Clinical presentation with anxiety, low mood	AG genotype for rs4680 (COMT V158M)	Reduced activity of COMT activity, leading to slightly higher levels of brain dopamine compared with people with other genotypes

Table 7.3 Functional blood biochemistry and saliva testing

Marker	Rationale	Result	Significance
Homocysteine	Family history of CVD and neurodegenerative disease, in addition to clinical presentation with anxiety and low mood	Several samples, never higher than 9 mmol/L 10 mmol/L would be a cause of concern in this client	Homocysteine levels within an optimal range confirm the need to pay attention to the clinical presentation and not just look for potentially deranged biochemistry
LDL cholesterol	Family history of CVD and neurodegenerative disease	Several samples ranging from 3.9 mmol/L at its highest to 3 mmol/L at its lowest, with a trend to be over 3.5 mmol/L	High LDL would not be significant or clinically actionable as a standalone marker, but with the APOE3/4 genotype, family history of neurodegeneration and concerning symptoms of mild cognitive impairment, it is a marker worth tackling
Four-point salivary cortisol and DHEA in saliva	Lethargy, fatigue, low mood	Assessed twice, in 2011 and 2017 Both samples showed low DHEA:Cortisol ratio, and the December 2017 sample showed cortisol high at the four sample points of the day, with evening cortisol significantly above optimum ranges (1.88 nmol/L, where the optimum range is up to 0.94 nmol/L)	Results are clear signs of autonomic dysregulation Given the similarities between samples, it is safe to say that the autonomic nervous system has been under chronic stress for quite some time See Chapter 3 for further discussion on this test

cont.

Marker	Rationale	Result	Significance
Thyroid function	Lethargy, fatigue, low mood	Based on several samples: free T4 rarely over 15 pmol/L (12.0–22.0 pmol/L) Free T3 mostly below 4 pmol/L (3.1–6.8 pmol/L)	This is one of the issues the client had sought professional support for originally

Table 7.4 Gastrointestinal assessment

Marker	Rationale	Result	Significance
Microbial diversity	Presence of ongoing GI symptoms	Several samples confirming low microbial association compared with a healthy cohort	Low microbial diversity has been associated with a number of conditions, including CVD and neurodegenerative diseases (Toribio-Mateas, 2018)
Faecal calprotectin	Localized inflammation of the GI	Several samples ranging from 102 mcg/L at its lowest to 144 mcg/L at its highest	Aside from GI inflammation (over 50 mcg/L it warrants further investigation and over 120 mcg/L confirms IBD), it shows intestinal permeability affecting gut–brain communication (Kelly *et al.*, 2015; Liu and Zhu, 2018; Maes, Kubera and Leunis, 2008; Obrenovich, 2018)

Eosinophil protein X (EPX)	Ongoing GI inflammation and discomfort	Measured twice, at 5.7 mcg/g both times Optimal range is ≤ 4.6 mcg/g	Indicates increased intraluminal release of eosinophil granule proteins, i.e. immune activation in the intestinal lumen, and typically a sign of subclinical inflammation (Peterson et al., 2016)
Pancreatic elastase 1	Bloating, slow digestion	Tested several times, ranging from 234 mcg/g at its highest to 134 mcg/g at its lowest Optimal range is > 200 mcg/g	Identifies mild exocrine pancreatic insufficiency (Domínguez-Muñoz et al., 2017)
Parasitology	Lethargy, fatigue, low mood	No parasites, yeast or pathogenic bacteria have ever been found in any of the samples	It can often be the case that clients with low energy have parasitic microorganisms in their gut, but that wasn't the case for GA

Interpretation

The practitioner decided to focus on the gut as the gateway system for the interpretation of the case, followed by consideration of some key genetic variants. An explanation is provided for of each of the factors considered when 'connecting the dots' of this case.

Microbial diversity

Microbial diversity was a key focus for the practitioner. Why? Because there is evidence that gut microbiota profiles in individuals suffering from low mood and depression show narrowing in microbial diversity (Dinan and Cryan, 2015), rendering the host more susceptible to infection and consequently negatively affecting innate immune function (Patterson *et al.*, 2014). The client's microbial composition was assessed by 16S sequencing stool test several times in the last seven years, and microbial (alpha) diversity association was consistently low compared with healthy cohorts, as provided by the testing laboratory (see Chapter 3). Additionally, recent studies have identified that subject biological age correlates with a decrease in stool microbial diversity (Maffei *et al.*, 2017) – that is, pathological ageing is associated with a narrowing in microbial diversity whereas healthy ageing correlates with a more diverse microbiota (Dinan and Cryan, 2017). Additionally, GA's dietary pattern had been limited to a few foods that she repeated constantly for years as she was fearful that stepping out of that 'comfort zone' would trigger UC symptoms. Results from a recent open-platform citizen science microbiome research project known as the 'American Gut' project (McDonald *et al.*, 2018) found emergent positive associations among the microbiome, metabolome (the collection of metabolites resulting from the interaction between the gut microbiota's genes and that of its host) and the diversity of plant-based foods consumed by participants. Based on more than 10,000 food frequency questionnaires, researchers concluded those people consuming a minimum of 30 different polyphenol-rich plant-based foods per week had the highest microbial diversity.

The significance of chronically raised faecal calprotectin

Faecal calprotectin (FC) is an established inflammatory marker used to assess the presence and severity of IBDs (Argollo *et al.*, 2017). Given its high sensitivity as a marker of inflammation in CD and UC, a negative result can safely spare most individuals with idiopathic gastrointestinal symptoms, as well as those with IBS, from having to undergo invasive investigations such as colonoscopies (Waugh *et al.*, 2013). Other markers such as C-reactive protein (CRP) and erythrocyte sedimentation rate (ESR) – both in serum – can provide additional clues to differentiate between IBD and IBS. FC levels correlate significantly with endoscopic disease activity in IBD and are useful in clinical practice for assessment of disease activity and/or remission (D'Haens *et al.*, 2012). Additionally, literature on FC agrees that results have good reproducibility (Mumolo *et al.*, 2018), and therefore clinicians can trust them to mean the same thing across the board.

Aside from its relevance as a marker in management of gastrointestinal health, so far emerging evidence suggests that FC could also be useful in the assessment of cognitive decline. A study on 22 Alzheimer's patients found almost three-quarters of AD patients presented with faecal calprotectin concentrations higher than normal (>50 mg/kg) (Leblhuber *et al.*, 2015). This is interpreted to be a sign of gastrointestinal permeability contributing to inflammation and neuroinflammation as well as affecting availability of key cognitive amino acids such as tryptophan.

APOE genotyping

Practitioners often have high expectations of genetic testing as a tool to help them accurately predict the optimal diets or risk of common diseases for their patients. The reality is that genetic data can only provide partial answers to complex health questions, like providing some of the missing pieces in a large jigsaw that is difficult to complete (Toribio-Mateas and Spector, 2017). What genetic data can provide a really useful insight into, however, is disease risk reduction, prevention and disease management, particularly when other markers that are involved in the development of a condition are assessed – for example, APOE and cholesterol levels, so that the practitioner knows whether the susceptibility conferred by the existence of the gene variant may be materializing functionally. GA's grandmother had developed late-onset Alzheimer's disease (LOAD). With that in mind and given her signs of cognitive impairment, GA's medical practitioner recommended APOE genotyping.

The human APOE gene exists in three common allelic variations: ε2, ε3 (the wild type) and ε4 (Myers *et al.*, 1996). There are six possible genotypic combinations, including three homozygous (ε2/ε2, ε3/ε3 and ε4/ε4) and three heterozygous (ε2/ε3, ε3/ε4 and ε2/ε4). The ε4 allele, resulting in the ApoE4 protein, has been shown to be associated with genetic risk factors for developing LOAD: ε4 heterozygotes are at 2–3 times more risk, and ε4 homozygotes have up to 12 times more risk than those with ε3 wildtype alleles (Kim, Basak and Holtzman, 2009). Furthermore, this genotype has been shown to be associated also with general cognitive decline in cognitively normal individuals with no symptoms of AD-related disorders (Caselli *et al.*, 2011, 2009). Only around 40% of individuals who develop LOAD possess an ε4 allele. For practitioners working with genetic data, this means that a ε4 variant can only provide susceptibility estimates of the likelihood of developing LOAD – that is, carrying the ε4 allele means greater risk (Farrer *et al.*, 1997; Ungar, Altmann and Greicius, 2014) but it doesn't necessarily guarantee that a person will develop the condition.

The catechol-O-methyltransferase gene: COMT

GA is – to a certain extent – a pathological worrier who fears uncertainty, particularly when it comes to how food might affect her bowel. However, taking into consideration the fact that the severity of her UC resulted in her being hospitalized, it is easy to see how her anxiety could be somewhat justified.

The COMT gene provides instructions for making an enzyme called catechol-O-methyltransferase which is particularly important in an area at the front of the brain called the prefrontal cortex, a region that is involved with personality, planning, inhibition of behaviours, abstract thinking, emotion and short-term (working) memory. To function efficiently, the prefrontal cortex requires dopamine and noradrenaline, and catechol-O-methyltransferase helps break these down so that they are present in adequate amounts. When this enzyme is hyperactivated, dopamine – responsible for drive or 'get up and go' – is disposed of too quickly, leaving a person feeling flat and potentially apathetic. Conversely, when activity of catechol-O-methyltransferase is reduced, higher levels of dopamine remain in the prefrontal cortex. In the shorter run, this can have a positive effect on the experience of reward (Wichers *et al.*, 2008), as well as verbal fluency and creativity (Zhang, Zhang and Zhang, 2014). In the longer run, the impaired ability to break down these catecholamines can result in higher risk of impulsivity, neuroticism and anxiety disorders (Gottschalk and Domschke, 2017; Soeiro-De-Souza *et al.*, 2013; Stein *et al.*, 2005).

Methylenetetrahydrofolate reductase (MTHFR) and anxiety

The 5,10-methylenetetrahydrofolate reductase (MTHFR) gene is responsible for the metabolism of folate. There is evidence of common polymorphisms in this gene, including MTHFR C677T and A1298C, and their association with anxiety disorders (Gilbody, Lewis and Lightfoot, 2007) as well as depression (Zintzaras, 2006). It is worth noting that not everyone who has these type of genetic variants presents with low folate or high homocysteine. Indeed, that is GA's case, whose bloods over the five years prior to writing this report never showed low folate or high homocysteine. (This is despite her having an even greater susceptibility due to the presence of a variant in another gene – the NBPF3 gene – which is associated with lower circulating levels of pyridoxine – vitamin B6.) The point highlighted here is that folate and vitamins B12 and B6 are part of the methyl donor subgroup of B vitamins (Sharma and Litonjua, 2014; Tanaka *et al.*, 2009). Even though these three markers were within normal levels in blood tests, the practitioner felt that sensible supplementation was warranted, due to the presence of her genetic variants and her clinical presentation of extreme fatigue and low mood. This will be discussed further in the next section.

Recommendations: Tackling a complex system

The practitioner agreed with GA that the focus should be on lifestyle and food, with only a few selected nutraceuticals that merited their use based on clinical evidence and previous experience of effectiveness in similar cases. The following sections detail the recommendations for each of the connected areas tackled as part of this case.

Stress and sleep

Gut sensitivity and motility had been a chronic feature in the client's life, as has the dysregulation of autonomic nervous function and the hypothalamic–pituitary axis through lack of cortisol homeostasis. Emotions such as stress play a substantial role in cognitive health (Wingenfeld and Otte, 2018) and are capable of disrupting brain–gut homeostasis (Pellissier and Bonaz, 2017). Recent evidence points to oncologic caregivers, both formal and informal (i.e. a paid carer or someone caring for their partner at home), presenting with higher overall perceived stress levels (including high anxiety, and higher perceived self-reported psychological stress rate) compared with caregivers of geriatric patients with chronic diseases (Aguiló *et al.*, 2018). GA cares for both a patient with cancer (her long-term partner) and an older friend in her 90s. When asked to rate her own stress levels by MYMOP, she rated them as 6 or 'as bad as they could be'. Her MYMOP score for sleep was also 6. She told her practitioner that she was getting a maximum of three hours' uninterrupted sleep per night and feeling exhausted in the morning. Chronic stress is known to contribute to the dysregulation of the hypothalamic–pituitary–adrenal system and to have a negative impact on sleep quality, which in the longer run has been seen to lead to sleep disturbance and depression as well as decreased brain-derived neurotrophic factor (BDNF) levels (Giese *et al.*, 2013; Schmitt, Holsboer-Trachsler and Eckert, 2016). BDNF belongs to a family of small secreted proteins with very well-researched positive effect on hippocampal synaptic plasticity, through which it promotes learning and memory, and enables resilience to exposure to glucocorticoids such as cortisol –that is, endurance to psychological stress (Leal, Bramham and Duarte, 2017).

Sleep disturbances and disorders have also been implicated in cardiovascular morbidity and mortality (Hall, Brindle and Buysse, 2018), and GA has a family history of CVD and carries some risk factor – both genetic (MTHFR and APOE polymorphisms) and biochemical (elevated LDL)

– which make a cardiovascular event a more tangible possibility, so it was decided to tackle the client's 'broken system' from the sleep angle first. To do that, the practitioner agreed with GA the introduction of anxiolytic botanicals with a long history of traditional use.

Bacopa monnieri and Gotu kola

In a randomized, double-blind, placebo-controlled clinical trial with a placebo run-in of six weeks and a treatment period of 12 weeks in patients of an average age of 73 years, 300 mg/day standardized *Bacopa monnieri* extract helped relieve anxiety and symptoms of depression (Calabrese *et al.*, 2008). The same dose had previously been shown to improve cognitive functions such as learning and memory in healthy participants compared with placebo (Stough *et al.*, 2001). More recent studies have supplemented *Bacopa* at slightly higher doses with positive effects on cognitive performance and anxiety (Sathyanarayanan *et al.*, 2013). *Bacopa monnieri* is a shrub used traditionally in Ayurveda for the balancing properties of its terpenoids, known as bacosides, which have been seen to lead to enhanced BDNF production and subsequent improvements in neuroplasticity (Sangiovanni *et al.*, 2017). In this practitioner's clinical experience it helps with sleep quality and reduction of anxiety in a 2–3-week time frame. Furthermore, *Bacopa monnieri* can work synergistically with Gotu kola (*Centella asiatica*), also known to attenuate anxiety and improve cognition (Jana *et al.*, 2010) as well as modulate mood (Wattanathorn *et al.*, 2008). In pre-clinical models, terpenoids in Gotu kola have been seen to increase hippocampal synaptic density and to improve memory and executive function.

Introducing Mediterranean diversity

Perhaps the most important recommendation of all was asking GA to focus on including a diversity of brightly coloured vegetables and fruit as part of her daily diet and to try not to repeat the same vegetables every day, but to rotate them. The rationale was to emulate the beneficial effect of dietary diversity seen in the Mediterranean diet (MD) on the gut microbiota.

Why is diet diversity so important? There is plenty of evidence pointing that way. For example, a recent study of 31 Spanish adults in the north of Spain found that participants with the closest adherence to a Mediterranean-style dietary pattern to be the most statistically significant and beneficial changes in a number of bacterial communities including overall higher abundance of *Bacteroidetes*, *Prevotellacea* and *Prevotella*, and a lower concentration of *Firmicutes* and *Lachnospiraceae*, all of which been found to display anti-inflammatory properties (Gutiérrez-Díaz *et al.*, 2016). The alterations in gut microbiota richness and spread triggered by the MD are consistent with previously reported clinical data on the effects of increased dietary fibre from vegetables, legumes and whole grains – meaning minimally processed – as well as phenolic compounds and carotenoids typically featured in MD foods such as seasonal and citrus fruits, leafy, pod and root vegetables, in addition to bulbs, such as onions, garlic, leeks, as well as red wine and coffee (González *et al.*, 2014; Tap *et al.*, 2015).

The same research team (2016) reported a link between the high diversity of dietary bioactive compounds in the MD and higher levels of a commensal bacteria group known as *Clostridium* cluster XVIa, particularly *Faecalibacterium prausnitzii*. This bundle of Firmicutes is known for their ability to colonize the mucin layer of the human colon, thereby aiding in the maintenance of gut homeostasis (Lopetuso *et al.*, 2013). It includes species such as *Eubacterium rectale*, *Papillibacter cinnamivorans*, *Eubacterium ventriosum*, *Butyrivibrio crossotus*, *Clostridium orbiscindens*, *Coprococcus eutactus*, *Roseburia intestinalis* and *Faecalibacterium prausnitzii* known to plays a major role in mediating the production of butyrate from fermentable dietary carbohydrates (El Aidy *et al.*, 2013; Van den Abbeele *et al.*, 2013). F. prausnitzii is considered to have strong anti-inflammatory properties (Lopez-Siles *et al.*, 2017). This is largely mediated by its ability to produce butyrate, thereby protecting the gut mucosa (Sokol *et al.* 2009), and for its ability to block pro-inflammatory cytokines such as NF-kappaB and IL-8 production (Sokol *et al.*, 2008). Low levels of F. prausnitzii, have been associated with a peripheral inflammatory state in patients with cognitive impairment and brain amyloidosis (Cattaneo *et al.*, 2017). Low levels of genus *Roseburia* microbes have been seen in patients with UC (Bajer *et al.*, 2017; Machiels *et al.*, 2014), as well as in those affected by constipation-predominant irritable bowel syndrome (C-IBS) (Gobert *et al.*, 2016). Figure 7.1 depicts the impact of dietary diversity on the gut–

brain axis. It is worth noting that the microbial ecosystem in the gut is extremely complex; individual microbes that are part of a group or family can sometimes be found to have effects that contradict those of the group they belong to. For example, *F. prausnitzii* or *Roseburia* are part of the Firmicutes phyla, but tend to behave differently compared with other Firmicutes.

Because of GA's attachment to the principles of the specific carbohydrate diet, she had been limiting the vegetables and fruit she consumed for years. Although there are anecdotal reports of benefit from this and other types of diets in IBD, there is no consistent clinical data to support their effectiveness as long-term dietary patterns. On that basis, the practitioner suggested to introduce new colours of the same vegetable as a first step forward – for example, red, white and green cabbage, green, red, yellow and orange peppers, different types of mushrooms, from oyster to shiitake, maitake, button, chestnut – increasing diversity by mindfully adding five or six portions (about 80 g each) of vegetables daily in total, with a new vegetable or a different colour of the same vegetable every couple of days.

Although the emerging evidence on the effects of dietary diversity on the microbiome and the human host has been focusing on plant-based foods, the practitioner believes there is also argument for protein diversity. Different meats and types of fish provide different amino acid profiles along with minerals and trace elements. Based on that principle, the client was asked to include a variety of good-quality meat cuts, organic if possible, and of wild-caught fish such as Alaskan salmon, mackerel, cod, coley or pollock, as well as tinned sardines, ideally in olive oil. In fact, as a clinician looking at GA's individual case through a wider-angle lens, the practitioner emphasized the role of olive oil as a simple yet extremely powerful food-based intervention that targets both the gut and the cardiovascular system. To illustrate this point, recent clinical evidence described how adding a mere 25 ml/day of olive oil infused with fresh thyme has been seen to improve the lipid profile of hypercholesterolemic individuals, and the cardioprotective effect is believed to be mediated by an increase in *Bifidobacteria* triggered by the phenolic compounds found in olive oil and thyme, both food items typically featured in Mediterranean dietary patterns (Martín-Peláez *et al.*, 2017).

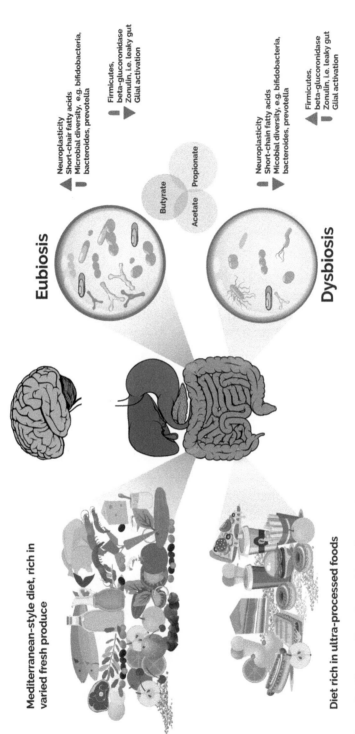

Eubiosis

Neuroplasticity
Short-chair fatty acids
Microbial diversity, e.g. bifidobacteria,
bacteroides, prevotella

Firmicutes,
beta-glucoronidase
Zonulin, i.e. leaky gut
Glial activation

Dysbiosis

Neuroplasticity
Short-chain fatty acids
Micobial diversity, e.g. bifidobacteria,
bacteroides, prevotella

Firmicutes,
beta-glucoronidase
Zonulin, i.e. leaky gut
Glial activation

Butyrate
Acetate
Propionate

Mediterranean-style diet, rich in
varied fresh produce

Diet rich in ultra-processed foods

Figure 7.1 Dietary diversity and its effect on the gut–brain axis (see online colour plate)
Source: Reproduced with permission from Toribio-Mateas (2018)

Red rice yeast

GA's medical practitioner had been keen for her to take statins in order to manage her LDL cholesterol levels, but GA had wanted to tackle this issue by means of nutrition and lifestyle. Because of the increased predisposition to cardiovascular and cerebrovascular events, the practitioner suggested a three-month course of red rice yeast, 400 mg/day, providing 1.6 mg monacolin K, a natural substance chemically identical to lovastatin, that has been recognized as responsible for its cholesterol-reducing properties (Nguyen, Karl and Santini, 2017). In the same way as lovastatin and other statins, monacolin K inhibits hydroxymethylglutaryl-coenzyme A (HMG CoA) reductase, the rate-limiting step in cholesterol synthesis, which also depletes coenzyme Q_{10} (CoQ_{10}) levels from the body. On that basis, and following recent clinical evidence of CoQ_{10} administration alongside red rice yeast (Mazza *et al.*, 2018), a supplement that contained 20 mg CoQ_{10} was recommended.

While red rice yeast works on exactly the same pathway as statins, in the author's clinical experience it is the very low dose of the 'natural statin' in red rice yeast that seems to enable the beneficial effects on LDL cholesterol reduction, but without the side effects experienced by those on lovastatin and other statins, such as muscle pain.

Fermented foods

Fermented foods provide a way to re-establish gut microbiota homeostasis that has been reported to be a relevant strategy to prevent or attenuate several conditions, not just gastrointestinal but also cardiovascular and metabolic disorders (Pimenta *et al.*, 2018). Given the practitioner's own clinical experience over the last few years, he was particularly keen on the use of kefir, a complex fermented dairy product created through the symbiotic fermentation of milk or sucrose-enriched water by lactic acid bacteria and yeasts contained within an exopolysaccharide and protein complex called a kefir grain (Bourrie, Willing and Cotter, 2016). Kefir is an excellent source of microbial diversity, providing up to 60 different species, including *Lactobacillus casei/paracasei*, *Lactobacillus harbinensis*, *Lactobacillus hilgardii*, *Bifidobacterium psychraerophilum/crudilactis*, *Saccharomyces cerevisiae* and *Dekkera bruxellensis* (Laureys and De Vuyst, 2014). Regular consumption of kefir and its exopolysaccharides has been associated with improved digestion and tolerance to lactose, as well as with antibacterial and hypocholesterolaemic effects, control of plasma glucose, antihypertensive effect, anti-inflammatory effect, antioxidant activity, anti-carcinogenic activity, anti-allergenic activity and healing effects (Lim *et al.*, 2017; Rosa *et al.*, 2017).

Kombucha, a fermented drink made from sugared black tea by a symbiotic colony of bacteria and yeast (SCOBY), is a natural source of short-chain fatty acids, enzymes and living microbes that has been seen to inhibit pathogenic bacteria such as *Escherichia coli*, *Vibrio cholerae*, *Shigella flexneri* and *Salmonella typhimurium* (Bhattacharya *et al.*, 2016).

GA was provided with instructions on how to make water kefir and kombucha at home and she was advised to drink up to two glasses (600 ml) of water kefir and one glass (300 ml) of kombucha daily. The practitioner suggested to start with 50 ml on day one and to build up by an additional 50 ml a day until reaching the suggested dose. Based on his own clinical experience, this gentle approach to introducing fermented foods works well with individuals with gut issues whose GI tract may be 'shocked' by the high amounts of live bacteria contained in kefir and kombucha, experiencing bloating and flatulence as a result, which can detract from compliance going forward. Even though these are food sources of probiotic microbes, they are extremely powerful and should be used sensibly. For clarity, the same applies to milk kefir and kefir made with milk substitute (e.g. coconut).

Methylated B vitamins

The idea that methylated B vitamins – for example, methylfolate, methylcobalamine – are superior has quickly spread among nutrition practitioners, particularly for clients like GA whose folate reductase activity is potentially limited by her genetic variants. In fact, the availability of nutrigenetic testing and the lack of precise clinical protocols has led to a variety of treatment strategies that rely on hypotheses and mechanistic studies (Oberg *et al.*, 2015), including supplementation with L-methylfolate with or without other B vitamins. Hyperbole aside, what is clear is that folate, folic acid and 5-methyltetrahydrofolate are not the same thing and that those with potentially detrimental MTHFR variants are more likely to benefit from methylated B-vitamin forms than the corresponding non-methylated versions. In this particular case, L-methylfolate was recommended to support the synthesis of the three major neurochemicals: serotonin, noradrenaline and dopamine – across the blood–brain barrier (Leahy, 2017) which has been seen to achieve significant improvements in self-reported depression symptoms and functioning in naturalistic settings (Shelton *et al.*, 2013) – that is, real-world settings like those nutrition practitioners operate in. As discussed previously, the client didn't present with raised homocysteine but reported some of the symptoms typically seen in cases of B-vitamin deficit or under-utilization, including fatigue, 'brain fog' and low mood. L-methylfolate or 5-MTHF also prevents the potential negative effects of unconverted or unmetabolized folic acid in the peripheral circulation (Scaglione and Panzavolta, 2014), which provides another reason for practitioners to consider this form of folate when looking at suitable options for a specific case.

GA has a COMT gene variant that makes her prone to experiencing the negative effects of dopamine recirculation. Why would methylfolate be an appropriate option for this client when this form of folate supports the synthesis of dopamine? The answer, as mentioned earlier, is not to 'treat the SNP' or 'second guess' a reaction based on genetic data or even on genetic data coupled with blood/urine biochemistry. The advice is to try, with the client's consent, assessing progress by means of the collection of patient-reported outcome measures like MYMOP scores. As evidence of the reactions to different types of B-vitamin supplements is scarce and too heterogenous to provide solid support to make a clinical decision (Anderson *et al.*, 2016), it is necessary to keep talking to the client to keep them engaged in the process and to find out how they feel appropriate adjustments can be made. Based on client reporting, changes may include increasing/decreasing the dose of the same form of the same nutrient or changing to another form altogether.

In this practitioner's clinical experience, it isn't unusual for individuals with a genetic predisposition to having high homocysteine to present with levels that are within an optimal range. This confirms the need for practitioners to pay attention to the clinical presentation and not issue recommendations based purely on laboratory tests. The methylated B-vitamin supplementation for GA included 200 mcg calcium L-methylfolate, 1000 mcg methylcobalamine and 20 mg pyridoxal-5-phosphate.

Progress and development

Sleep
After 500 mg Gotu kola and 500 mg *Bacopa monnieri* daily for a month, GA described her sleep as 'the best she's had in years' and rated it as a 2 in the follow-up MYMOP (see Table 7.5). This is an improvement of four points, having been rated 'as bad as it could be' at 6 only four weeks earlier.

Dietary diversity
Introducing diversity can be daunting for someone whose repertoire of foods is limited because of fear of triggering symptoms. Using a tool like the '50 food chart' as shown in Figure 7.2 (Toribio-Mateas, 2018) can be a very useful way for practitioners to assess where the starting point of a particular client is with regard to diversity. For someone who has no issues getting up to 25 or more foods in a week, pushing it a bit harder and introducing different foods altogether is likely to be easy.

For someone who is more limited in their food diversity, using 'baby steps' and introducing the same food in different colours – for example, red, yellow and green peppers, red and white cabbage – is an easy way to increase nutrient density, improving the likelihood of compliance and without overwhelming the client. Being more mindful of the variety of colours in her basket was the advice given to GA, a recommendation that she was able to implement fairly easily over the course of a few weeks, finally reaching close to 50 different foods.

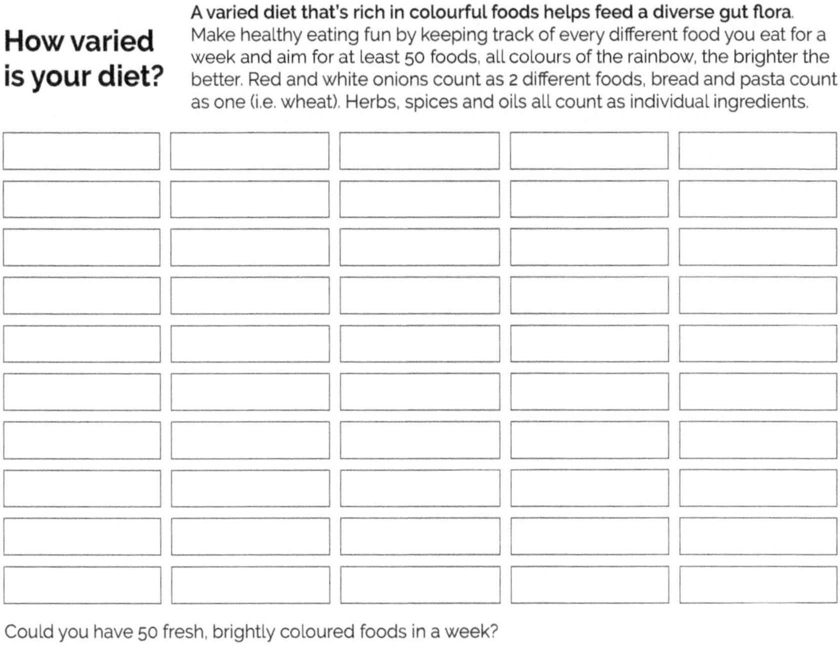

How varied is your diet?

A varied diet that's rich in colourful foods helps feed a diverse gut flora. Make healthy eating fun by keeping track of every different food you eat for a week and aim for at least 50 foods, all colours of the rainbow, the brighter the better. Red and white onions count as 2 different foods, bread and pasta count as one (i.e. wheat). Herbs, spices and oils all count as individual ingredients.

Could you have 50 fresh, brightly coloured foods in a week?

Figure 7.2 The practitioner's '50-food challenge' chart

This an example of a simple but powerful data collection tool used in clinical practice to engage with clients in a light-hearted way so that they report back to their practitioner on their dietary diversity.

Source: Reproduced with permission from Toribio-Mateas (2018)

Red rice yeast

Within three months of supplementation with 400 mg/day, providing 1.6 mg monacolin K and 20 mg/day CoQ_{10}, GA's LDL cholesterol levels had decreased from 3.6 to 3 mmol/L.

Fermented foods

The client really liked the idea of making both water kefir and kombucha at home as part of her 'taking back control of her health'. GA followed the instructions and staged the introduction of both by limiting the amount to 50 ml a day until reaching the recommended two glasses (600 ml) of water kefir and one glass (300 ml) of kombucha every day. She mixed the water kefir and the kombucha and diluted them with filtered water which she drank throughout the day. When asked to described how her gut felt, she said she had had the best bowel motions since she remembered. No MYMOP score was taken for this, but GA agreed that her gut health had contributed to her general feeling of wellbeing, which had improved from an initial 6 to a follow-up score of 3 (see Table 7.5).

Methylated B vitamins

The client believes these have contributed to her improved energy and her ability to think more clearly. This is reflected in her MYMOP score for energy, which has gone from 6 (as bad as it could be) to 3 (see Table 7.5). The practitioner did not document a MYMOP score for foggy thinking, but GA confirmed that her cognitive function has improved, even if her stressful situation at home was still ongoing. However, a MYMOP score of 3 was recorded for anxiety (see Table 7.5). That is a reduction of three points from the initial rating of 6 four weeks prior to the follow-up. There is some evidence that methylated B vitamins provide relief for depressive and anxiety symptoms and improvement of quality of life in adults with depression (Anderson *et al.*, 2016; Fava and Mischoulon, 2009; Lewis *et al.*, 2013; Papakostas, Cassiello and Iovieno, 2012).

The improved sleep duration and quality has quite possibly had a knock-on effect on energy. However, the client feels (in her own words) that 'the B vitamins are doing something' and, on that basis, the practitioner recommended ongoing daily supplementation at the same dose for at least another six months. Table 7.5 summarizes the improvements in the MYMOP questionnaire discussed above.

Table 7.5 Post-intervention MYMOP questionnaire for GA

Concern	Rating	Makes difficult or prevents
Anxiety	0 1 2 ③ 4 5 6	Makes day-to-day life difficult
Fatigue	0 1 2 ③ 4 5 6	Shopping, house chores
Sleep	0 1 2 ③ 4 5 6	Makes day-to-day life difficult
General feeling of wellbeing	0 1 2 ③ 4 5 6	

These follow-up scores were taken eight weeks into the dietary and supplement recommendations.

Follow-up testing was not undertaken for the gastrointestinal function markers or salivary cortisol due to cost issues. In the practitioner's experience this highlights the necessity for focusing on clinical presentation and the usefulness of a validated PROM such as MYMOP. Comparison of before and after symptom ratings and the application of critical thinking helps to establish what body systems are implicated in the changes in scoring.

Although it is always reassuring to add data to a patient's clinical file, it may sometimes be not absolutely necessary, particularly when self-reported wellbeing has increased.

Discussion and reflection

This case provides a great example of a clinical scenario where several systems are affected and how this can be both exciting and daunting for a systems-oriented practitioner. The practitioner even chose not to tackle some other less systemic/more localized symptoms reported by the client in order to keep this complexity within manageable parameters. One such symptom was ongoing idiopathic itching, particularly in the back, which seems to be responding well to a diamine oxidase (DAO) supplement to manage histamine breakdown in the gut. For situations where a bioactive compound is difficult to source from food and/or requires a drastic change in dietary habits – for example, a low-histamine diet – practitioners should focus on patient preferences. A low-histamine diet was discussed with GA as a first-line intervention but was seen as too cumbersome by the client who expressed a preference for trying a supplement instead. Methylated B vitamins may also have helped with regard to methylation of histamine.

Why would complexity be daunting, you might wonder. Well, in the author's own experience in clinical education, practitioners can sometimes spend excessive time and resources – both theirs and their clients' – trying to answer the many questions posed by the multiple systems involved in the clinical problem they are up against. As an analogy, when trying to answer a black-or-white-type question – for example, 'Is the client pregnant?' – answers are also either black or white.

This is typical of pathology-related questions where the answer is yes or no, positive or negative – just as you cannot be 'a little pregnant'. The same would apply to being infected by the HIV virus. Answers for these two 'yes/no' clinical questions are either positive or negative. But in systems-biology-based clinical practice, many of the questions do not lend themselves to black/white, yes/no answers. Practitioners tend to operate somewhere between certainty and chaos (Innes, Campion and Griffiths, 2005), making sense of complexity based on a number of partial answers and a range of markers, and marrying those up with their clients' clinical presentation. [Editor's note: See Chapter 2 for a deeper discussion on complexity in clinical practice.]

Tests are just like pieces in a jigsaw. They help the practitioner to get 'the bigger picture' and go deep into a specific area of interest, as needed. For example, in GA's case, a dysfunctional gut microbiota is just one of the many factors contributing to her loss of overall homeostasis. The client's clinical presentation has been chronically characterized by severe gastrointestinal symptoms, which gives the practitioner a way into a broken system that she can relate to. Referring to the prior point on time and resource effectiveness, finding a relatable starting point makes it easier for a systems-oriented practitioner to negotiate how to tackle a case. Biological anthropologists Edes and Crews would see GA's disturbed gut ecosystem as the type of physiological and somatic dysregulation that results from ongoing exposure to 'stressors and senescent processes accumulated over the person's lifespan' (Edes and Crews, 2017, p.44). In other words, her chronic gastrointestinal dysregulation hasn't taken place in isolation. It has simply added to what is referred to in literature as allostatic load, a concept defined by McEwen and Stellar as 'the cost of chronic exposure to fluctuating or heightened neural or neuroendocrine responses resulting from repeated or chronic environmental challenge that an individual reacts to as being particularly stressful' (McEwen and Stellar, 1993, p.2093).

In this particular case, the most tangible manifestation of the excessive allostatic load materialized as extreme anxiety, leading to poor sleep quality and lack of energy, which, in turn, led to her inability to think clearly, or 'foggy thinking', and some memory loss typically seen in mild cognitive impairment. Working on those areas as layers superimposed on to a core intervention – that is, the gut – has resulted in a satisfactory overall improvement. But GA's case could have been tackled differently, and successfully, by another practitioner using the same systems-oriented approach but getting into the system from another angle. GA's case illustrates how practitioners should always combine their clinical insight and expertise with good-quality scientific evidence and the results of any tests they may choose to use based on that evidence, in order to provide creative solutions that support complex clinical scenarios, thereby helping their clients achieve better health outcomes.

Q&A

AW: I know you are a fan of the Mediterranean diet. We know it has been defined in some of the studies you mention in your case, but there is also a lot of misunderstanding around this. For example, some claim the EatWell Guide (formerly the EatWell Plate) is a version of the Mediterranean diet. Can you explain how you define it for your clients, how you coach and mentor someone to introduce it (over and above the 50 foods, which is one key element)?

MTM: I know there are various different definitions of the Mediterranean diet. I like to think of it as a 'pattern' rather than a 'diet'. As such, it features high sources of dietary fibre with high unsaturated fatty acids relative to saturated fatty acids and is low glycaemic load – that is, it includes foods with lower glycaemic indices that tend to promote favourable insulin responses and postprandial blood glucose profiles, enhancing appropriate appetite regulation. It is also rich in a diversity of dietary polyphenols. The diversity in structure and function of polyphenols could influence a variety of metabolic pathways, such as inhibition of lipogenesis, stimulation of catabolic pathways, reduction of chronic inflammation and upregulation of uncoupling proteins (a measure of healthy mitochondrial function) (Guo *et al.*, 2016).

AW: Reflecting on the case, is there anything you would do differently?

MTM: Quite probably. I am a fairly creative practitioner so I am always open to possibilities. However, in my clinical experience, the gut is an 'easy' point of entry into most people's systems. If I was to use just one single intervention out of all the things I did for GA, I would have started with the increase in dietary diversity first and foremost.

AW: Was there any other advice you gave to GA regarding sleep, such as light or temperature, or was it purely the supplements and diet change that improved her sleep so rapidly?

MTM: Yes, I certainly gave her wider recommendations to improve sleep. For me it's about comfortable sleep conditions, including the mattress, the duvet or blankets, but most of all about the light. Particularly where the hypothalamus–pituitary–adrenal (HPA) axis is involved, avoiding exposure to light during the night – for example, a window with no curtains close to a streetlight or lights on during the night. A room that is totally blacked out during sleeping hours is ideal and can make a great contribution to improved sleep quality.

AW: I know you are keen to introduce greater evidence-based practice into personalized nutrition, recognizing that evidence comes from many different sources. I love how you use a combination of sources in this case. What is your advice to a less experienced practitioner on how to develop that clinical insight?

MTM: Start always by looking at the highest sources of evidence – that is, randomized controlled trials (RCTs) and pooled data from systematic reviews or meta-analysis. Failing the availability of those, then look into cohort studies or even single case studies like those in this book. Be mindful of your intervention's likelihood to cause harm. If you are recommending increasing how much broccoli someone eats, you're unlikely to harm them, although this may make a few people more uncomfortable in situations where gut dysbiosis and sulphate-reducing bacteria may lead to an increase in bloating. So even if there was no RCT documenting exactly how to use broccoli in clinical practice, you could be pretty sure you'd be safe. The nastiest thing your client can experience is flatulence, which will clear after they reduce the amount of broccoli they eat. But when you're recommending individual nutrients, sometimes at high dose, that could potentially lead to issues that you hadn't anticipated. For example, you could argue that *Bacopa* and Gotu kola are natural, and hence safe. However, I would not feel comfortable recommending their use at dosages that are ten times what has been seen to be safe and effective in a clinical trial. If there was no clinical data for either of these botanicals, I would always err on the side of caution and use them as close to a food-type use as possible – for example, as a tea instead of as a high-dosage supplement. The same applies to probiotics. I feel much more comfortable working with food-based ferments than with supplements, although if a certain microbial strain has proven clinical efficacy for a specific condition, I would be only too happy to recommend it too. In general, I would just call for common sense in how we approach nutrition, and for steady use of resources that provide access to good-quality clinical data, such as PubMed or Nutrition Evidence.

BOX 7.1 CLINICAL DATA RESOURCES FOR PERSONALIZED NUTRITION PRACTICE

Nutrition Evidence is a database created to support evidence-based practice in nutrition and lifestyle medicine. It is produced by BANT and it is open access. It can be found at www.nutrition-evidence.com.

Pubmed is available to all – www.ncbi.nlm.nih.gov/pubmed.

References

Aguiló, S., García, E., Arza, A., Garzón-Rey, J.M., Aguiló, J., 2018. Evaluation of chronic stress indicators in geriatric and oncologic caregivers: A cross-sectional study. *Stress* 21, 36–42. https://doi.org/10.1080/10253890.2017.1391211

Anderson, S., Panka, J., Rakobitsch, R., Tyre, K., Pulliam, K., 2016. Anxiety and methylenetetrahydrofolate reductase mutation treated with s-adenosyl methionine and methylated B vitamins. *Integrative Medicine* 15, 48–52.

Argollo, M., Fiorino, G., Hindryckx, P., Peyrin-Biroulet, L., Danese, S., 2017. Novel therapeutic targets for inflammatory bowel disease. *Journal of Autoimmunity* 85, 103–116. https://doi.org/10.1016/j.jaut.2017.07.004

Awoyemi, A., Trøseid, M., Arnesen, H., Solheim, S., Seljeflot, I., 2018. Markers of metabolic endotoxemia as related to metabolic syndrome in an elderly male population at high cardiovascular risk: A cross-sectional study. *Diabetology and Metabolic Syndrome* 10, 59. https://doi.org/10.1186/s13098-018-0360-3

Bajer, L., Kverka, M., Kostovcik, M., Macinga, P. *et al.*, 2017. Distinct gut microbiota profiles in patients with primary sclerosing cholangitis and ulcerative colitis. *World Journal of Gastroenterology* 23, 4548–4558. https://doi.org/10.3748/wjg.v23.i25.4548

Basso, P.J., Câmara, N.O.S., Sales-Campos, H., 2018. Microbial-based therapies in the treatment of inflammatory bowel disease – an overview of human studies. *Frontiers in Pharmacology* 9, 1571. https://doi.org/10.3389/fphar.2018.01571

Battson, M.L., Lee, D.M., Jarrell, D.K., Hou, S. *et al.*, 2018a. Suppression of gut dysbiosis reverses Western diet-induced vascular dysfunction. *American Journal of Physiology – Endocrinology and Metabolism* 314, E468–E477. https://doi.org/10.1152/ajpendo.00187.2017

Battson, M.L., Lee, D.M., Weir, T.L., Gentile, C.L., 2018b. The gut microbiota as a novel regulator of cardiovascular function and disease. *Journal of Nutritional Biochemistry* 56, 1–15. https://doi.org/10.1016/j.jnutbio.2017.12.010

Bhattacharya, D., Bhattacharya, S., Patra, M.M., Chakravorty, S. *et al.*, 2016. Antibacterial activity of polyphenolic fraction of kombucha against enteric bacterial pathogens. *Current Microbiology* 73, 885–896. https://doi.org/10.1007/s00284-016-1136-3

Bourrie, B.C.T., Willing, B.P., Cotter, P.D., 2016. The microbiota and health promoting characteristics of the fermented beverage kefir. *Frontiers in Microbiology* 7, 647. https://doi.org/10.3389/fmicb.2016.00647

Bu, J., Wang, Z., 2018. Cross-talk between gut microbiota and heart via the routes of metabolite and immunity. *Gastroenterology Research and Practice* 2018, 6458094. https://doi.org/10.1155/2018/6458094

Buford, T.W., 2017. (Dis)Trust your gut: The gut microbiome in age-related inflammation, health, and disease. *Microbiome* 5, 80. https://doi.org/10.1186/s40168-017-0296-0

Calabrese, C., Gregory, W.L., Leo, M., Kraemer, D., Bone, K., Oken, B., 2008. Effects of a standardized *Bacopa monnieri* extract on cognitive performance, anxiety, and depression in the elderly: A randomized, double-blind, placebo-controlled trial. *Journal of Alternative and Complementary Medicine* 14, 707–713. https://doi.org/10.1089/acm.2008.0018

Caputi, V., Marsilio, I., Filpa, V., Cerantola, S. *et al.*, 2017. Antibiotic-induced dysbiosis of the microbiota impairs gut neuromuscular function in juvenile mice. *British Journal of Pharmacology* 174, 3623–3639. https://doi.org/10.1111/bph.13965

Caselli, R.J., Dueck, A.C., Locke, D.E.C., Hoffman-Snyder, C.R. *et al.*, 2011. Longitudinal modeling of frontal cognition in APOE ε4 homozygotes, heterozygotes, and noncarriers. *Neurology* 76, 1383–1388. https://doi.org/10.1212/WNL.0b013e3182167147

Caselli, R.J., Dueck, A.C., Osborne, D., Sabbagh, M.N. *et al.*, 2009. Longitudinal modeling of age-related memory decline and the APOE epsilon4 effect. *New England Journal of Medicine* 361, 255–263. https://doi.org/10.1056/NEJMoa0809437

Cattaneo, A., Cattane, N., Galluzzi, S., Provasi, S. *et al.*, 2017. Association of brain amyloidosis with pro-inflammatory gut bacterial taxa and peripheral inflammation markers in cognitively impaired elderly. *Neurobiology of Aging* 49, 60–68. https://doi.org/10.1016/j.neurobiolaging.2016.08.019

D'Haens, G., Ferrante, M., Vermeire, S., Baert, F. *et al.*, 2012. Fecal calprotectin is a surrogate marker for endoscopic lesions in inflammatory bowel disease. *Inflammatory Bowel Diseases* 18, 2218–2224. https://doi.org/10.1002/ibd.22917

Dinan, T.G., Cryan, J.F., 2017. Gut instincts: Microbiota as a key regulator of brain development, ageing and neurodegeneration. *Journal of Physiology* 595, 489–503. https://doi.org/10.1113/JP273106

Dinan, T.G., Cryan, J.F., 2015. The impact of gut microbiota on brain and behaviour: Implications for psychiatry. *Current Opinion in Clinical Nutrition and Metabolic Care* 18, 552–558. https://doi.org/10.1097/MCO.0000000000000221

Domínguez-Muñoz, J.E., D Hardt, P., Lerch, M.M., Löhr, M.J., 2017. Potential for screening for pancreatic exocrine insufficiency using the fecal elastase-1 test. *Digestive Diseases and Sciences* 62, 1119–1130. https://doi.org/10.1007/s10620-017-4524-z

Drossman, D.A., 2016. Functional gastrointestinal disorders: History, pathophysiology, clinical features and Rome IV. *Gastroenterology*. https://doi.org/10.1053/j.gastro.2016.02.032

Drossman, D.A., Hasler, W.L., 2016. Rome IV-Functional GI Disorders: Disorders of gut–brain interaction. *Gastroenterology* 150, 1257–1261. https://doi.org/10.1053/j.gastro.2016.03.035

Edes, A.N., Crews, D.E., 2017. Allostatic load and biological anthropology. *American Journal of Physical Anthropology* 162 Suppl 63, 44–70. https://doi.org/10.1002/ajpa.23146

El Aidy, S., Van den Abbeele, P., Van de Wiele, T., Louis, P., Kleerebezem, M., 2013. Intestinal colonization: How key microbial players become established in this dynamic process: Microbial metabolic activities and the interplay between the host and microbes. *BioEssays* 35, 913–923. https://doi.org/10.1002/bies.201300073

Farrer, L.A., Cupples, L.A., Haines, J.L., Hyman, B. et al,, 1997. Effects of age, sex, and ethnicity on the association between apolipoprotein E genotype and Alzheimer disease. A meta-analysis. APOE and Alzheimer Disease Meta Analysis Consortium. *JAMA* 278, 1349–1356.

Fava, M., Mischoulon, D., 2009. Folate in depression: Efficacy, safety, differences in formulations, and clinical issues. *Journal of Clinical Psychiatry* 70, Suppl 5, 12–17. https://doi.org/10.4088/JCP.8157su1c.03

Giese, M., Unternaehrer, E., Brand, S., Calabrese, P., Holsboer-Trachsler, E., Eckert, A., 2013. The interplay of stress and sleep impacts BDNF level. *PloS ONE* 8, e76050. https://doi.org/10.1371/journal.pone.0076050

Gilbody, S., Lewis, S., Lightfoot, T., 2007. Methylenetetrahydrofolate reductase (MTHFR) genetic polymorphisms and psychiatric disorders: A HuGE review. *American Journal of Epidemiology* 165, 1–13. https://doi.org/10.1093/aje/kwj347

Gobert, A.P., Sagrestani, G., Delmas, E., Wilson, K.T. et al., 2016. The human intestinal microbiota of constipated-predominant irritable bowel syndrome patients exhibits anti-inflammatory properties. *Scientific Reports* 6, 39399. https://doi.org/10.1038/srep39399

González, S., Fernández, M., Cuervo, A., Lasheras, C., 2014. Dietary intake of polyphenols and major food sources in an institutionalised elderly population. *Journal of Human Nutrition and Dietetics* 27, 176–183. https://doi.org/10.1111/jhn.12058

Gottschalk, M.G., Domschke, K., 2017. Genetics of generalized anxiety disorder and related traits. *Dialogues in Clinical Neuroscience* 19, 159–168.

Guo, X., Tresserra-Rimbau, A., Estruch, R., Martínez-González, M.A. et al., 2016. Effects of polyphenol, measured by a biomarker of total polyphenols in urine, on cardiovascular risk factors after a long-term follow-up in the PREDIMED Study. *Oxidative Medicine and Cellular Longevity* 2016, 2572606. https://doi.org/10.1155/2016/2572606

Gutiérrez-Díaz, I., Fernández-Navarro, T., Sánchez, B., Margolles, A., González, S., 2016. Mediterranean diet and faecal microbiota: A transversal study. *Food and Function* 7, 2347–2356. https://doi.org/10.1039/c6fo00105j

Hall, M.H., Brindle, R.C., Buysse, D.J., 2018. Sleep and cardiovascular disease: Emerging opportunities for psychology. *American Psychologist* 73, 994–1006. https://doi.org/10.1037/amp0000362

Hold, G.L., Smith, M., Grange, C., Watt, E.R., El-Omar, E.M., Mukhopadhya, I., 2014. Role of the gut microbiota in inflammatory bowel disease pathogenesis: What have we learnt in the past 10 years? *World Journal of Gastroenterology* 20, 1192–1210. https://doi.org/10.3748/wjg.v20.i5.1192

Horvath, I., Jia, X., Johansson, P., Wang, C. *et al.*, 2016. Pro-inflammatory S100A9 Protein as a robust biomarker differentiating early stages of cognitive impairment in Alzheimer's disease. *ACS Chemical Neuroscience* 7, 34–39. https://doi.org/10.1021/acschemneuro.5b00265

Innes, A.D., Campion, P.D., Griffiths, F.E., 2005. Complex consultations and the 'edge of chaos.' *British Journal of General Practice* 55, 47–52.

Jana, U., Sur, T.K., Maity, L.N., Debnath, P.K., Bhattacharyya, D., 2010. A clinical study on the management of generalized anxiety disorder with Centella asiatica. *Nepal Medical College Journal* 12, 8–11.

Kelly, J.R., Kennedy, P.J., Cryan, J.F., Dinan, T.G., Clarke, G., Hyland, N.P., 2015. Breaking down the barriers: The gut microbiome, intestinal permeability and stress-related psychiatric disorders. *Frontiers in Cellular Neuroscience* 9, 392. https://doi.org/10.3389/fncel.2015.00392

Kim, J., Basak, J.M., Holtzman, D.M., 2009. The role of apolipoprotein E in Alzheimer's disease. *Neuron* 63, 287–303. https://doi.org/10.1016/j.neuron.2009.06.026

Knox, N.C., Forbes, J.D., Van Domselaar, G., Bernstein, C.N., 2019. The gut microbiome as a target for IBD treatment: Are we there yet? *Current Treatment Options in Gastroenterology*. https://doi.org/10.1007/s11938-019-00221-w

Lääveri, T., Antikainen, J., Pakkanen, S.H., Kirveskari, J., Kantele, A., 2016. Prospective study of pathogens in asymptomatic travellers and those with diarrhoea: Aetiological agents revisited. *Clinical Microbiology and Infection* 22, 535–541. https://doi.org/10.1016/j.cmi.2016.02.011

Lau, K., Srivatsav, V., Rizwan, A., Nashed, A. *et al.*, 2017. Bridging the gap between gut microbial dysbiosis and cardiovascular diseases. *Nutrients* 9. https://doi.org/10.3390/nu9080859

Laureys, D., De Vuyst, L., 2014. Microbial species diversity, community dynamics, and metabolite kinetics of water kefir fermentation. *Applied and Environmental Microbiology* 80, 2564–2572. https://doi.org/10.1128/AEM.03978-13

Leahy, L.G., 2017. Vitamin B supplementation: What's the right choice for your patients? *Journal of Psychosocial Nursing and Mental Health Services* 55, 7–11. https://doi.org/10.3928/02793695-20170619-02

Leal, G., Bramham, C.R., Duarte, C.B., 2017. BDNF and hippocampal synaptic plasticity. *Vitamins and Hormones* 104, 153–195. https://doi.org/10.1016/bs.vh.2016.10.004

Leblhuber, F., Geisler, S., Steiner, K., Fuchs, D., Schütz, B., 2015. Elevated fecal calprotectin in patients with Alzheimer's dementia indicates leaky gut. *Journal of Neural Transmission* 122, 1319–1322. https://doi.org/10.1007/s00702-015-1381-9

Lewis, J.E., Tiozzo, E., Melillo, A.B., Leonard, S. *et al.*, 2013. The effect of methylated vitamin B complex on depressive and anxiety symptoms and quality of life in adults with depression. *ISRN Psychiatry* 2013, 621453. https://doi.org/10.1155/2013/621453

Lim, J., Kale, M., Kim, D.-H., Kim, H.-S. *et al.*, 2017. Antiobesity effect of exopolysaccharides isolated from kefir grains. *Journal of Agricultural and Food Chemistry* 65, 10011–10019. https://doi.org/10.1021/acs.jafc.7b03764

Liu, L., Zhu, G., 2018. Gut–brain axis and mood disorder. *Frontiers in Psychiatry* 9, 223. https://doi.org/10.3389/fpsyt.2018.00223

Lopetuso, L.R., Scaldaferri, F., Petito, V., Gasbarrini, A., 2013. Commensal Clostridia: Leading players in the maintenance of gut homeostasis. *Gut Pathogens* 5, 23. https://doi.org/10.1186/1757-4749-5-23

Lopez-Siles, M., Duncan, S.H., Garcia-Gil, L.J., Martinez-Medina, M., 2017. *Faecalibacterium prausnitzii*: From microbiology to diagnostics and prognostics. *ISME Journal* 11, 841–852. https://doi.org/10.1038/ismej.2016.176

Ma, J., Li, H., 2018. The role of gut microbiota in atherosclerosis and hypertension. *Frontiers in Pharmacology* 9, 1082. https://doi.org/10.3389/fphar.2018.01082

Machiels, K., Joossens, M., Sabino, J., De Preter, V. *et al.*, 2014. A decrease of the butyrate-producing species *Roseburia hominis* and *Faecalibacterium prausnitzii* defines dysbiosis in patients with ulcerative colitis. *Gut* 63, 1275–1283. https://doi.org/10.1136/gutjnl-2013-304833

Maes, M., Kubera, M., Leunis, J.-C., 2008. The gut–brain barrier in major depression: Intestinal mucosal dysfunction with an increased translocation of LPS from gram negative enterobacteria (leaky gut) plays a role in the inflammatory pathophysiology of depression. *Neuro Endocrinology Letters* 29, 117–124.

Maffei, V.J., Kim, S., Blanchard, E., Luo, M. *et al.*, 2017. Biological aging and the human gut microbiota. *Journals of Gerontology Series A* 72, 1474–1482. https://doi.org/10.1093/gerona/glx042

Marchesi, J.R., Ravel, J., 2015. The vocabulary of microbiome research: A proposal. *Microbiome* 3, 31. https://doi.org/10.1186/s40168-015-0094-5

Martín-Peláez, S., Mosele, J.I., Pizarro, N., Farràs, M. *et al.*, 2017. Effect of virgin olive oil and thyme phenolic compounds on blood lipid profile: Implications of human gut microbiota. *European Journal of Nutrition* 56, 119–131. https://doi.org/10.1007/s00394-015-1063-2

Mazza, A., Lenti, S., Schiavon, L., Di Giacomo, E. *et al.*, 2018. Effect of Monacolin K and COQ_{10} supplementation in hypertensive and hypercholesterolemic subjects with metabolic syndrome. *Biomedicine and Pharmacotherapy* 105, 992–996. https://doi.org/10.1016/j.biopha.2018.06.076

McDonald, D., Hyde, E., Debelius, J.W., Morton, J.T. *et al.*, 2018. American Gut: An open platform for citizen science microbiome research. *mSystems* 3. https://doi.org/10.1128/mSystems.00031-18

McEwen, B.S., Stellar, E., 1993. Stress and the individual: Mechanisms leading to disease. *Archives of Internal Medicine* 153, 2093–2101.

Mumolo, M.G., Bertani, L., Ceccarelli, L., Laino, G. *et al.*, 2018. From bench to bedside: Fecal calprotectin in inflammatory bowel diseases clinical setting. *World Journal of Gastroenterology* 24, 3681–3694. https://doi.org/10.3748/wjg.v24.i33.3681

Myers, R.H., Schaefer, E.J., Wilson, P.W., D'Agostino, R. *et al.*, 1996. Apolipoprotein E epsilon4 association with dementia in a population-based study: The Framingham study. *Neurology* 46, 673–677.

Nagpal, R., Yadav, H., Marotta, F., 2014. Gut microbiota: The next-gen frontier in preventive and therapeutic medicine? *Frontiers in Medicine* 1, 15. https://doi.org/10.3389/fmed.2014.00015

Nguyen, T., Karl, M., Santini, A., 2017. Red yeast rice. *Foods* 6. https://doi.org/10.3390/foods6030019

Nissilä, E., Korpela, K., Lokki, A.I., Paakkanen, R. *et al.*, 2017. C4B gene influences intestinal microbiota through complement activation in patients with paediatric-onset inflammatory bowel disease. *Clinical and Experimental Immunology* 190, 394–405. https://doi.org/10.1111/cei.13040

Oberg, E., Givant, C., Fisk, B., Parikh, C., Bradley, R., 2015. Epigenetics in clinical practice: Characterizing patient and provider experiences with MTHFR polymorphisms and methylfolate. *Journal of Nutrigenetics and Nutrigenomics* 8, 137–150. https://doi.org/10.1159/000440700

Obrenovich, M.E.M., 2018. Leaky gut, leaky brain? *Microorganisms* 6. https://doi.org/10.3390/microorganisms6040107

Papakostas, G.I., Cassiello, C.F., Iovieno, N., 2012. Folates and S-adenosylmethionine for major depressive disorder. *Canadian Journal of Psychiatry* 57, 406–413. https://doi.org/10.1177/070674371205700703

Paterson, C., 2004. Seeking the patient's perspective: A qualitative assessment of EuroQol, COOP-WONCA charts and MYMOP. *Quality of Life Research* 13, 871–881. https://doi.org/10.1023/B:QURE.0000025586.51955.78

Paterson, C., 1996. Measuring outcomes in primary care: A patient generated measure, MYMOP, compared with the SF-36 health survey. *BMJ* 312, 1016–1020.

Paterson, C., Britten, N., 2000. In pursuit of patient-centred outcomes: A qualitative evaluation of the 'Measure Yourself Medical Outcome Profile'. *Journal of Health Services Research and Policy* 5, 27–36. https://doi.org/10.1177/135581960000500108

Patterson, E., Cryan, J.F., Fitzgerald, G.F., Ross, R.P., Dinan, T.G., Stanton, C., 2014. Gut microbiota, the pharmabiotics they produce and host health. *Proceedings of the Nutrition Society* 73, 477–489. https://doi.org/10.1017/S0029665114001426

Pellissier, S., Bonaz, B., 2017. The place of stress and emotions in the irritable bowel syndrome. *Vitamins and Hormones* 103, 327–354. https://doi.org/10.1016/bs.vh.2016.09.005

Peterson, C.G.B., Lampinen, M., Hansson, T., Lidén, M., Hällgren, R., Carlson, M., 2016. Evaluation of biomarkers for ulcerative colitis comparing two sampling methods: Fecal markers reflect colorectal inflammation both macroscopically and on a cellular level. *Scandinavian Journal of Clinical and Laboratory Investigation* 76, 393–401. https://doi.org/10.1080/00365513.2016.1185145

Pimenta, F.S., Luaces-Regueira, M., Ton, A.M., Campagnaro, B.P. *et al.*, 2018. Mechanisms of action of kefir in chronic cardiovascular and metabolic diseases. *Cell Physiology and Biochemistry* 48, 1901–1914. https://doi.org/10.1159/000492511

Porter, C.K., Olson, S., Hall, A., Riddle, M.S., 2017. Travelers' diarrhea: An update on the incidence, etiology, and risk in military deployments and similar travel populations. *Military Medicine* 182, 4–10. https://doi.org/10.7205/MILMED-D-17-00064

Pruenster, M., Vogl, T., Roth, J., Sperandio, M., 2016. S100A8/A9: From basic science to clinical application. *Pharmacology and Therapeutics* 167, 120–131. https://doi.org/10.1016/j.pharmthera.2016.07.015

Qiao, Y.Q., Cai, C.W., Ran, Z.H., 2016. Therapeutic modulation of gut microbiota in inflammatory bowel disease: More questions to be answered. *Journal of Digestive Diseases* 17, 800–810. https://doi.org/10.1111/1751-2980.12422

Richards, E.M., Pepine, C.J., Raizada, M.K., Kim, S., 2017. The gut, its microbiome, and hypertension. *Current Hypertension Reports* 19, 36. https://doi.org/10.1007/s11906-017-0734-1

Rosa, D.D., Dias, M.M.S., Grześkowiak, Ł.M., Reis, S.A., Conceição, L.L., Peluzio, M. do C.G., 2017. Milk kefir: Nutritional, microbiological and health benefits. *Nutrition Research Reviews* 30, 82–96. https://doi.org/10.1017/S0954422416000275

Sangiovanni, E., Brivio, P., Dell'Agli, M., Calabrese, F., 2017. Botanicals as modulators of neuroplasticity: Focus on BDNF. *Neural Plasticity* 2017, 5965371. https://doi.org/10.1155/2017/5965371

Sartor, R.B., Wu, G.D., 2017. Roles for intestinal bacteria, viruses, and fungi in pathogenesis of inflammatory bowel diseases and therapeutic approaches. *Gastroenterology* 152, 327-339.e4. https://doi.org/10.1053/j.gastro.2016.10.012

Sathyanarayanan, V., Thomas, T., Einöther, S.J.L., Dobriyal, R., Joshi, M.K., Krishnamachari, S., 2013. Brahmi for the better? New findings challenging cognition and anti-anxiety effects of Brahmi (*Bacopa monniera*) in healthy adults. *Psychopharmacology* 227, 299–306. https://doi.org/10.1007/s00213-013-2978-z

Scaglione, F., Panzavolta, G., 2014. Folate, folic acid and 5-methyltetrahydrofolate are not the same thing. *Xenobiotica* 44, 480–488. https://doi.org/10.3109/00498254.2013.845705

Schmitt, K., Holsboer-Trachsler, E., Eckert, A., 2016. BDNF in sleep, insomnia, and sleep deprivation. *Annals of Medicine* 48, 42–51. https://doi.org/10.3109/07853890.2015.1131327

Sharma, S., Litonjua, A., 2014. Asthma, allergy, and responses to methyl donor supplements and nutrients. *Journal of Allergy and Clinical Immunology* 133, 1246–1254. https://doi.org/10.1016/j.jaci.2013.10.039

Shelton, R.C., Sloan Manning, J., Barrentine, L.W., Tipa, E.V., 2013. Assessing effects of l-methylfolate in depression management: Results of a real-world patient experience trial. *Primary Care Companion for CNS Disorders* 15. https://doi.org/10.4088/PCC.13m01520

Soeiro-De-Souza, M.G., Stanford, M.S., Bio, D.S., Machado-Vieira, R., Moreno, R.A., 2013. Association of the COMT Met[158] allele with trait impulsivity in healthy young adults. *Molecular Medicine Reports* 7, 1067–1072. https://doi.org/10.3892/mmr.2013.1336

Sokol, H., Pigneur, B., Watterlot, L., Lakhdari, O. et al., 2008. *Faecalibacterium prausnitzii* is an anti-inflammatory commensal bacterium identified by gut microbiota analysis of Crohn disease patients. *Proceedings of the National Academy of Sciences of the USA* 105, 16731–16736. https://doi.org/10.1073/pnas.0804812105

Sokol, H., Seksik, P., Furet, J.P., Firmesse, O., Nion-Larmurier, I. et al., 2009. Low counts of *Faecalibacterium prausnitzii* in colitis microbiota. *Inflammatory Bowel Diseases* 15, 1183–1189. https://doi.org/10.1002/ibd.20903

Stefano, G.B., Samuel, J., Kream, R.M., 2017. Antibiotics may trigger mitochondrial dysfunction inducing psychiatric disorders. *Medical Science Monitor* 23, 101–106.

Stein, M.B., Fallin, M.D., Schork, N.J., Gelernter, J., 2005. COMT polymorphisms and anxiety-related personality traits. *Neuropsychopharmacology* 30, 2092–2102. https://doi.org/10.1038/sj.npp.1300787

Stough, C., Lloyd, J., Clarke, J., Downey, L.A. et al., 2001. The chronic effects of an extract of *Bacopa monniera* (Brahmi) on cognitive function in healthy human subjects. *Psychopharmacology* 156, 481–484.

Suskind, D.L., Wahbeh, G., Cohen, S.A., Damman, C.J. et al., 2016. Patients perceive clinical benefit with the specific carbohydrate diet for inflammatory bowel disease. *Digestive Diseases and Sciences* 61, 3255–3260. https://doi.org/10.1007/s10620-016-4307-y

Tack, J., Drossman, D.A., 2017. What's new in Rome IV? *Neurogastroenterology and Motility* 29. https://doi.org/10.1111/nmo.13053

Tanaka, T., Scheet, P., Giusti, B., Bandinelli, S. et al., 2009. Genome-wide association study of vitamin B6, vitamin B12, folate, and homocysteine blood concentrations. *American Journal of Human Genetics* 84, 477–482. https://doi.org/10.1016/j.ajhg.2009.02.011

Tap, J., Furet, J.-P., Bensaada, M., Philippe, C. et al., 2015. Gut microbiota richness promotes its stability upon increased dietary fibre intake in healthy adults. *Environmental Microbiology* 17, 4954–4964. https://doi.org/10.1111/1462-2920.13006

Toribio-Mateas, M., 2018. Harnessing the power of microbiome assessment tools as part of neuroprotective nutrition and lifestyle medicine interventions. *Microorganisms* 6. https://doi.org/10.3390/microorganisms6020035

Toribio-Mateas, M.A., Spector, T.D., 2017. Could food act as personalized medicine for chronic disease? *Personalized Medicine* 14, 193–196. https://doi.org/10.2217/pme-2016-0017

Ungar, L., Altmann, A., Greicius, M.D., 2014. Apolipoprotein E, gender, and Alzheimer's disease: An overlooked, but potent and promising interaction. *Brain Imaging and Behavior* 8, 262–273. https://doi.org/10.1007/s11682-013-9272-x

Van den Abbeele, P., Belzer, C., Goossens, M., Kleerebezem, M. et al., 2013. Butyrate-producing *Clostridium* cluster XIVa species specifically colonize mucins in an *in vitro* gut model. *ISME Journal* 7, 949–961. https://doi.org/10.1038/ismej.2012.158

Wang, C., Iashchishyn, I.A., Pansieri, J., Nyström, S. et al., 2018. S100A9-driven amyloid-neuroinflammatory cascade in traumatic brain injury as a precursor state for Alzheimer's disease. *Scientific Reports* 8, 12836. https://doi.org/10.1038/s41598-018-31141-x

Wattanathorn, J., Mator, L., Muchimapura, S., Tongun, T. et al., 2008. Positive modulation of cognition and mood in the healthy elderly volunteer following the administration of *Centella asiatica*. *Journal of Ethnopharmacology* 116, 325–332. https://doi.org/10.1016/j.jep.2007.11.038

Waugh, N., Cummins, E., Royle, P., Kandala, N.-B. et al., 2013. Faecal calprotectin testing for differentiating amongst inflammatory and non-inflammatory bowel diseases: Systematic review and economic evaluation. *Health Technology Assessment* 17, xv–xix, 1–211. https://doi.org/10.3310/hta17550

Wichers, M., Aguilera, M., Kenis, G., Krabbendam, L. et al., 2008. The catechol-O-methyl transferase Val158Met polymorphism and experience of reward in the flow of daily life. *Neuropsychopharmacology* 33, 3030–3036. https://doi.org/10.1038/sj.npp.1301520

Wingenfeld, K., Otte, C., 2018. Mineralocorticoid receptor function and cognition in health and disease. *Psychoneuroendocrinology*. https://doi.org/10.1016/j. psyneuen.2018.09.010

Yin, J., Liao, S.-X., He, Y., Wang, S. *et al.*, 2015. Dysbiosis of gut microbiota with reduced trimethylamine-N-oxide level in patients with large-artery atherosclerotic stroke or transient ischemic attack. *Journal of the American Heart Association* 4. https://doi. org/10.1161/JAHA.115.002699

Zhang, S., Zhang, M., Zhang, J., 2014. Association of COMT and COMT-DRD2 interaction with creative potential. *Frontiers in Human Neuroscience* 8, 216. https://doi.org/10.3389/ fnhum.2014.00216

Zhou, Y., Xu, Z.Z., He, Y., Yang, Y. *et al.*, 2018. Gut microbiota offers universal biomarkers across ethnicity in inflammatory bowel disease diagnosis and infliximab response prediction. *mSystems* 3. https://doi. org/10.1128/mSystems.00188-17

Zintzaras, E., 2006. C677T and A1298C methylenetetrahydrofolate reductase gene polymorphisms in schizophrenia, bipolar disorder and depression: A meta-analysis of genetic association studies. *Psychiatric Genetics* 16, 105–115. https://doi. org/10.1097/01.ypg.0000199444.77291.e2

8

A Personalized Nutrition Approach to Suspected Metabolic Syndrome

Practitioner: Jo Gamble

Additional contribution to case write-up: Angela Walker

Introduction

This case features a female in her 50s hoping to lose weight, reduce blood pressure and improve menopause symptoms. We will see how investigations revealed elevated blood lipids, abdominal adiposity, systemic inflammation and elevated thyroid antibodies. The client had a cluster of symptoms typically seen in metabolic syndrome and where the underlying pathophysiology is thought to be related to insulin resistance (Kahn *et al.*, 2005). Taking a personalized nutrition approach led to simple but profound lifestyle changes, which were achievable for her and which she embraced and enjoyed. Over a relatively short time, she saw fundamental improvements which reversed her symptoms and improved her quality of life, even during periods of extreme stress. What is more, with the support of her endocrinologist, she was able to avoid prescription medication.

Initial case presentation

SD is a 56-year-old female. Her husband had recently been diagnosed with lymphoma, which prompted SD to see a personalized nutrition practitioner for her own health. She has one daughter in her 30s.

SD is a music teacher working three days a week in a school. As her classes are often during lunch breaks, she regularly missed lunch.

Key presenting symptoms and conditions were:

- high blood pressure
- weight gain, particularly around the middle
- symptoms of menopause (hot flushes and night sweats).

Medical and health history

SD had significantly heavy bleeding from menarche aged 11. Oral contraception was used during her early 20s before falling pregnant. She did not restart oral contraception due to high blood pressure (BP). She had two dilation and curettages followed by a full-term pregnancy.

Age 37, an endometrial ablation was undertaken to reduce menstrual bleeding. Menstruation ceased at age 54. In menopause SD experienced hot flushes and night sweats for which she self-prescribed the herbs black cohosh and sage and sought the support of a homoeopath. Some relief was experienced, but symptoms still persisted.

Age 55, she noticed a groin pain. Investigations led to an ultrasound which found no abnormality in the liver, gallbladder, kidneys, spleen or pancreas. The ultrasound revealed two fibroids (2.5 cm and 4.5 cm).

From her early 20s until mid-40s her weight was 65 kg +/- 1.5 kg. Weight started to increase from her late 40s. She now weighed 74.2 kg and found it difficult to lose weight. She was currently a dress size 18 and her target was to be a dress size 12 (estimated target weight 63–65 kg).

SD reported a regular, daily bowel movement. She experienced some bloating and discomfort in her abdomen, but this was not a concern for her and was only elicited during specific questions.

Apart from the above SD would describe her health as generally good.

Physical examination (conducted during initial consultation)

- BP: 166/75, systolic (high).
- Pulse: 97 bpm (high normal given normal range of 60–100 bpm).
- Height: 165 cm.
- Waist-to-hip ratio: 1:1 indicative of central adiposity.
- Body mass index (BMI): 27.29 overweight.

BMI alone does not indicate the *location* of body fat and is therefore not, on its own, considered the best indicator of overweight (Després, 2012). In this case, the high waist-to-hip ratio does suggest central adiposity and therefore supports the overweight description given by her BMI.

Tests brought to initial consultation

Total cholesterol 7 mmol/L (reference range, below 5.2 mmol/l). Her doctor had advised her to avoid saturated fats and provided a handout which listed fatty foods to be avoided: fatty cuts of meat and meat products, such as sausages and pies, butter, ghee, lard, cream, sour cream, crème fraîche and ice cream. These foods had not featured highly in her historical diet. No formal diagnosis was given.

Family history

- Mother had a heart bypass surgery age 72.
- Father had a stroke age 74.
- Both parents were alive but in declining health.
- Daughter has rheumatoid arthritis.

Medications

SD was prescribed ramipril 5 mg and candesartan 4 mg for hypertension one year prior but discontinued due to side effects after just a few months. No medications were currently taken.

Diet

Since her husband's recent diagnosis, the family had switched from a diet high in refined carbohydrates and processed food and low vegetable intake (2–3 daily portions), to one that was richer in vegetables (five daily portions) and salads, and where all meals were cooked from scratch. It was a mainly organic diet. She had switched from cows' dairy to goats' dairy (personal preference) and from margarine-type spread to organic butter. These changes had occurred in the past three months. Prior to that, her diet was high in ready meals, takeaways, simple sugars – what can be termed a 'typical Western diet'. While working, she would eat small sugary treats from the school staff room or canteen. Dinner was eaten post 8.30 pm, breakfast at 7.30–8.00 am.

- **Current dietary negatives:** Frequently eats lunch in a hurry or skips it; lunch bought at school is largely based around white carbohydrates such as a jacket potato and quick-fix high sugar bars on the run.
- **Current dietary strengths:** Organic; three servings of oily fish per week; the evening meal was home-cooked with fresh ingredients.

Lifestyle and other history factors

- First husband died, leaving SD a single mother with a young daughter.
- Second, current husband had a recent cancer diagnosis.
- Although SD was on her feet for much of the day, she neither currently nor previously undertook any formal or structured exercise.
- Lives in very close proximity to a major airport, in an air-quality monitoring area.
- While SD found it easy to fall asleep, she was waking two or three times in the night due to hot flushes and then struggling to fall back to sleep. Total sleep hours were 5–6 per night. Did not feel refreshed on waking.

Summary of SD's goals

- To reduce dress size from 18 to 12 (estimated to be equivalent to 10 kg weight loss).

- To have no more symptoms of menopause.
- To reduce blood pressure without medication.

Initial interpretation

The practitioner used a functional matrix approach (based on the Institute of Functional Medicine model) to review potential contributory underlying factors in SD's case to help inform decision making.

Digestion and assimilation

- SD experienced modest bloating. Her previous diet, high stress load and poor sleep are all factors that may lead to reduced microbial diversity. Dietary diversity (which is expanded on in Chapter 7) is associated with improved systemic health (McDonald *et al.*, 2018). Specifically in relation to SD's case, a potential reduced microbial diversity could be an underlying factor in systemic inflammation, given that certain bacteria strains, which flourish as dietary diversity stimulates microbial diversity, may be associated with anti-inflammation properties (Gutiérrez-Díaz *et al.*, 2016).
- Gastrointestinal dysbiosis involving reduced diversity has been associated with hypertension (J. Li *et al.*, 2017; Yan *et al.*, 2017).

Communication: Hypothalamus–pituitary–adrenal (HPA) axis and hypothalamus–pituitary–thyroid (HPT) axis

- A high stress load and sleep deprivation may indicate dysregulation of the HPA response. Through activation of the HPA axis, the hypersecretion of stress system mediators may increase insulin and decrease growth hormone and sex steroids, leading to increased visceral accumulation of fat and loss of muscle mass (Nicolaides *et al.*, 2015).
- Dysregulation of the HPA axis and the impact of that on the sex hormones (Oyola and Handa, 2017) may be a factor in poor

sleep. Disordered sleep is thought to contribute to hypertension, although the mechanism is not fully understood (Thomas and Calhoun, 2017).

- Prolonged stress activation may suppress thyroid-stimulating hormone and the activation of inactive thyroxine to active triiodothyronine in peripheral tissues (Nicolaides *et al.*, 2015).
- Could thyroid hypofunction be a contributory factor in weight gain? Could dysregulation of the HPA axis be a contributory factor in weight gain and visceral adiposity, as well as sleep disruption and hypertension?

Glucose and insulin metabolism

- Sugar cravings and skipped meals could indicate imbalances in blood sugar control.
- Central obesity is associated with insulin resistance (Arner *et al.*, 2010; Moon *et al.*, 2019).
- Vitamin D deficiency may be a risk factor in accelerating insulin resistance (Szymczak-Pajor and Śliwińska, 2019). Given SD's sedentary (indoor-based) lifestyle and location, she may have suboptimal vitamin D levels.
- Is insulin resistance a factor for SD? And if so, what are the contributory diet and lifestyle factors?

Immune system

- Hypertrophy of adipose cells leads to the upregulation of inflammation, altered free fatty acid metabolism and altered release of adipokines (cytokines released by adipose tissue) which can drive hunger signals, systemic inflammation and systemic insulin resistance (Després, 2012; Ouchi *et al.*, 2011).
- There is mechanistic evidence that vitamin D status may alter the balance between pro- and anti-inflammatory cytokines and hence influence insulin action, lipid metabolism and adipose tissue function and structure (Garbossa and Folli, 2017). A

systematic review of immune cell studies concluded that the evidence is consistent for the anti-inflammatory role of vitamin D (Calton *et al.*, 2015).

- Can it be assumed/confirmed that SD is in an inflammatory state? What might be the underlying factors driving inflammation: gastrointestinal dysbiosis, abdominal obesity, HPA activation, toxicant factors, vitamin D status?

Cardiovascular system

- SD is known to have high cholesterol. While that alone may not be cause for concern, along with abdominal obesity and hypertension there is a pattern of accumulating risk factors for cardiovascular disease (CVD). Furthermore, if present, systemic inflammation would be an additional risk factor.
- Low vitamin D status is associated with hypertension (Burgaz *et al.*, 2011; Ke *et al.*, 2015) and is thought to play a role in CVD (Lee *et al.*, 2008).

Detoxification and biotransformation

- Living within 10 km of an airport was shown to increase pollution levels and hospitalization rates for respiratory and heart-related admissions (Schlenker and Walker, 2011). Benzene, one of the volatile hydrocarbons, while now highly controlled, can be found in jet fuel and has been reported at higher than threshold-limit levels in those exposed to airports and aeroplanes (Egeghy *et al.*, 2003; Pleil, Smith and Zelnick, 2000). Benzene exposure was found in animal models to increase CVD risk (Abplanalp *et al.*, 2017) and induce insulin resistance (Abplanalp *et al.*, 2019).
- Environmental toxins are believed to have endocrine-disrupting properties and as such may be a driver of weight gain and metabolic disturbances (Janesick and Blumberg, 2016).
- Could a high toxicant load be a contributory factor for SD's health concerns?

The practitioner recommended further investigations via the following tests:

- **Hs-CRP and fibrinogen:** To help understand the systemic inflammation status.
- **Homocysteine:** To further understand cardiovascular (CV) health. Elevated blood levels of homocysteine, a marker of hypomethylation, has been associated with CVD: homocysteine may compromise arterial structure and function due to its adverse effects on the CV endothelium and smooth-muscle cells (Ganguly and Alam, 2015; Lai and Kan, 2015; Wang and Jin, 2017).
- **Advanced lipid profile:** While SD's primary medical practitioner had tested total cholesterol, they were not able to offer further lipid testing. The practitioner explained what is available with advanced lipid tests (which are discussed more fully in Chapter 3) which SD was willing to undertake to better understand her risk factors in the knowledge these could be discussed with her medical practitioner.
- **Comprehensive thyroid testing (total thyroid, TSH, T4, T3, reverse T3, thyroid antibodies):** While TSH (and perhaps T4) would have been available from SD's medical practitioner, the practitioner explained that comprehensive testing would help understand underlying root causes, and SD agreed to go ahead with this.
- **Vitamin D:** Given its potential role in inflammation, insulin resistance and hypertension.

A four-point salivary cortisol test and a comprehensive stool test (to assess HPA axis and digestive function respectively) were considered but deemed lower priorities and for financial reasons were not ordered. The practitioner hoped that dietary changes would be sufficient to increase microbial diversity (which was suspected to be low). SD was clear that she was under stress, so testing to support that was perhaps unnecessary since she had the motivation and commitment to address her stress.

Initial recommendations

While waiting for test results, the practitioner gave SD initial recommendations for diet and supplements. These recommendations were made on the basis that she had a high familial risk of CVD, high blood pressure, central adiposity, suspected inflammation and insulin resistance.

Diet recommendations

A modified Mediterranean diet (MD), with a macronutrient ratio of approximately 25/30/45 (protein/fat/carbohydrate), with a focus on the *quality* of the macronutrients, was recommended. The main foods containing fat in SD's diet were butter, goats' dairy (cheese and yoghurt), oily fish and some of the packaged 'food on the go' that she currently ate. SD was asked to replace at least 50% of her butter with olive oil, to continue eating oily fish three times a week, to reduce goats dairy by 25% (using beans and lentils as replacement protein source where dishes used cheese) and to use nuts or seeds and fruit as alternative snacks on the go. This would help to switch the emphasis to unsaturated rather than saturated fats. With regard to carbohydrates, refined carbohydrates such as white pasta and white bread were replaced with wholegrain varieties such as brown rice and wholegrain bread.

SD was asked to focus on adding vegetables to her meals, initially by adding one extra vegetable portion (80 g) at each lunch and dinner. SD was currently eating five portions of vegetables a day so adding two portions per day would lead to seven per day. She was asked to focus on vegetables grown above the ground (rather than the starchier below-the-ground vegetables).

Based on a meta-analysis, the MD is thought to be protective for CVD (Sofi *et al.*, 2010). A MD-style diet plus olive oil was shown in an RCT to reduce the incidence of major CD events in a populate age 50–80 years compared with a low-fat diet (Estruch *et al.*, 2018). A prospective cohort study showed that reducing saturated fat and replacing it with polyunsaturated fats (PUFAs) and unrefined carbohydrates reduced CVD risk (Li *et al.*, 2015). While dietary assessment in the study was self-reported, it is one of the first studies to discriminate between the type of carbohydrates consumed and to show that the type of carbohydrate, as well as the type of fat consumed, may have an impact on CVD risk. While low-carbohydrate diets have received interest with regard to weight loss and insulin resistance (Box 8.1), the totality of evidence seems to support the *quality* of macronutrients to be of equal importance to the *quantity* of macronutrients (ratios). Furthermore, in the absence of advanced lipid testing results (which had been ordered) a modified MD was felt to be more appropriate for SD.

The MD was modified to include ground flaxseed and sesame, and to use tofu as a protein source at least once a week and edamame beans in stir fries. As well as offering a plant-based protein source and fibre, these foods contain phytoestrogens which may have a modest effect on reducing the severity of hot flushes in menopausal women (Lewis *et al.*, 2006). Although some animal studies have shown that phytoestrogen intake stimulates oestrogen-dependent breast cancers (Allred *et al.*, 2001), it has been argued that animals metabolize phytoestrogens differently from humans and that studies consistently show a modest benefit of phytoestrogens in post-menopausal women (Messina, 2016). Although some studies have shown no effect of soy protein on menopausal symptoms (St Germain *et al.*, 2001), a meta-analysis of 15 studies concluded that phytoestrogens can reduce the frequency of hot flushes and their side effects, although there was heterogeneity in the dosage used (Chen, Lin and Liu, 2015).

Intake of dietary phytoestrogens was associated with a lower likelihood of hypertension in a cohort study of adults living in a Mediterranean area (Godos *et al.*, 2018). In an animal model, the soy phytoestrogen genistein reversed pulmonary hypertension and prevented right heart failure, thought to be via downregulation of oestrogen receptor-β expression (Matori *et al.*, 2012). Systematic reviews and meta-analysis data suggest that circa 25–30 g soy protein daily may reduce LDL cholesterol by approximately 6% (Anderson and Bush, 2011; Harland and Haffner, 2008). Although it is noted that SD was not going to be consuming this amount of daily soy protein, this was not the only rationale for adding soy protein to her diet.

SD was advised to eat three meals a day, including lunch, and avoid snacking; It was suggested she took food from home on weekdays to avoid the canteen choices.

Xenoestrogens such as bisphenol A (BPA) are thought to be associated with CVD (Lang *et al.*, 2008) and may potentially act as an obesogen (Rubin, Schaeberle and Soto, 2019) and a risk factor for type 2 diabetes (Hwang *et al.*, 2018). The practitioner asked SD to start reducing exposure to BPA. Previously, most foods were wrapped or stored in plastic. These were now to be avoided along with BPA-lined cans, plastic water bottles and paper coffee cups. Proximity to an airport may increase the overall toxicant load and hence all steps to reduce the toxicant load from other sources should be beneficial alongside dietary changes to enhance resources to support detoxification. With this in mind, SD was advised to choose smaller types of oily fish such as sardine, mackerel and salmon, rather than tuna or swordfish which may contain higher levels of mercury (EDF, 2013). While seafood may also contain microplastic contamination (Smith *et al.*, 2018), the practitioner felt the overall benefit of fish in providing dietary variety, protein and PUFAs justified inclusion in SD's diet.

> ## BOX 8.1 LOW-CARBOHYDRATE DIETS, WEIGHT LOSS AND INSULIN RESISTANCE
>
> Low-carbohydrate diets have received significant interest in the scientific and lay media. Two well-designed studies published recently provide interesting insight.
>
> Ebbeling and colleagues (2018) asked participants (BMI >25) to complete a run-in period consuming 60% of energy needs to achieve a 12% weight loss. They were then assigned to one of three groups for 20 weeks of weight maintenance with the following macronutrient ratios: 60% carbohydrate (CHO) diet, 40% CHO or 20% CHO; fat ratios were correspondingly 20%, 40%, 60%; 35% of the fat intake was saturated fats. Protein intake was fixed at 20%. The primary output measure was total energy expenditure (TEE), a metabolic effect that might support sustained weight loss. TEE was significantly greater in the low-CHO than high-CHO groups.

The low-carbohydrate diet had a greater effect on TEE in those who had the highest pre-weight-loss insulin secretion.

The DIETfit study (Gardner *et al.*, 2018) compared either a low-fat or a low-carbohydrate diet, with no limitation on total energy (calorie) but guidance given on food *quality,* to find an *individual* level of fat or carbohydrate intake that was sustainable. Examples of quality of food instructions were to choose lean grass-fed or pasture-raised meat and sustainable fish; to use whole unrefined grains and vegetables; to prepare their own food at home using fresh seasonal ingredients; and to avoid processed foods, added sugar, trans fats or refined white flour. Weight loss was the primary outcome measured. There was no significant weight-loss difference between the study arms. In both groups fasting insulin and glucose fell with no significant difference between groups. LDL was significantly lower in the low-fat group than low-CHO while TRIG and HDL were significantly improved for the low-CHO compared with the low-fat group.

A conclusion from evaluation of both studies is that a low-fat or low-CHO diet can support weight loss and reduce insulin when the *quality* of the carbohydrates and fats is considered; that the impact on lipid profiles may vary depending on low-fat or low-carbohydrate; and that a low-carbohydrate diet may lead to a greater reduction in insulin secretion.

Lifestyle recommendations

Sedentary behaviour is thought to increase CVD risk (Young *et al.*, 2016) and SD was open to becoming more active. SD was encouraged to attend a yoga class starting with a 60-minute weekly class. This type of activity has been shown in a review of 35 studies to significantly reduce stress and anxiety (Li and Goldsmith, 2012). A systematic review and meta-analysis looked at the effect of yoga compared with active and inactive controls on older adults, concluding that yoga improved strength, balance and flexibility as well as health-related quality-of-life scores (Sivaramakrishnan *et al.*, 2019).

Supplement recommendations

Table 8.1 outlines the recommended supplements, based on the understanding that they would be reviewed on test results.

Table 8.1 Summary of initial supplements and doses

Supplement	Dose
EPA/DHA	2 g QD
Cinnamon extract	500 mg BID
Chromium	600 mcg BID
Alpha lipoic acid	300 mg BID

Chromium has been shown to improves blood glucose, insulin, cholesterol and HbA1c in type 2 diabetes, via increased insulin binding, increased insulin receptor number and increased insulin receptor phosphorylation (Anderson, 1998). Cinnamon at 3–6 g a day was effective at lowering postprandial blood glucose in healthy adults (Kizilaslan and Erdem, 2019). A water-soluble cinnamon extract at 500 g per day led to a significant decrease in fasting blood glucose and systolic blood pressure and a significant increase in lean muscle mass compared with the control group after 12 weeks, in individuals with pre-diabetes and metabolic syndrome (Ziegenfuss *et al.*, 2006).

Alpha lipoic acid (ALA) is thought to increase insulin sensitivity by activating AMP-activated protein kinase (AMPK), a regulator of cellular energy metabolism, in skeletal muscle (Lee *et al.*, 2005). ALA at 400 mg per day improved insulin sensitivity in 32 subjects with obesity and PCOS compared with controls (Genazzani *et al.*, 2018). Following a stroke, patients were given 600 mg ALA per day for 12 weeks; significant improvements were reported in blood pressure and fasting blood glucose but not in fasting insulin levels (Mohammadi *et al.*, 2018).

Long-chain omega 3 fatty acids have been shown to reduce NF-kappaB activity and increase PPAR-y, thereby exerting an anti-inflammatory effect (Calder, 2017). In a clinical trial they increased plaque stability in those with CVD (Cawood *et al.*, 2010).

Laboratory results

Table 8.2 summarizes the laboratory test results.

Table 8.2 Summary of test results compared with reference ranges and, where appropriate, optimal ranges

Analyte	Client's result*	Reference range (optimal range where available*)
25 hydroxy vitamin D nmol/L	23 (L)	75–200
Total thyroxine nmol/L	76.1 (LN)	58–154 (77–150)
TSH mIU/L	10.8 (H)	0.4–4.0 (1.0–2.0)
Free thyroxine pmol/L	10.5 (LN)	10–22 (12–20)
Free T3 (FT3) pmol/L	6.45 (HN)	2.8–6.5 (3.4–6.0)
FT4:FT3 ratio	1.6 (L)	2.0–4.5 (2.5–4.0)
Reverse T3 pmol/L	0.21	0.14–0.54 (0.14–0.52)
Thyroglobulin IU/L	87.1 (H)	0–40
Peroxidase IU/L	188 (H)	0–35
LDL cholesterol nmol/L	4.47 (H)	< 2.59
HDL cholesterol nmol/L	1.32	> 1.01
Triglycerides nmol/L	3.14 (H)	< 1.69
Total cholesterol nmol/L	7.24 (H)	< 5.17
LDL particle # nmol/L	2865 (H)	< 1000
HDL particle # □mol/L	39.9	> 34.9
LDL size	20.1 Small Pattern B (H)	Large, Pattern A
Lipoprotein (a) □mol/L	0.07	< 1.07

Hs-CRP mg/L	4.78 (H)	< 1.00
Lp-PLA2 ng/mL	126	< 200
Fibrinogen ▢mol/L	9.6	5.8-12.9
Insulin Resistance Score	77–0 (H)	< 27
Homocysteine ▢mol/L	8	3.7–10.4

* Where optimal reference ranges are given, these are shown. L denotes low, H denotes high, LN denotes low normal and HN denotes high normal i.e. within reference range but outside of optimal reference range.

Interpretation of the results in clinical context

Vitamin D, low

Serum concentration of 25 hydroxyvitamin D is a biomarker for vitamin D status and at 25 nmol/L is considered low. As outlined above, vitamin D deficiency may be a factor driving inflammation, insulin resistance and hypertension.

Raised TSH, low normal T4, high thyroid antibodies

Raised TSH and low normal T4 are suggestive of hypothyroidism. Of course, as a personalized nutrition practitioner no diagnosis was made and SD was referred to her medical practitioner. Elevated thyroid antibodies indicate an autoimmune process.

Low thyroid function could be a factor in SD's weight gain/difficulty losing weight. Thyroid hormone influences lipid synthesis, metabolism and mobilization; low thyroid function can be a factor in high total cholesterol and LDL cholesterol (Pearce, 2012). Infections, toxicants, cytokines and hormonal imbalance are all factors which can trigger thyroid antibody elevations (Fröhlich and Wahl, 2017). Furthermore, there is emerging evidence that environmental toxicants such as BPA can trigger autoimmunity (Kharrazian, 2014; Vojdani, 2014).

Hs-CRP, elevated

CRP is a protein elevated in response to inflammatory conditions and, according to meta-analysis, hs-CRP is an independent risk factor for atherosclerosis (Y. Li *et al.*, 2017). Inflammation might be an underlying factor in autoimmunity, central obesity and suspected insulin resistance.

LDL-C, lipid particles, triglycerides, total cholesterol, all elevated; LDL size pattern B

Advanced lipid testing extends beyond the standard total cholesterol, low-density lipoprotein cholesterol (LDL-C), high-density lipoprotein cholesterol (HDL-C) and triglycerides, and allows a look at the numbers and sizes of the lipoproteins, the cholesterol-carrying particles, as well as other atherogenic molecules. More information on this can be found in Chapter 3.

Where there is discordance (inconsistency) between particle number, particle size and LDL cholesterol, the risk attributed to LDL-C alone can be over- or under-estimated (Allaire *et al.*, 2017; Mora, Buring and Ridker, 2014; Sniderman *et al.*, 2014). For SD, there is consistency as both LDL-C and LDL particle number are elevated. Furthermore, her particle sizes tend towards the smaller denser pattern, which also carries increased risk of CVD (Blake *et al.*, 2002; Gentile *et al.*, 2008).

This confirms to the practitioner that CVD disease risk is genuine and helps clarify priorities for nutrition recommendations. Elevated triglycerides are thought to be a factor contributing to insulin resistance (Kim *et al.*, 2007). The insulin resistance score is an algorithm calculated by the laboratory and based on LDL particle number, LDL particle size, HDL particle number and cholesterol measures.

Of note, lipoprotein-a (Lp(a)) is a genetic risk factor for CVD with a positive association for CVD risk, especially when LDL-C is high. SD's Lp(a) level was within range. Homocysteine was also within normal ranges.

The practitioner wrote to SD's medical practitioner (with her permission) sharing the test results, and SD was advised to request an appointment to discuss the results.

Revisions to client recommendations

Summary of dietary recommendations

- Reduce eating window to ten hours by eating dinner earlier and breakfast later.
- All carbohydrates to be low-glycaemic varieties – for example, beans, wholegrain bread, long-grain rice.
- Maximum size for a grain portion to be no bigger than the palm of the hand.
- Evening meal to be based around a protein served with leafy green and other non-starchy vegetables (i.e. relatively lower in carbohydrates).
- Increase vegetable servings to 7–9 per daily (a serving is 80 g), with a minimum of 50% of the plate to be based around non-starchy vegetables or salads. Eat a wide range of different-coloured vegetables.
- Reduce animal protein and replace with plant protein such as tofu, lentils, beans and other pulses. Reduce chicken and meat to twice a week, wild fish (and smaller species), three times a week, eggs up to six per week, vegetable proteins for all other meals; limit portion size to a maximum of the palm of one hand.

SD's dietary recommendations could be described as a modified MD with an increased fasting window. The impact of these specific recommendations will be to increase fibre and foods containing plant sterols as well as lowering the overall glycaemic load of the diet.

Rationale for recommendations

A Mediterranean diet is likely to be rich in a diversity of dietary polyphenols, which may influence a number of metabolic pathways such as reduction of chronic inflammation, inhibition of lipogenesis and stimulation of catabolic pathways (Guo *et al.*, 2016).

A diet high in plant sterols such as soy, viscous fibre such as psyllium and almonds (which are all included in SD's recommended diet) was as effective in reducing LDL-C and hs-CRP over four weeks as a low-fat diet plus statin protocol (Jenkins, 2003). The same diet (high in plant sterols and viscous fibre) has been shown consistently in follow-up clinical studies to reduce inflammation and improve blood lipids (Jenkins *et al.*, 2010; S.S. Li *et al.*, 2017; Ramprasath *et al.*, 2014).

In a cohort analysis, replacing animal protein with plant protein was associated with lower CV mortality and all-cause mortality (Song *et al.*, 2016).

Late-evening meals increased the glucose response to the evening meal and following breakfast, and therefore a relative reduction of carbohydrates at dinner and extending the overnight fast may help reduce triglyceride levels (Sato *et al.*, 2011). Furthermore, the natural reduction in refined sugars from this approach should support a reduction in triglyceride, given that, in a prospective cohort study, those consuming the highest quantity of foods with added sugars had a significantly higher blood triglyceride level (Sonestedt *et al.*, 2015).

A number of human studies have demonstrated the potential for intermittent feeding,[4] meaning eating contained to a fixed window of hours (in SD's case, ten hours) to improve weight loss, improve insulin sensitivity, improve glucose response, reduce LDL-C and hs-CRP (Carlson *et al.*, 2007; Harvie *et al.*, 2011; LeCheminant *et al.*, 2013; Patterson *et al.*, 2015; Stote *et al.*, 2007).

Lifestyle

Sleep debt has been shown to decrease glucose tolerance and activate the sympathetic nervous system (Spiegel, Leproult and Van Cauter, 1999) and reduce insulin sensitivity (Buxton *et al.*, 2010). Although laboratory studies were conducted on young healthy males, it is believed that insufficient sleep is a potential risk factor for obesity and insulin resistance in more recent systematic reviews (Reutrakul and Van Cauter, 2018),

SD was unaware of the association and found it motivating as this was a habit she could address. SD recognized that she was very active before bed, and was coached on spending 15 minutes' relaxation time before bed and to avoid blue light from screens and devices that can

---

4   Here, the term 'intermittent feeding' is preferred to 'intermittent fasting' as the former focuses on time *to eat*, whereas the latter focuses on *not eating*.

suppress melatonin production (Wood *et al.*, 2013). She committed to going to bed 45 minutes earlier to increase sleep hours.

SD was enjoying her yoga class and was keen to add more physical activity. It was agreed to introduce a walk, initially twice a week for ten minutes, and to build to three times a week and 30 minutes. Adding exercise (either resistance or aerobic) to dietary changes led to great fat mass loss in a controlled study on 249 older, overweight adults (Beavers *et al.*, 2017).

While resistance training was considered (and will be discussed later), walking was recommended at this stage as it was something SD could do without any equipment. She was advised to walk at a pace that would increase her heart rate and rate of breathing as a guide to ensuring there was an aerobic element to the walk.

SD was feeling less stressed since embarking on her nutrition and lifestyle changes. She had learned about diaphragmatic breathing through her yoga class. When the practitioner discussed further ways to support her stress reduction, daily use of breathing exercises was quickly identified by SD as something she would enjoy. Breathing exercises have been shown in primary studies to increase heartrate variability and reduce pulse rate as measures of an improved stress response (Mejía-Mejía, Torres and Restrepo, 2018) and to improve systolic blood pressure (Zhang *et al.*, 2017). SD was willing to listen to meditation and mindfulness sound files on a digital app. A systematic review concluded that meditation can reduce physiological markers of stress (Pascoe *et al.*, 2017).

Supplement recommendations
Revised supplement recommendations are shown in Table 8.3.

Table 8.3 Revised supplement recommendations

Supplement	Dose
EPA/DHA	2 g QD
Chromium	1000 mcg QD

cont.

Supplement	Dose
D3	4000 IU QD
Magnesium as glycinate	400 mg QD
CoQ$_{10}$ as ubiquinol	300 mg QD
Alpha lipoic acid	150 mg QID
Thyroid glandular	300 mg QD
Lactobacillus rhamnosus GG	15 billion CFU QD

ALA, EPA/DHA and chromium were continued and cinnamon stopped. Magnesium was added; magnesium supplementation has been shown to improve intracellular magnesium levels and improve insulin-mediated glucose take-up (Barbagallo *et al.*, 2003).

A systematic review of vitamin D supplementation in those with CVD concluded that vitamin D supplementation may improve glycaemic control, HDL cholesterol and CRP levels (but not triglycerides or total and LDL cholesterol) (Ostadmohammadi *et al.*, 2019). While large-scale cross-sectional studies show an inverse relation between vitamin D supplementation and improvements in hypertension (Legarth *et al.*, 2018), RCTs remain inconclusive (Bernini *et al.*, 2013), which, according to Legarth and colleagues (2018) may be due to suboptimal study design. A systematic review and meta-analysis on vitamin D status and CVD risk factors concluded that vitamin D supplementation may help reduce hypertension, dyslipidaemia and inflammation, and therefore protect against CVD (Mirhosseini, Rainsbury and Kimball, 2018). Since SD had a low 25 hydroxy vitamin D finding, there was a clear rationale to add a vitamin D supplementation.

CoQ$_{10}$ was added to support antioxidant systems (Mancini *et al.*, 2013), given SD's elevated blood lipids and inflammation markers. CoQ$_{10}$ and magnesium are vital for mitochondria function, and while no tests were undertaken to measure their status in SD, given her historical diet it is reasonable to suspect low levels. With a systems biology approach to thyroid function, supporting mitochondria ATP helps maintain energy-dependent processes vital to thyroid function such as iodine uptake; perfusion patterns of the thyroid have been shown to respond to magnesium and CoQ_{10} supplementation (Moncayo and Moncayo, 2017, 2015).

The rationale for glandular supplements is based on traditional use. Organ meats and offal have been a traditional feature of diets until recently. A case study report documents their successful use in a patient very similar to SD (Wellwood and Rardin, 2014). This practitioner has experiential evidence from her own clinic for their effective and safe short-term use in similar situations.

Lactobacillus rhamnosus GG was shown in a small RCT of patients with inflammation on the gastrointestinal tract to reduce expression of inflammation markers (Pagnini *et al.*, 2018). This was added with the goal of supporting a systemic reduction in inflammation.

Client motivation

While SD was rather shocked by her test results, she found them highly motivating for the dietary and lifestyle changes that were recommended. SD was clear on the goals she wanted to achieve (see above). The practitioner helped to educate her on how the new habits might be expected to influence both symptoms and the biomarkers from testing. Achievable targets were agreed with regard to dietary and lifestyle changes.

Case management

SD had follow-up appointments every eight weeks for ten months. She successfully adhered to the recommendations, following a modified MD.

Her medical practitioner had referred her to an endocrinologist who diagnosed Hashimoto's thyroiditis. SD was given a prescription for thyroxine and statins but decided not to take them and to continue with the personalized nutrition programme for a few more months. The medical practitioner was happy for SD to continue with the diet and lifestyle programme and to monitor the effect of that on the other out-of-range test results.

After four months she had lost 16 lb (7 kg) in weight and three inches around her waist, reducing her waist-to-hip ratio to 0.82. A follow-up with the endocrinologist confirmed normalization of her vitamin D (84 nmol/L) and TSH (3.68 mIU/L). The endocrinologist was happy with the results and agreed continuation of the programme without pharmaceuticals.

SD's menopausal symptoms had reduced; she had hot flushes and night sweats much less frequently.

The practitioner recommended some adjustments to SD's programme:

- To join a gym and start taking classes which would involve resistance as well as aerobic training. A systematic review and meta-analysis looking at the impact of training on glycaemic control (measured by HbA1c) in a non-diabetic population concluded that the characteristics of training that led to a greater effect were that it was supervised, included resistance training and involved over 150 minutes per week (Cavero-Redondo *et al.*, 2018). Reviews and meta-analysis of the effect of training on glycaemic control in patients with diabetes reached similar findings in terms of the preference for supervised training and at least 150 minutes per week of aerobic and resistance training (Nery *et al.*, 2017; Pan *et al.*, 2018).
- Increase in intermittent feeding, extending the overnight fast to 16 hours two to three days a week.
- Focus on the following foods as containing phytonutrients with specific potential benefits for CV health: tomatoes, green leafy vegetables, citrus fruits, soy proteins, green and black tea, grapes, extra-virgin olive oil, oily fish, dark chocolate, pomegranate, nuts and seeds (whole and in oil form) (Alissa and Ferns, 2012).

Selected supplements were used, focusing on one of three main areas: providing cofactors for hormone balance, blood lipid metabolism or inflammation support. These were not used at the same time; the length of time used is given in Table 8.4. *Lactobacillus* GG was reduced to 10 billion CFU per day; EPA/DHA, chromium, ALA, magnesium and

CoQ$_{10}$ were continued. Vitamin D dose was reduced to 800 IU per day. The glandular was stopped.

Table 8.4 Additional supplements used during the follow-up period

Supplement	Dose	Time used
Cofactors for hormone balance		
B complex	1000 mcg (folic acid, B9) 1000 mcg (B12) 50 mg (B6) 300 mg (B5) (All QD)	6 months
Improve lipid metabolism		
Niacin	1 g QD for 1 week 2 g QD for weeks 2–4	4 weeks
NAC	1.5 g BID on empty stomach	3 months
Red yeast rice	1200 mg BID	4 months
Plant sterols	3 g QD	3 months
EGCG	200 mg BID	2 months
Berberine	400 mg TID	8 weeks
Inflammation support		
Curcumin with bioperine	1 g BID	3 months

The B complex was added to provide one-carbon nutrients for methylation (Ulrich *et al.*, 2012), important for hormone metabolism and signalling (Kabat *et al.*, 2008). There are some indications that folic acid (B9, a one-carbon nutrient) may lower LDL-C (Vijayakumar *et al.*, 2017).

Curcumin modulates multiple cell-signalling pathways involved in inflammation (Gupta, Patchva and Aggarwal, 2012). Improvements in beta cell function and insulin sensitivity were seen in pre-diabetic patients given 750 mg curcuminoid for nine months compared with controls in an RCT, with minimal adverse reactions (Chuengsamarn *et al.*, 2012).

Berberine has been shown to improve insulin sensitivity (Zhang *et al.*, 2008), and through modulation of AMPK, berberine has been shown to dampen all primary pro-inflammatory cellular signalling (Jeong *et al.*, 2009). Epiogallocatechin-3-gallate taken in a supplement or in green tea was shown to help reduce body weight in an eight-week controlled trial in obese and overweight subjects (Basu *et al.*, 2010).

Studies on red yeast rice consistently show it to lower LDL-C (Pirro *et al.*, 2017). Safety issues have been raised with red yeast rice as some preparations can contain mycotoxins; care is always taken to use only reputable, practitioner-grade products.

A meta-analysis of 11 studies found niacin supplementation to be effective in improving outcomes for those with CVD, although a direct impact was not consistently shown with LDL-C (Lavigne and Karas, 2013). Niacin can cause unpleasant side effects of flushing and so care is taken when using it. Apple pectin may moderate the flushing effect (Moriarty *et al.*, 2013); eating an apple at the same time may therefore reduce flushing. SD did not experience any flushing with niacin.

N-acetyl-L-cysteine (NAC) is a thiol compound. It acts as a scavenger of free radicals and as an antioxidant by restoring the pool of intracellular glutathione-S-transferase activity. NAC supplementation has been shown to improve peripheral insulin sensitivity and reduce oxidative stress associated with elevated blood lipids (Dludla *et al.*, 2018).

Intake of plant sterols may reduce LDL cholesterol concentrations by 5–15%, through interfering with cholesterol absorption (AbuMweis, Barake and Jones, 2008). Their dietary use has also been discussed above.

Lifestyle

Sadly, SD's mother died during this period and the impact of grief as well as caring for her widowed father meant her stress response remained activated. SD continued to use the breathing exercises and meditation tools and reported finding these 'helpful' in managing her stress response.

At ten months, the thyroid and advanced lipid tests were repeated. The results are shown in Table 8.5.

Table 8.5 Comparison of initial and follow-up laboratory tests with comments

Analyte	Lab 1	Lab 2	Comment
TSH	10.8	3.68	Now considered normal by GP ranges
Free t4	10.5	11.6	Still low, but improved
Thyroglobulin	87.1	< dl	Now undetectable
Anti-TPO	188	33	Normal although top end of normal range limit
LDL-C	4.47	3.98	Improvement although still elevated
Triglycerides	3.14	2.08	Improvement although still elevated
Total cholesterol	7.24	6.08	Improvement although still elevated
LDL particle #	2865	2061	Improvement although still elevated
LDL size	20.1	21	An increase into the optimal zone
Hs-CRP	4.78	2.69	Improvement although still elevated
Insulin resistance score	77	54	Improvement although still elevated

SD was delighted to see the results: they gave her objective 'black and white' evidence of the physical improvement she felt in her own body. SD had now lost a total of 10.8 kg, was a size 14, and had a waist-to-hip ratio of 0.8 which is optimal for woman and suggests a significant reduction is abdominal adiposity. She barely noticed menopause symptoms. Blood pressure was consistently 120/80 which was within normal range.

Eating was now established in a window of eight to ten hours, and a low-GI, phytonutrient-rich diet was established and honoured daily. She was exercising twice weekly in the gym with a mixture of aerobic and resistance supervised training, as well as a weekly yoga class and daily walks, all of which she was happy to continue.

Discussion and conclusion

The door was opened to SD to pay more attention to her health due to her husband's diagnosis. SD was anticipating help with weight loss, blood pressure reduction and improvement in menopausal symptoms. What she perhaps had not fully realized is that through a personalized nutrition approach the practitioner undertakes to identify the underlying factors. Recognizing that the body is a complex adaptive and dynamic system, the personalized nutrition practitioner looks for root causes. In the search for factors involved in high blood pressure, menopausal symptoms and weight gain, the practitioner identified systemic inflammation, thyroid imbalance, specifically with an autoimmune response, and a blood lipids picture that highlighted her CVD risk.

In this personalized nutrition approach, simple changes to SD's diet, targeted supplements and lifestyle appear to have had an impact on a number of underlying areas of imbalance.

A Mediterranean-style diet formed the basis of SD's dietary recommendations. While low-carbohydrate diets have received a deserving amount of interest for weight loss, the practitioner selected a Mediterranean-style diet, which is also well evidenced for CVD and has other components that should support some of the other underlying factors identified in her case.

The MD will likely have impacted her at a multitude of levels. The addition of 25 ml/day olive oil infused with thyme has been shown to improve blood lipids in hypercholesterolemic individuals, thought to be due to the phenolic compounds of the olive oil and thyme increasing *Bifidobacteria* species in the microbiome (Martín-Peláez *et al.*, 2017). The microbiome has emerged as an important factor in obesity and its related metabolic diseases; in obese individuals the Firmicutes species can tend to be over-represented while the Bacteroidetes species are under-represented (Johnson *et al.*, 2017).

A cross-sectional study in healthy adults found those eating a Mediterranean-style diet had a statistically high number of *Bacteroidetes*, *Prevotellacea* and *Prevotella*, and a lower concentration of *Firmicutes* and *Lachnospiraceae* (Gutiérrez-Díaz *et al.*, 2016) – the microbiome profile which tends to be associated with optimal body weight.

A Mediterranean-style diet is naturally lower on the glycemic index as it replaces refined grains with wholegrains, includes whole fruits and vegetables, and avoids refined sugar (Davis *et al.*, 2015). Furthermore, as a traditional diet it has a good safety record.

The practitioner tailored the diet. First, she made it easy for SD to implement the diet, with simple instructions and a phased approach, initially focusing on simple switches in the types of fats used and the types of carbohydrates used. Based on her clinical experience, this makes it much easier and motivating for a client to adapt.

As time went on, the practitioner started to recommend a focus on foods for their specific phytonutrients. Table 8.6 highlights specific phytonutrients with a cardioprotective effect and the foods in which they are found (Alissa and Ferns, 2012). Furthermore, these phytonutrients are reported to induce Nrf2, a transcription factor that protects against oxidative stress (Hodges and Minich, 2015).

Table 8.6 Foods focused on for SD and their cardioprotective phytonutrients

Foods	Phytonutrients with a cardioprotective effect
Tomatoes	Lycopene
Green leafy vegetables	Carotenoids
Citrus fruits and vegetables	Vitamin C
Soy proteins	Genistein, daidzein
Green and black tea	Tea polyphenols

cont.

Foods	Phytonutrients with a cardioprotective effect
Grapes	Anthocyanins
Fish	Omega 3 fatty acids
Extra-virgin olive oil	Polyphenolics and oleic acid
Dark chocolate	Flavonoids
Pomegranate	Polyphenols
Nuts seeds and oils	Vitamin E, tocopherol, tocotrienols

Source: Adapted from Alissa and Fernss (2012)

Intermittent feeding was introduced. While evidence on fasting from human studies is still emerging, there is growing evidence that modified fasting regimens, without calorie restriction, promote weight loss and improve metabolic health (Patterson *et al.*, 2015). In animal models it can be shown that that intermittent feeding decreases obesity through manipulation of the microbiome (G. Li *et al.*, 2017). Fasting may also lead to a correction of increased intestinal permeability – and therefore reduce postprandial endotoxemia, antigenic exposure and inflammation (Kelly, Colgan and Frank, 2012).

Targeted supplements included vitamin D. While low vitamin D is associated with blood pressure (BP) and metabolic syndrome, systematic reviews have shown that supplementation of vitamin D does resolve hypertension alone (Beveridge *et al.*, 2015; Legarth *et al.*, 2018). But is it realistic to expect a single intervention to 'resolve' something as complex and systemic as BP? In SD's case, she had a low baseline vitamin D level, plus she has signs of insulin resistance and inflammation which are also linked to low vitamin D status (as previously discussed). It can be hypothesized that bringing vitamin D status to normal levels may have had a positive influence across inflammation, insulin resistance *and* hypertension.

Over time, SD was able to increase exercise and structured classes. Exercise has been shown to increase muscle sensitivity to insulin due to translocation of GLUT4 glucose transporters to the cell surface

(Turcotte and Fisher, 2008). Increased muscle sensitivity to insulin may lead to lower fasting insulin and glucose levels. Resistance training has a number of positive metabolic benefits: it reduces visceral fat, increases peripheral glucose uptake, reduces TNFalpha and increases muscle mass (Flack *et al.*, 2010). Cohort analysis from the Women's Health study found a j-shaped association for strength (resistance) training and all-cause mortality – in other words, a moderate amount (approximately 145 minutes per week) of strength training was associated with a lower risk of mortality independent of aerobic activity (Kamada *et al.*, 2017). Resistance training in healthy adults over 50 improved health-related quality of life according to a meta-analysis (Hart and Buck, 2019). Resistance training, however, was not recommended initially, but was introduced later when SD had started to see initial improvements. This reflects an interpretation of the evidence within a personal context which can and should be accommodated in a personalized nutrition setting.

This case attempts to demonstrate the essence of personalized nutrition: that simple changes to diet, tailored supplements and lifestyle, tailored to the individual, based on their current capabilities and preferences, and designed to address their individual underlying factors, should have a profound effect on symptoms, quality of life, chronic disease risk factors and longer-term health outcomes. What is more, SD was empowered to take back control of her own health.

Q&A

AW: In personalized nutrition we recognize that each individual can only make changes at their own pace. How do you coach your clients on dietary change? I know when we spoke you used the term 'simple and achievable'. Can you share some specific tips on how you did this with SD?

JG: I believe a big part of my work is in the education and empowerment of my clients. In this case, SD already had the desire to make changes due to her husband's diagnosis. The functional testing results helped to guide me and to educate her on what was needed to tailor a diet for her. I then worked with her on realistic and simple steps she could make. The diet evolved with each consultation. I would listen to her report on her progress, both in terms of symptoms and how she had implemented the dietary recommendations, and recommend refinements such as specific vegetables and fruits and the stages of intermittent feeding. With this approach, I find clients are able to build confidence in their ability to make lifestyle changes that initially may seem quite daunting.

AW: On reflection, is there anything you would do differently in this case?

JG: In an ideal world I would have included a comprehensive stool test in the initial testing. Cost was the major reason this wasn't included; as a family, they were undertaking a lot of functional testing at the same time, so cost was an issue. However, I'm not sure it would have hugely altered the recommendations I made as progress was maintained at a steady rate and more comprehensive gastrointestinal issues didn't seem to arise for SD, as can sometimes happen if clients become normalized to underlying digestive symptoms. Her modest bloating did improve, which I suspect was due to dietary changes and the introduction of *Lactobacillus rhamnosus*.

AW: Dialogue with a patient's general practitioner (GP) is so important in clinical work. How did you share information and engage with SD's GP? Do you have a standard letter format? Do you share full test results or summarize findings? Any tips on how to handle this?

JG: I absolutely agree and in this case I had several letters of correspondence going back and forth. Typically, I start off with a client by asking the GP to authorize any bloods that may be beneficial for us based on the client's presenting symptoms. In this case, I sent the doctor a letter requesting key bloodwork to be undertaken and monitored going forward, saving the client the cost of repeated private testing. I don't tend to send full reports of functional tests to the doctor, as some markers are not typically reported in conventional medicine. Therefore,

I tend to add screenshots of key markers that would be beneficial for us to share as part of bridging the gap towards collaborative medicine.

References

Abplanalp, W., DeJarnett, N., Riggs, D.W., Conklin, D.J. *et al.*, T.E., 2017. Benzene exposure is associated with cardiovascular disease risk. *PloS ONE* 12, e0183602. https://doi.org/10.1371/journal.pone.0183602

Abplanalp, W.T., Wickramasinghe, N.S., Sithu, S.D., Conklin, D.J. *et al.*, 2019. Benzene exposure induces insulin resistance in mice. *Toxicological Sciences* 167, 426–437. https://doi.org/10.1093/toxsci/kfy252

AbuMweis, S.S., Barake, R., Jones, P.J.H., 2008. Plant sterols/stanols as cholesterol lowering agents: A meta-analysis of randomized controlled trials. *Food and Nutrition Research* 52. https://doi.org/10.3402/fnr.v52i0.1811

Alissa, E.M., Ferns, G.A., 2012. Functional foods and nutraceuticals in the primary prevention of cardiovascular diseases. *Journal of Nutrition and Metabolism*. https://doi.org/10.1155/2012/569486

Allaire, J., Vors, C., Couture, P., Lamarche, B., 2017. LDL particle number and size and cardiovascular risk: Anything new under the sun? *Current Opinion in Lipidology* 28, 261–266. https://doi.org/10.1097/MOL.0000000000000419

Allred, C.D., Ju, Y.H., Allred, K.F., Chang, J., Helferich, W.G., 2001. Dietary genistin stimulates growth of estrogen-dependent breast cancer tumors similar to that observed with genistein. *Carcinogenesis* 22, 1667–1673.

Anderson, J.W., Bush, H.M., 2011. Soy protein effects on serum lipoproteins: A quality assessment and meta-analysis of randomized, controlled studies. *Journal of the American College of Nutrition* 30, 79–91.

Anderson, R.A., 1998. Chromium, glucose intolerance and diabetes. *Journal of the American College of Nutrition* 17, 548–555.

Arner, E., Westermark, P.O., Spalding, K.L., Britton, T. *et al.*, 2010. Adipocyte turnover: relevance to human adipose tissue morphology. *Diabetes* 59, 105–109. https://doi.org/10.2337/db09-0942

Barbagallo, M., Dominguez, L.J., Galioto, A., Ferlisi, A. *et al.*, 2003. Role of magnesium in insulin action, diabetes and cardio-metabolic syndrome X. *Molecular Aspects of Medicine* 24, 39–52.

Basu, A., Sanchez, K., Leyva, M.J., Wu, M. *et al.*, 2010. Green tea supplementation affects body weight, lipids, and lipid peroxidation in obese subjects with metabolic syndrome. *Journal of the American College of Nutrition* 29, 31–40.

Beavers, K.M., Ambrosius, W.T., Rejeski, W.J., Burdette, J.H. *et al.*, 2017. Effect of exercise type during intentional weight loss on body composition in older adults with obesity. *Obesity* 25, 1823–1829. https://doi.org/10.1002/oby.21977

Bernini, G., Carrara, D., Bacca, A., Carli, V. *et al.*, 2013. Effect of acute and chronic vitamin D administration on systemic renin angiotensin system in essential hypertensives and controls. *Journal of Endocrinological Investigation* 36, 216–220. https://doi.org/10.1007/BF03347275

Beveridge, L.A., Struthers, A.D., Khan, F., Jorde, R. *et al.*, 2015. Effect of vitamin D supplementation on blood pressure: A systematic review and meta-analysis incorporating individual patient data. *JAMA Internal Medicine* 175, 745–754. https://doi.org/10.1001/jamainternmed.2015.0237

Blake, G.J., Otvos, J.D., Rifai, N., Ridker, P.M., 2002. Low-density lipoprotein particle concentration and size as determined by nuclear magnetic resonance spectroscopy as predictors of cardiovascular disease in women. *Circulation* 106, 1930–1937. https://doi.org/10.1161/01.CIR.0000033222.75187.B9

Burgaz, A., Orsini, N., Larsson, S.C., Wolk, A., 2011. Blood 25-hydroxyvitamin D concentration and hypertension: A meta-analysis. *Journal of Hypertension* 29, 636–645. https://doi.org/10.1097/HJH.0b013e32834320f9

Buxton, O.M., Pavlova, M., Reid, E.W., Wang, W., Simonson, D.C., Adler, G.K., 2010. Sleep restriction for 1 week reduces insulin sensitivity in healthy men. *Diabetes* 59, 2126–2133. https://doi.org/10.2337/db09-0699

Calder, P.C., 2017. Omega-3 fatty acids and inflammatory processes: From molecules to man. *Biochemical Society Transactions* 45, 1105–1115. https://doi.org/10.1042/BST20160474

Calton, E.K., Keane, K.N., Newsholme, P., Soares, M.J., 2015. The impact of vitamin D levels on inflammatory status: A systematic review of immune cell studies. *PLoS ONE* 10. https://doi.org/10.1371/journal.pone.0141770

Carlson, O., Martin, B., Stote, K.S., Golden, E. *et al.*, 2007. Impact of reduced meal frequency without caloric restriction on glucose regulation in healthy, normal weight middle-aged men and women. *Metabolism* 56, 1729–1734. https://doi.org/10.1016/j.metabol.2007.07.018

Cavero-Redondo, I., Peleteiro, B., Álvarez-Bueno, C., Artero, E.G., Garrido-Miguel, M., Martinez-Vizcaíno, V., 2018. The effect of physical activity interventions on glycosylated haemoglobin (HbA1c) in non-diabetic populations: A systematic review and meta-analysis. *Sports Medicine* 48, 1151–1164. https://doi.org/10.1007/s40279-018-0861-0

Cawood, A.L., Ding, R., Napper, F.L., Young, R.H. *et al.*, 2010. Eicosapentaenoic acid (EPA) from highly concentrated n-3 fatty acid ethyl esters is incorporated into advanced atherosclerotic plaques and higher plaque EPA is associated with decreased plaque inflammation and increased stability. *Atherosclerosis* 212, 252–259. https://doi.org/10.1016/j.atherosclerosis.2010.05.022

Chen, M.-N., Lin, C.-C., Liu, C.-F., 2015. Efficacy of phytoestrogens for menopausal symptoms: A meta-analysis and systematic review. *Climacteric* 18, 260–269. https://doi.org/10.3109/13697137.2014.966241

Chuengsamarn, S., Rattanamongkolgul, S., Luechapudiporn, R., Phisalaphong, C., Jirawatnotai, S., 2012. Curcumin extract for prevention of type 2 diabetes. *Diabetes Care* 35, 2121–2127. https://doi.org/10.2337/dc12-0116

Davis, C., Bryan, J., Hodgson, J., Murphy, K., 2015. Definition of the Mediterranean diet: A literature review. *Nutrients* 7, 9139–9153. https://doi.org/10.3390/nu7115459

Després, J.-P., 2012. Body fat distribution and risk of cardiovascular disease. *Circulation* 126, 1301–1313. https://doi.org/10.1161/CIRCULATIONAHA.111.067264

Dludla, P.V., Dias, S.C., Obonye, N., Johnson, R., Louw, J., Nkambule, B.B., 2018. A systematic review on the protective effect of *N*-acetyl cysteine against diabetes-associated cardiovascular complications. *American Journal of Cardiovascular Drugs* 18, 283–298. https://doi.org/10.1007/s40256-018-0275-2

Ebbeling, C.B., Feldman, H.A., Klein, G.L., Wong, J.M.W. *et al.*, 2018. Effects of a low carbohydrate diet on energy expenditure during weight loss maintenance: Randomized trial. *BMJ* 363, k4583. https://doi.org/10.1136/bmj.k4583

EDF, 2013. Mercury in seafood. Accessed on 26/05/2019 at http://seafood.edf.org/mercury-seafood

Egeghy, P.P., Hauf-Cabalo, L., Gibson, R., Rappaport, S.M., 2003. Benzene and naphthalene in air and breath as indicators of exposure to jet fuel. *Occupational and Environmental Medicine* 60, 969–976.

Estruch, R., Ros, E., Salas-Salvadó, J., Covas, M.-I. *et al.*, 2018. Primary prevention of cardiovascular disease with a Mediterranean diet supplemented with extra-virgin olive oil or nuts. *New England Journal of Medicine* 378, e34. https://doi.org/10.1056/NEJMoa1800389

Flack, K.D., Davy, K.P., Hulver, M.W., Winett, R.A., Frisard, M.I., Davy, B.M., 2010. Aging, resistance training, and diabetes prevention. *Journal of Aging Research* 2011. https://doi.org/10.4061/2011/127315

Fröhlich, E., Wahl, R., 2017. Thyroid autoimmunity: Role of anti-thyroid antibodies in thyroid and extra-thyroidal diseases. *Frontiers in Immunology* 8. https://doi.org/10.3389/fimmu.2017.00521

Ganguly, P., Alam, S.F., 2015. Role of homocysteine in the development of cardiovascular disease. *Nutrition Journal* 14. https://doi.org/10.1186/1475-2891-14-6

Garbossa, S.G., Folli, F., 2017. Vitamin D, sub-inflammation and insulin resistance. A window on a potential role for the interaction between bone and glucose metabolism. *Reviews in Endocrine Metabolic Disorders* 18, 243–258. https://doi.org/10.1007/s11154-017-9423-2

Gardner, C.D., Trepanowski, J.F., Del Gobbo, L.C., Hauser, M.E. *et al.*, 2018. Effect of low-fat vs low-carbohydrate diet on 12-month weight loss in overweight adults and the association with genotype pattern or insulin secretion: The DIETFITS randomized clinical trial. *JAMA* 319, 667–679. https://doi.org/10.1001/jama.2018.0245

Genazzani, A.D., Shefer, K., Della Casa, D., Prati, A. *et al.*, 2018. Modulatory effects of alpha-lipoic acid (ALA) administration on insulin sensitivity in obese PCOS patients. *Journal of Endocrinological Investigation* 41, 583–590. https://doi.org/10.1007/s40618-017-0782-z

Gentile, M., Panico, S., Jossa, F., Mattiello, A. *et al.*, 2008. Small dense LDL particles and metabolic syndrome in a sample of middle-aged women. *Clinica Chimica Acta* 388, 179–183. https://doi.org/10.1016/j.cca.2007.10.033

Godos, J., Bergante, S., Satriano, A., Pluchinotta, F.R., Marranzano, M., 2018. Dietary phytoestrogen intake is inversely associated with hypertension in a cohort of adults living in the Mediterranean area. *Molecules* 23. https://doi.org/10.3390/molecules23020368

Guo, X., Tresserra-Rimbau, A., Estruch, R., Martínez-González, M.A. *et al.*, 2016. Effects of polyphenol, measured by a biomarker of total polyphenols in urine, on cardiovascular risk factors after a long-term follow-up in the PREDIMED study. *Oxidative Medicine and Cellular Longevity* 2016, 2572606. https://doi.org/10.1155/2016/2572606

Gupta, S.C., Patchva, S., Aggarwal, B.B., 2012. Therapeutic roles of curcumin: Lessons learned from clinical trials. *AAPS Journal* 15, 195–218. https://doi.org/10.1208/s12248-012-9432-8

Gutiérrez-Díaz, I., Fernández-Navarro, T., Sánchez, B., Margolles, A., González, S., 2016. Mediterranean diet and faecal microbiota: A transversal study. *Food and Function* 7, 2347–2356. https://doi.org/10.1039/c6fo00105j

Harland, J.I., Haffner, T.A., 2008. Systematic review, meta-analysis and regression of randomised controlled trials reporting an association between an intake of circa 25 g soya protein per day and blood cholesterol. *Atherosclerosis* 200, 13–27. https://doi.org/10.1016/j.atherosclerosis.2008.04.006

Hart, P.D., Buck, D.J., 2019. The effect of resistance training on health-related quality of life in older adults: Systematic review and meta-analysis. *Health Promotion Perspectives* 9, 1–12. https://doi.org/10.15171/hpp.2019.01

Harvie, M.N., Pegington, M., Mattson, M.P., Frystyk, J. *et al.*, 2011. The effects of intermittent or continuous energy restriction on weight loss and metabolic disease risk markers: A randomized trial in young overweight women. *International Journal of Obesity* 2005 35, 714–727. https://doi.org/10.1038/ijo.2010.171

Hodges, R.E., Minich, D.M., 2015. Modulation of metabolic detoxification pathways using foods and food-derived components: A scientific review with clinical application. *Journal of Nutrition and Metabolism* 2015. https://doi.org/10.1155/2015/760689

Hwang, S., Lim, J.-E., Choi, Y., Jee, S.H., 2018. Bisphenol A exposure and type 2 diabetes mellitus risk: A meta-analysis. *BMC Endocrine Disorders* 18, 81. https://doi.org/10.1186/s12902-018-0310-y

Janesick, A.S., Blumberg, B., 2016. Obesogens: An emerging threat to public health. *American Journal of Obstetrics and Gynecology* 214, 559–565. https://doi.org/10.1016/j.ajog.2016.01.182

Jenkins, D.J.A., 2003. Effects of a Dietary portfolio of cholesterol-lowering foods vs lovastatin on serum lipids and C-reactive protein. *JAMA* 290, 502. https://doi.org/10.1001/jama.290.4.502

Jenkins, D.J.A., Chiavaroli, L., Wong, J.M.W., Kendall, C. *et al.*, 2010. Adding monounsaturated fatty acids to a dietary portfolio of cholesterol-lowering foods in hypercholesterolemia. *CMAJ* 182, 1961–1967. https://doi.org/10.1503/cmaj.092128

Jeong, H.W., Hsu, K.C., Lee, J.-W., Ham, M. *et al.*, 2009. Berberine suppresses proinflammatory responses through AMPK activation in macrophages. *American Journal of Physiology – Endocrinology and Metabolism* 296, E955–E964. https://doi.org/10.1152/ajpendo.90599.2008

Johnson, E.L., Heaver, S.L., Walters, W.A., Ley, R.E., 2017. Microbiome and metabolic disease: Revisiting the bacterial phylum Bacteroidetes. *Journal of Molecular Medicine* 95, 1–8. https://doi.org/10.1007/s00109-016-1492-2

Kabat, G.C., Miller, A.B., Jain, M., Rohan, T.E., 2008. Dietary intake of selected B vitamins in relation to risk of major cancers in women. *British Journal of Cancer* 99, 816–821. https://doi.org/10.1038/sj.bjc.6604540

Kahn, R., Buse, J., Ferrannini, E., Stern, M., 2005. The metabolic syndrome: Time for a critical appraisal. Joint statement from the American Diabetes Association and the European Association for the Study of Diabetes. *Diabetologia* 48, 1684–1699. https://doi.org/10.1007/s00125-005-1876-2

Kamada, M., Shiroma, E.J., Buring, J.E., Miyachi, M., Lee, I.-M., 2017. Strength training and all-cause, cardiovascular disease, and cancer mortality in older women: A cohort study. *Journal of the American Heart Association* 6. https://doi.org/10.1161/JAHA.117.007677

Ke, L., Mason, R.S., Kariuki, M., Mpofu, E., Brock, K.E., 2015. Vitamin D status and hypertension: A review. *Integrated Blood Pressure Control* 8, 13–35. https://doi.org/10.2147/IBPC.S49958

Kelly, C.J., Colgan, S.P., Frank, D.N., 2012. Of microbes and meals: The health consequences of dietary endotoxemia. *Nutrition in Clinical Practice* 27, 215–225. https://doi.org/10.1177/0884533611434934

Kharrazian, D., 2014. The potential roles of bisphenol A (BPA) pathogenesis in autoimmunity. *Autoimmune Diseases* 2014, 743616. https://doi.org/10.1155/2014/743616

Kim, D.-S., Jeong, S.-K., Kim, H.-R., Kim, D.-S., Chae, S.-W., Chae, H.-J., 2007. Effects of triglyceride on ER stress and insulin resistance. *Biochemical and Biophysical Research Communications* 363, 140–145. https://doi.org/10.1016/j.bbrc.2007.08.151

Kizilaslan, N., Erdem, N.Z., 2019. The effect of different amounts of cinnamon consumption on blood glucose in healthy adult individuals. *International Journal of Food Science* 2019, 4138534. https://doi.org/10.1155/2019/4138534

Lai, W.K.C., Kan, M.Y., 2015. Homocysteine-induced endothelial dysfunction. *Annals of Nutrition and Metabolism* 67, 1–12. https://doi.org/10.1159/000437098

Lang, I.A., Galloway, T.S., Scarlett, A., Henley, W.E. *et al.*, 2008. Association of urinary bisphenol A concentration with medical disorders and laboratory abnormalities in adults. *JAMA* 300, 1303–1310. https://doi.org/10.1001/jama.300.11.1303

Lavigne, P.M., Karas, R.H., 2013. The current state of niacin in cardiovascular disease prevention: A systematic review and meta-regression. *Journal of the American College of Cardiology* 61, 440–446. https://doi.org/10.1016/j.jacc.2012.10.030

LeCheminant, J.D., Christenson, E., Bailey, B.W., Tucker, L.A., 2013. Restricting night-time eating reduces daily energy intake in healthy young men: A short-term cross-over study. *British Journal of Nutrition* 110, 2108–2113. https://doi.org/10.1017/S0007114513001359

Lee, J.H., O'Keefe, J.H., Bell, D., Hensrud, D.D., Holick, M.F., 2008. Vitamin D deficiency an important, common, and easily treatable cardiovascular risk factor? *Journal of the American College of Cardiology* 52, 1949–1956. https://doi.org/10.1016/j.jacc.2008.08.050

Lee, W.J., Song, K.-H., Koh, E.H., Won, J.C. *et al.*, 2005. Alpha-lipoic acid increases insulin sensitivity by activating AMPK in skeletal muscle. *Biochemical and Biophysical Research Communications* 332, 885–891. https://doi.org/10.1016/j.bbrc.2005.05.035

Legarth, C., Grimm, D., Wehland, M., Bauer, J., Krüger, M., 2018. The impact of vitamin D in the treatment of essential hypertension. *International Journal of Molecular Sciences* 19. https://doi.org/10.3390/ijms19020455

Lewis, J.E., Nickell, L.A., Thompson, L.U., Szalai, J.P., Kiss, A., Hilditch, J.R., 2006. A randomized controlled trial of the effect of dietary soy and flaxseed muffins on quality of life and hot flashes during menopause. *Menopause* 13, 631–642. https://doi.org/10.1097/01.gme.0000191882.59799.67

Li, A.W., Goldsmith, C.-A.W., 2012. The effects of yoga on anxiety and stress. *Alternative Medicine Review* 17, 21–35.

Li, G., Xie, C., Lu, S., Nichols, R.G. *et al.*, 2017. Intermittent fasting promotes white adipose browning and decreases obesity by shaping the gut microbiota. *Cell Metabolism* 26, 672–685.e4. https://doi.org/10.1016/j.cmet.2017.08.019

Li, J., Zhao, F., Wang, Y., Chen, J., Tao, J. et al., 2017. Gut microbiota dysbiosis contributes to the development of hypertension. *Microbiome* 5, 14. https://doi.org/10.1186/s40168-016-0222-x

Li, S.S., Blanco Mejia, S., Lytvyn, L., Stewart, S.E. et al., 2017. Effect of plant protein on blood lipids: A systematic review and meta-analysis of randomized controlled trials. *Journal of the American Heart Association* 6. https://doi.org/10.1161/JAHA.117.006659

Li, Y., Hruby, A., Bernstein, A.M., Ley, S.H. et al., 2015. Saturated fats compared with unsaturated fats and sources of carbohydrates in relation to risk of coronary heart disease: A prospective cohort study. *Journal of the American College of Cardiology* 66, 1538–1548. https://doi.org/10.1016/j.jacc.2015.07.055

Li, Y., Zhong, X., Cheng, G., Zhao, C. et al., 2017. Hs-CRP and all-cause, cardiovascular, and cancer mortality risk: A meta-analysis. *Atherosclerosis* 259, 75–82. https://doi.org/10.1016/j.atherosclerosis.2017.02.003

Mancini, A., Raimondo, S., Di Segni, C., Persano, M. et al., 2013. Thyroid hormones and antioxidant systems: Focus on oxidative stress in cardiovascular and pulmonary diseases. *International Journal of Molecular Sciences* 14, 23893–23909. https://doi.org/10.3390/ijms141223893

Martín-Peláez, S., Mosele, J.I., Pizarro, N., Farràs, M. et al., 2017. Effect of virgin olive oil and thyme phenolic compounds on blood lipid profile: Implications of human gut microbiota. *European Journal of Nutrition* 56, 119–131. https://doi.org/10.1007/s00394-015-1063-2

Matori, H., Umar, S., Nadadur, R.D., Sharma, S. et al., 2012. Genistein, a soy phytoestrogen, reverses severe pulmonary hypertension and prevents right heart failure in rats. *Hypertension* 1979 60, 425–430. https://doi.org/10.1161/HYPERTENSIONAHA.112.191445

McDonald, D., Hyde, E., Debelius, J.W., Morton, J.T. et al., 2018. American Gut: An open platform for citizen science microbiome research. *mSystems* 3. https://doi.org/10.1128/mSystems.00031-18

Mejía-Mejía, E., Torres, R., Restrepo, D., 2018. Physiological coherence in healthy volunteers during laboratory-induced stress and controlled breathing. *Psychophysiology* 55, e13046. https://doi.org/10.1111/psyp.13046

Messina, M., 2016. Soy and health update: Evaluation of the clinical and epidemiologic literature. *Nutrients* 8. https://doi.org/10.3390/nu8120754

Mirhosseini, N., Rainsbury, J., Kimball, S.M., 2018. Vitamin D supplementation, serum 25(OH)D concentrations and cardiovascular disease risk factors: A systematic review and meta-analysis. *Frontiers in Cardiovascular Medicine* 5, 87. https://doi.org/10.3389/fcvm.2018.00087

Mohammadi, V., Khorvash, F., Feizi, A., Askari, G., 2018. Does alpha-lipoic acid supplementation modulate cardiovascular risk factors in patients with stroke? A randomized, double-blind clinical trial. *International Journal of Preventive Medicine* 9, 34. https://doi.org/10.4103/ijpvm.IJPVM_32_17

Moncayo, R., Moncayo, H., 2015. The WOMED model of benign thyroid disease: Acquired magnesium deficiency due to physical and psychological stressors relates to dysfunction of oxidative phosphorylation. *BBA Clinical* 3, 44–64. https://doi.org/10.1016/j.bbacli.2014.11.002

Moncayo, R., Moncayo, H., 2017. Applying a systems approach to thyroid physiology: Looking at the whole with a mitochondrial perspective instead of judging single TSH values or why we should know more about mitochondria to understand metabolism. *BBA Clinical* 7, 127–140. https://doi.org/10.1016/j.bbacli.2017.03.004

Moon, H.U., Ha, K.H., Han, S.J., Kim, H.J., Kim, D.J., 2019. The association of adiponectin and visceral fat with insulin resistance and β-cell dysfunction. *Journal of Korean Medical Science* 34, e7. https://doi.org/10.3346/jkms.2019.34.e7

Mora, S., Buring, J.E., Ridker, P.M., 2014. Discordance of low-density lipoprotein (LDL) cholesterol with alternative LDL-related measures and future coronary events. *Circulation* 129, 553–561. https://doi.org/10.1161/CIRCULATIONAHA.113.005873

Moriarty, P.M., Backes, J., Dutton, J.-A., He, J., Ruisinger, J.F., Schmelzle, K., 2013. Apple pectin for the reduction of niacin-induced flushing. *Journal of Clinical Lipidology* 7, 140–146. https://doi.org/10.1016/j. jacl.2012.11.005

Nery, C., Moraes, S.R.A.D., Novaes, K.A., Bezerra, M.A., Silveira, P.V.D.C., Lemos, A., 2017. Effectiveness of resistance exercise compared to aerobic exercise without insulin therapy in patients with type 2 diabetes mellitus: A meta-analysis. *Brazilian Journal of Physical Therapy* 21, 400–415. https://doi.org/10.1016/j.bjpt.2017.06.004

Nicolaides, N.C., Kyratzi, E., Lamprokostopoulou, A., Chrousos, G.P., Charmandari, E., 2015. Stress, the stress system and the role of glucocorticoids. *Neuroimmunomodulation* 22, 6–19. https://doi.org/10.1159/000362736

Ostadmohammadi, V., Milajerdi, A., Ghayour-Mobarhan, M., Ferns, G. *et al.*, 2019. The effects of vitamin D supplementation on glycemic control, lipid profiles and C-reactive protein among patients with cardiovascular disease: A systematic review and meta-analysis of randomized controlled trials. *Current Pharmaceutical Design* 25, 2. https://doi.org/10.2174/1381612825666190 308152943

Ouchi, N., Parker, J.L., Lugus, J.J., Walsh, K., 2011. Adipokines in inflammation and metabolic disease. *Nature Reviews Immunology* 11, 85–97. https://doi.org/10.1038/nri2921

Oyola, M.G., Handa, R.J., 2017. Hypothalamic-pituitary–adrenal and hypothalamic-pituitary–gonadal axes: Sex differences in regulation of stress responsivity. *Stress* 20, 476–494. https://doi.org/10.1080/10253890 .2017.1369523

Pagnini, C., Corleto, V.D., Martorelli, M., Lanini, C. *et al.*, 2018. Mucosal adhesion and anti-inflammatory effects of Lactobacillus rhamnosus GG in the human colonic mucosa: A proof-of-concept study. *World Journal of Gastroenterology* 24, 4652–4662. https://doi.org/10.3748/wjg.v24.i41.4652

Pan, B., Ge, L., Xun, Y.-Q., Chen, Y.-J. *et al.*, 2018. Exercise training modalities in patients with type 2 diabetes mellitus: A systematic review and network meta-analysis. *International Journal of Behavioral Nutrition and Physical Activity* 15, 72. https://doi. org/10.1186/s12966-018-0703-3

Pascoe, M.C., Thompson, D.R., Jenkins, Z.M., Ski, C.F., 2017. Mindfulness mediates the physiological markers of stress: Systematic review and meta-analysis. *Journal of Psychiatric Research* 95, 156–178. https://doi. org/10.1016/j.jpsychires.2017.08.004

Patterson, R.E., Laughlin, G.A., Sears, D.D., LaCroix, A.Z. *et al.*, 2015. Intermittent fasting and human metabolic health. *Journal of the Academy of Nutrition and Dietetics* 115, 1203–1212. https://doi.org/10.1016/j. jand.2015.02.018

Pearce, E.N., 2012. Update in lipid alterations in subclinical hypothyroidism. *Journal of Clinical Endocrinology and Metabolism* 97, 326–333. https://doi.org/10.1210/jc.2011-2532

Pirro, M., Vetrani, C., Bianchi, C., Mannarino, M.R., Bernini, F., Rivellese, A.A., 2017. Joint position statement on 'Nutraceuticals for the treatment of hypercholesterolemia' of the Italian Society of Diabetology (SID) and of the Italian Society for the Study of Arteriosclerosis (SISA). *Nutrition, Metabolism and Cardiovascular Diseases* 27, 2–17. https:// doi.org/10.1016/j.numecd.2016.11.122

Pleil, J.D., Smith, L.B., Zelnick, S.D., 2000. Personal exposure to JP-8 jet fuel vapors and exhaust at air force bases. *Environmental Health Perspectives* 108, 183–192.

Ramprasath, V.R., Jenkins, D.J., Lamarche, B., Kendall, C.W. *et al.*, 2014. Consumption of a dietary portfolio of cholesterol lowering foods improves blood lipids without affecting concentrations of fat soluble compounds. *Nutrition Journal* 13. https://doi. org/10.1186/1475-2891-13-101

Reutrakul, S., Van Cauter, E., 2018. Sleep influences on obesity, insulin resistance, and risk of type 2 diabetes. *Metabolism, Clinical and Experimental* 84, 56–66. https:// doi.org/10.1016/j.metabol.2018.02.010

Rubin, B.S., Schaeberle, C.M., Soto, A.M., 2019. The Case for BPA as an obesogen: Contributors to the controversy. *Frontiers in Endocrinology* 10, 30. https://doi.org/10.3389/fendo.2019.00030

Sato, M., Nakamura, K., Ogata, H., Miyashita, A. et al., 2011. Acute effect of late evening meal on diurnal variation of blood glucose and energy metabolism. *Obesity Research and Clinical Practice* 5, e220–e228. https://doi.org/10.1016/j.orcp.2011.02.001

Schlenker, W., Walker, R., 2011. Airports, air pollution, and contemporaneous health. *Review of Economic Studies* 83. https://doi.org/10.1093/restud/rdv043

Sivaramakrishnan, D., Fitzsimons, C., Kelly, P., Ludwig, K. et al., 2019. The effects of yoga compared to active and inactive controls on physical function and health related quality of life in older adults – systematic review and meta-analysis of randomised controlled trials. *International Journal of Behavioral Nutrition and Physical Activity* 16, 33. https://doi.org/10.1186/s12966-019-0789-2

Smith, M., Love, D.C., Rochman, C.M., Neff, R.A., 2018. Microplastics in seafood and the implications for human health. *Current Environmental Health Reports* 5, 375–386. https://doi.org/10.1007/s40572-018-0206-z

Sniderman, A.D., Lamarche, B., Contois, J.H., de Graaf, J., 2014. Discordance analysis and the Gordian Knot of LDL and non-HDL cholesterol versus apoB. *Current Opinion in Lipidology* 25, 461–467. https://doi.org/10.1097/MOL.0000000000000127

Sofi, F., Abbate, R., Gensini, G.F., Casini, A., 2010. Accruing evidence on benefits of adherence to the Mediterranean diet on health: An updated systematic review and meta-analysis. *American Journal of Clinical Nutrition* 92, 1189–1196. https://doi.org/10.3945/ajcn.2010.29673

Sonestedt, E., Hellstrand, S., Schulz, C.-A., Wallström, P. et al., 2015. The association between carbohydrate-rich foods and risk of cardiovascular disease is not modified by genetic susceptibility to dyslipidemia as determined by 80 validated variants. *PLoS ONE* 10. https://doi.org/10.1371/journal.pone.0126104

Song, M., Fung, T.T., Hu, F.B., Willett, W.C. et al., 2016. Association of animal and plant protein intake with all-cause and cause-specific mortality. *JAMA Internal Medicine* 176, 1453–1463. https://doi.org/10.1001/jamainternmed.2016.4182

Spiegel, K., Leproult, R., Van Cauter, E., 1999. Impact of sleep debt on metabolic and endocrine function. *Lancet* 354, 1435–1439. https://doi.org/10.1016/S0140-6736(99)01376-8

St Germain, A., Peterson, C.T., Robinson, J.G., Alekel, D.L., 2001. Isoflavone-rich or isoflavone-poor soy protein does not reduce menopausal symptoms during 24 weeks of treatment. *Menopause* 8, 17–26.

Stote, K.S., Baer, D.J., Spears, K., Paul, D.R. et al., 2007. A controlled trial of reduced meal frequency without caloric restriction in healthy, normal-weight, middle-aged adults. *American Journal of Clinical Nutrition* 85, 981–988.

Szymczak-Pajor, I., Śliwińska, A., 2019. Analysis of association between vitamin D deficiency and insulin resistance. *Nutrients* 11. https://doi.org/10.3390/nu11040794

Thomas, S.J., Calhoun, D., 2017. Sleep, insomnia, and hypertension: Current findings and future directions. *Journal of the American Society of Hypertension* 11, 122–129. https://doi.org/10.1016/j.jash.2016.11.008

Turcotte, L.P., Fisher, J.S., 2008. Skeletal muscle insulin resistance: Roles of fatty acid metabolism and exercise. *Physical Therapy* 88, 1279–1296. https://doi.org/10.2522/ptj.20080018

Ulrich, C.M., Toriola, A.T., Koepl, L.M., Sandifer, T. et al., 2012. Metabolic, hormonal and immunological associations with global DNA methylation among postmenopausal women. *Epigenetics* 7, 1020–1028. https://doi.org/10.4161/epi.21464

Vijayakumar, A., Kim, E., Kim, H., Choi, Y.J., Huh, K.B., Chang, N., 2017. Effects of folic acid supplementation on serum homocysteine levels, lipid profiles, and vascular parameters in post-menopausal Korean women with type 2 diabetes mellitus. *Nutrition Research and Practice* 11, 327–333. https://doi.org/10.4162/nrp.2017.11.4.327

Vojdani, A., 2014. A potential link between environmental triggers and autoimmunity. *Autoimmune Diseases* 2014. https://doi.org/10.1155/2014/437231

Wang, W.-M., Jin, H.-Z., 2017. Homocysteine: A potential common route for cardiovascular risk and DNA methylation in psoriasis. *Chinese Medical Journal* 130, 1980–1986. https://doi.org/10.4103/0366-6999.211895

Wellwood, C., Rardin, S., 2014. Adrenal and thyroid supplementation outperforms nutritional supplementation and medications for autoimmune thyroiditis. *Integrated Medicine: A Clinician's Journal* 13, 41–47.

Wood, B., Rea, M.S., Plitnick, B., Figueiro, M.G., 2013. Light level and duration of exposure determine the impact of self-luminous tablets on melatonin suppression. *Applied Ergonomics* 44, 237–240. https://doi.org/10.1016/j.apergo.2012.07.008

Yan, Q., Gu, Y., Li, X., Yang, W. *et al.*, 2017. Alterations of the gut microbiome in hypertension. *Frontiers in Cellular and Infection Microbiology* 7, 381. https://doi.org/10.3389/fcimb.2017.00381

Young, D.R., Hivert, M.-F., Alhassan, S., Camhi, S.M. *et al.*, 2016. Sedentary behavior and cardiovascular morbidity and mortality: A science advisory from the American Heart Association. *Circulation* 134, e262-279. https://doi.org/10.1161/CIR.0000000000000440

Zhang, Y., Li, X., Zou, D., Liu, W. *et al.*, 2008. Treatment of type 2 diabetes and dyslipidemia with the natural plant alkaloid berberine. *Journal of Clinical Endocrinology and Metabolism* 93, 2559–2565. https://doi.org/10.1210/jc.2007-2404

Zhang, Z., Wang, B., Wu, H., Chai, X., Wang, W., Peng, C.-K., 2017. Effects of slow and regular breathing exercise on cardiopulmonary coupling and blood pressure. *Medical and Biological Engineering and Computing* 55, 327–341. https://doi.org/10.1007/s11517-016-1517-6

Ziegenfuss, T.N., Hofheins, J.E., Mendel, R.W., Landis, J., Anderson, R.A., 2006. Effects of a water-soluble cinnamon extract on body composition and features of the metabolic syndrome in pre-diabetic men and women. *Journal of the International Society of Sports Nutrition* 3, 45–53. https://doi.org/10.1186/1550-2783-3-2-45

9

Gastrointestinal Health and the Gut–Brain Axis

Practitioner: Elspeth Stewart

Additional contribution to case write-up: Angela Walker

Introduction

In this case a detailed evaluation and support for gastrointestinal function led to improvements in neurological and digestive symptoms. This case demonstrates the gut–brain link, whereby the microbiota in the gastrointestinal tract interact with their host through pathways of the immune, neuroendocrine and nervous systems.

Initial case presentation

AB is a 42-year old woman, with a partner and no children. Twelve years prior to attending the practitioner's clinic, AB had experienced severe sudden-onset neurological symptoms including double vision, brain fog and dizziness. She saw a neurologist within three days of onset who diagnosed inflammation in the brain, which he indicated may potentially be a sign of early-stage multiple sclerosis (MS). A chemotherapy-based treatment was suggested, which the client declined. There were no test results from that period to refer back to and AB had not maintained a relationship with any neurologist after the initial flare-up.

Over the subsequent 12 years, AB had explored many avenues to support and improve her health. She had read around the topic of the gut–brain connection and self-prescribed a loosely Palaeo-style diet (see Box 9.1) and an extensive supplement programme (see Table 9.1). She reported improvements in her health from these actions but was now seeking personalized nutrition help as she felt improvements had stalled.

BOX 9.1 PALAEOLITHIC DIET DEFINITIONS

A Palaeolithic-style diet (PD) includes the consumption of meats, vegetables, eggs, nuts, seeds, fruits and oils from olive, walnut, flaxseed, avocado, macadamia and coconut. It excludes grains, legumes, dairy, refined sugar, processed foods, refined vegetable oils and salt. Potatoes are excluded due to their lectin content (Cordain *et al.*, 2000). It is proposed that the included foods are those that Palaeolithic man would have eaten, and, furthermore, that the excluded foods are those that have been introduced during the industrialization of agriculture – hence, the PD includes only foods that humans have genetically evolved to eat (Cordain *et al.*, 2005). Loren Cordain has published a number of peer-reviewed papers on the Palaeolithic-style diet and his website offers a useful resource for practitioners and clients (https://thepaleodiet.com). Compared with the low-FODMAP diet, used in Chapter 4, the PD (featured in Chapters 6, 9 and 11) could be said to be less defined and more open to interpretation in the lay media. There is clinical support, however, behind the diet. A summary of clinical trials that have examined the impact of the PD compared with other diets can be found in Wahls *et al.* (2018).

Symptoms at initial consultation

AB's list of symptoms at the initial consultation were as follows:

- persistent fatigue
- loss of strength in leg muscles with minimal exercise (e.g. a short walk), with recovery after a ten-minute rest
- vertigo and difficulties with balance and coordination
- difficulties with concentration and focus at times ('brain fog')
- migraines (onset within past two years)
- gastrointestinal bloating and flatulence
- constipation
- food intolerances
- sinus congestion and post-nasal drip
- insomnia.

AB worked full-time but had no additional energy for a social life or to exercise. She depended on taxis to commute to work and any appointments. While AB described her previous neurological symptoms (such as brain fog, inability to concentrate) as considerably improved compared with the initial flare-up, it was clear that her remaining symptoms around fatigue, digestion and physical health still significantly impacted her quality of life.

Health history

Figure 9.1 shows a timeline of AB's health history to assist the practitioner in the case analysis. Key events from her health history not already mentioned include food and sun sensitivities in childhood, periods of acne and several antibiotic courses while a teenager and in her 20s for various infections.

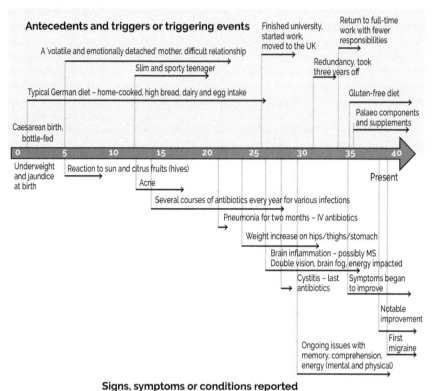

Figure 9.1 Timeline of AB's health history

Medication history

AB was taking no medications at the initial consultation but had taken the following medications in the past:

- cyproterone acetate and ethinylestradiol combination oestrogenic and antiandrogen contraceptive pill
- annual flu vaccinations
- over-the-counter decongestants (phenylephrine)
- high antibiotic intake throughout teens and 20s for various infections
  - most notably IV drip in early 20s for pneumonia.

Supplementation

AB was taking a number of supplements outlined in Table 9.1, all of which were self-prescribed. Full detail on the formulas can be found in Appendix 9.1. While AB was comfortable with this level of supplementation and seemed to tolerate them well, when a client arrives in clinic with this level of current supplementation, it raises the following questions:

- Are they all relevant/necessary?
- Are they suitable forms/brands/therapeutic dosages? (For example, vitamin D dosage was higher than this practitioner would have recommended.)
- Are there any contraindications or combined products taking levels of nutrients too high?
- How to incorporate additional or alternative supplements if indicated from clinical analysis.

Table 9.1 Supplements at initial consultation

Supplement	Dose per day
Probiotic	*Lactobacillus acidophilus* 25 bn CFU *Bifidobacterium* 25 bn CFU
L-glutamine	1000 mg
L-glutathione	150 mg
L-cysteine hydrochloride	600 mg
Vitamin C (as ascorbic acid)	1500 mg
B complex	See Appendix 9.1 for formula and dose
Bromelain	400 mg
Omega EPA/DHA	See Appendix 9.1 for formula and dose
Ginkgo Biloba	600 mg
Magnesium (from magnesium l-threonate)	144 mg
CoQ$_{10}$	200 mg
Quercetin	500 mg

cont.

Supplement	Dose per day
Vitamin C and K complex	See Appendix 9.1 for formula and dose
Turmeric	500 mg
Vitamin D3	10,000 IU
Multivitamin	See Appendix 9.1 for formula and dose Taking every other day, alternating with the multimineral
Multimineral	See Appendix 9.1 for formula and dose Taking every other day, alternating with the multivitamin
Magnesium (as citrate)	As required at night if sore calf muscles – up to 450 mg

Current diet

AB had self-prescribed a gluten-exclusion diet for six years and felt this improved her symptoms. Soon after going gluten-free, she implemented what she described as a Palaeolithic-style diet (PD) (see Box 9.1) which she also felt was helpful. Over the intervening years she had relaxed some areas of the PD (reintroducing dairy and some grains) and then one year prior to visiting the practitioner she reinstated a stricter diet as some symptoms had started to return, eliminating all grains again and also eliminating nightshade family vegetables. She continued to eat some dairy products. Although mindful of refined carbohydrate intake, she still had what could be described as 'a sweet tooth', eating dark chocolate most days, sometimes a sorbet, and drinking one to two glasses of wine two to three times a week. Honey was used as a sweetener.

Lifestyle factors and environmental exposures

AB finished university, relocated to a new city and country, and started working in a high-pressure environment in the same year as the neurological flare-up. She also reported having a difficult relationship with her mother. All are factors that may influence the individual's stress response.

Investigations

Previous tests brought to the initial consultation

AB had a recent vitamin D test, with total 25-hydroxy vitamin D of 160 nmol/L (reference range 75–200 nmol/L). Her ongoing supplementation of vitamin D (10,000 IU QD) was therefore above recommended levels (Bischoff-Ferrari *et al.*, 2006).

Prior IgG (all class) food sensitivity tests showed a high number of elevated IgG reactions (38 'highly reactive' foods) including elevated IgG antibodies to wheat, gluten (gliadin), buckwheat, corn and eggs (white and yolk). IgG antibodies to food (discussed further in Chapter 3) represent a delayed immune response to food. Large immune complexes can be formed from IgG antibodies (class 1, 2 and 3) which bind to complement and stimulate inflammation.

While conventional gliadin antibody testing is not sensitive, specific or accurate for true gluten allergy (coeliac disease) identification (Rashtak *et al.*, 2008), the client was already on a self-imposed gluten-exclusion diet which, as previously stated, she believed to be beneficial. A large number of IgG elevations may represent a situation of increased intestinal permeability, allowing larger food particles that would normally stay within the intestinal lumen to pass across the gastrointestinal barrier into the bloodstream (Karakuła-Juchnowicz *et al.*, 2017). This was a factor which led the practitioner to recommend further digestive function testing.

Digestive function testing

The practitioner suspected that dysfunction in the microbiome and intestinal barrier and immune function could be involved in this case and recommended digestive investigations via comprehensive stool, small intestinal bacterial overgrowth (SIBO) and intestinal permeability tests. The breadth of functional testing in this area aimed to provide a deeper evaluation of some of the underlying factors involved.

Gut permeability profile – six-hour PEG urine collection

The results of the six-hour polyethylene glycol (PEG) test are shown in Figure 9.2. The test is described in Chapter 3. In the results below, it can be seen that PEG molecules between 330 and 550 molecular weight have reached the urine at a higher proportion than would be expected in an optimally functioning intestinal barrier. This indicates increased intestinal permeability in the gastrointestinal tract.

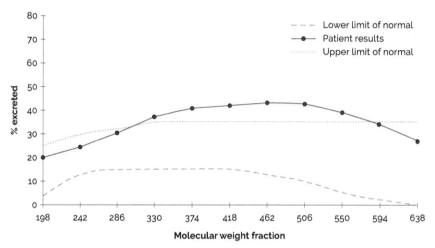

Figure 9.2 PEG six-hour urine collection result (see online colour plate)

Comment: Increased gut permeability to PEG from molecular weight 330 to molecular weight 550

Breath hydrogen and methane profile for SIBO

The use of hydrogen and methane breath tests for identification of small intestinal bacterial overgrowth (SIBO) is discussed in Chapter 3. The SIBO test showed no fermentation occurring until 120 minutes, which indicates fermentation in the lower colon only. This is a normal finding.

Comprehensive stool analysis with parasitology

The practitioner ordered a culture methodology stool test, which is discussed in more detail in Chapter 3. Figure 9.3 shows an excerpt from the test result. For the semi-quantified results in this test 1+ is low and 4+ is high. For beneficial bacteria one hopes to see +3 or +4; for pathogenic the target is none. As discussed in Chapter 3, the interpretation is based on overall patterns rather than a single result. A summary of the results from the test are as follows:

- Secretory IgA (sIgA) was below the reference range. sIgA is the first line of antigen-specific immune defence and prevents pathogens as well as commensal bacteria from crossing the epithelial surface (Kaetzel, 2014).
- *Lactobacillus* species and *Enterococcus* species levels were low, depicted by the 1+ and 2+ semi-quantifiable results from the culture methodology test. The other beneficial bacteria were reported at more optimal levels of +4.
- Modest levels of yeast albeit commensal yeast (two strains of *Candida* plus *Rhodotorula mucilaginosa*) at the semi-quantifiable level of +1.
- Bacteria species which potentially represent microbial imbalance; *Alpha haemolytic strep*, *Bacillus* and *Gamma haemolytic strep* were reported at semi-quantifiable levels of 3+, 2+ and 2+ respectively.
- Taken together, the above points support an interpretation of dysbiosis within the microbiome (see Box 9.2). Although the evidence is still emerging, there are studies which show differences in microbiota populations in those with irritable bowel syndrome and other functional bowel disorders (Distrutti *et al.*, 2016; Simrén *et al.*, 2013). Alterations in microbiota populations have also been reported in patients with MS compared with controls (Chen *et al.*, 2016).
- While the reliable markers for inflammation in the intestinal tract, lactoferrin and calprotectin, were in normal range, lysozyme was elevated. Elevated lysozyme has been found in patients with inflammatory bowel disease (van der Sluys Veer *et al.*, 1998). More recently, it has been shown that Paneth cells in the intestine secrete lysozyme to counter a bacterial infection (Bel *et al.*, 2017). While no specific infections (pathogenic bacteria or parasites) were reported in the stool test, it is possible that the lysozyme was elevated in response to the commensal bacteria and yeasts (dysbiosis). The elevated lysozyme supports the interpretation that microbial dysbiosis is an issue for AB.

- Markers for digestion and absorption, short-chain fatty acid ratios (not shown in Figure 9.3), were within range and no red blood cells or occult blood detected.
- No parasites identified (two stool samples were provided which increases confidence in parasitology findings using culture methods) (CDC, 2018).

BOX 9.2 DYSBIOSIS – WHAT DOES IT MEAN?

Dysbiosis refers to an alteration in the normal commensal gut microbiota so that homeostasis is disturbed. This could involve an increase in pathogenic bacteria. It also includes any situation of disturbed homeostasis within the microbiota. In this case, no pathogenic bacteria were identified, but there was an overall pattern of low beneficial bacteria relative to commensal bacterial and yeast, in addition to indications of a disturbed immune response. Placing this in clinical context, the more 'subtle' dysbiosis helps explain the client's symptoms and corresponds to the health timeline.

A functional matrix, based on the Institute of Functional Medicine 2011 model, was used by the practitioner to order her analysis of the case. As shown in Figure 9.4, AB's matrix notes are clustered primarily around assimilation, structural integrity, communication and energy.

Reviewing the client's case history, the practitioner noted a caesarean birth, bottle feeding after birth and a history of antibiotic use for childhood infections, all of which have been associated with impairments to the microbiome in later life (Belkaid and Hand, 2014; Karkman, Lehtimäki and Ruokolainen, 2017). The evidence is emerging (currently based on animal studies) that the microbiome influences the stress response and that microbiota may have a role in changing behaviour and brain function (Foster, Rinaman and Cryan, 2017). There is also a relationship in the opposite direction: human studies have demonstrated how acute stress can increase intestinal permeability (Vanuytsel et al., 2014). Furthermore, a hyperactive stress response can be 'primed' by early psychological stressors (Godoy et al., 2018).

A difficult relationship with her mother represents a potential early psychological stressor in AB's case. It is possible this 'primed' her stress response to react acutely in the high-pressure environment of her new job shortly before her neurological flare-up. Perhaps this played a role in her intestinal permeability and, combined with a disturbed microbiome, influenced the central nervous system.

BACTERIOLOGY CULTURE

Expected/beneficial flora	Commensal (imbalanced) flora	Dysbiotic flora
4+ Bacteroides fragilis group	3+ Alpha haemolytic strep	
4+ Bifidobacterium spp.	2+ Bacillus spp.	
4+ Escherichia coli	2+ Gamma haemolytic strep	
1+ Lactobacillus spp.		
2+ Enterococcus spp.		
2+ Clostridium spp.		
NG = no growth		

YEAST CULTURE

Normal flora	Dysbiotic flora
1+ Candida intermedia	
1+ Candida lambica	
1+ Rhodotorula mucilaginosa	

INFLAMMATION

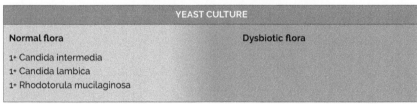

	Within	Outside	Reference range	
Lactoferrin	< 0.5		< 7.3	Lactoferrin and calprotectin are reliable markers for differentiating organic inflammation (IBD) from function symptoms (IBS) and for management of IBD. Monitoring levels of faecal lactoferrin and calprotectin can play an essential role in determining effectiveness of therapy, are good predictors of IBD remission, and can indicate a low risk of relapse. Lysozyme is an enzyme secreted at the site of inflammation in the GI tract and elevated levels have been identified in IBD patients. White blood cells (WBC) and mucus in the stool can occur with bacterial and parasitic infections, with mucosal irritation, and inflammatory bowel diseases such as Crohn's disease or ulcerative colitis.
Calprotectin	< 10		≤ 50 µg/g	
Lysozyme		687	≤ 600 ng/mL	
White blood cells	None		None–rare	
Mucus	Neg		Neg	

IMMUNOLOGY

	Within	Outside	Reference range	
Secretory IgA		46.6	51–204 mg/dL	Secretory IgA (sIgA) is secreted by mucosal tissue and represents the first line of defense of the GI mucosa and is central to the normal function of the GI tract as an immune barrier. Elevated levels of sIgA have been associated with an unregulated immune response.

Figure 9.3 Except from the comprehensive stool test (see online colour plate)

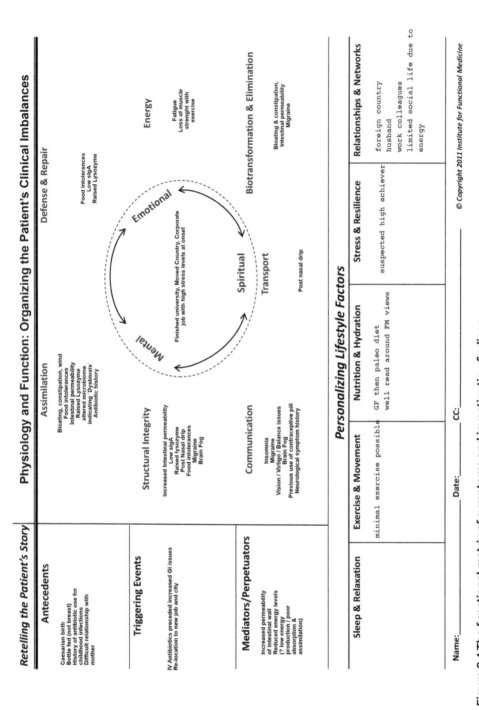

Figure 9.4 The functional matrix of symptoms and investigation findings

Source: Reproduced with permission from Institute for Functional Medicine (2011)

While a historical interpretation cannot be confirmed or disproved, it does help the practitioner to understand the potential factors involved and therefore where to focus recommendations. It played another important role; in explaining these theories to AB, it helped her to understand how her situation may have unfolded and build confidence in the approach that would be taken. This is an example of the narrative between the practitioner and client that is discussed in Chapter 2.

The practitioner elected to focus on the follow initial goals:

- support intestinal membrane health
- support intestinal immune health
- support a balanced microbiota.

This approach is often referred to as a 5R programme (Remove, Replace, Reinoculate, Repair, Rebalance). The approach is typically used by practitioners as a framework to personalize a protocol for a client where suspected gastrointestinal dysfunction is present.

The decision to focus initially on supporting gastrointestinal health was taken because gastrointestinal function may be the underlying driver for other symptoms or imbalances. In addressing these factors, the practitioner believed the programme would support assimilation and structural integrity and provide the necessary foundations for AB's health to improve. Once improvements to digestive health had been achieved, other remaining symptoms would be reviewed and addressed, as deemed appropriate from Figure 9.4.

Given the suspicion around AB's heightened stress response system and the role this could have played as a triggering factor, it was important to address this through the recommendations. As the next section will show, the practitioner elected to support this through lifestyle interventions rather than using specific supplements. This decision was taken partly to minimize additional supplements and partly on the basis that AB had already taken steps towards reducing her stress load and balancing her stress response with relaxation techniques.

Initial management plan

A personalized 5R programme for AB was designed, summarized in Table 9.2.

Diet

The dietary recommendations were as follows:

- Minimize foods containing simple sugars. For AB, this included wine, chocolate, sorbet, honey and a reduction in her fruit sugars.
- Continue to avoid gluten. AB reported a preference and belief that any deviation from gluten avoidance led to worsening of symptoms. This was sufficient justification for the practitioner to maintain gluten avoidance at this stage. The subject would be reviewed at a later stage.
- AB was including some white rice prior to seeing the practitioner. The practitioner encouraged her to keep this in her diet rather than exclude it to ensure she had sufficient carbohydrate options. The goal was to expand on plant-based dietary options, aiding microbial diversity. Rice may increase Firmicutes phylum, which includes *Lactobacillus* species. which were known to be low (Sheflin *et al.*, 2017). Rice would not be considered part of a PD, but the practitioner is tailoring the diet to be appropriate for AB's current needs.
- Increase vegetable intake, providing specific recommendations and guidance as follows:
  - Aim for 50% of the plate or more to be vegetables, choosing a variety of different-coloured vegetables to increase microbial diversity and eubiosis (Toribio-Mateas, 2018). Chapter 7 contains a wider discussion on the effect of dietary variety on the microbiome.
  - Use root vegetables as carbohydrate options for meals – for example, beetroots, carrots, turnips, sweet potatoes.
  - Eat 2–3 portions per day of brassica vegetables, a source of sulforaphane as well as fibre, folates and sulphur, which

are useful micronutrients for detoxification pathways and support microbiome diversity. Brassicas have also been linked to protection of inflammation in the brain, highlighting a potential role in gut–brain axis (Gu *et al.*, 2010).

- Nightshade vegetables were reintroduced as no benefit was experienced while excluded.

- A protein source was recommended with each meal so that 25–30% of the area of the plate contained protein.

- In order to keep the diet as diverse as possible, it was agreed to continue to eliminate only foods where AB felt she had a definite symptomatic reaction. Cow's milk did not appear to cause symptoms (and IgG antibodies were not elevated to cow's milk) and remained in AB's diet, providing cheese as a convenient protein source for some meals. Eggs were excluded as AB felt she had a symptomatic reaction to them and elevated IgG antibodies had been reported. Fish and meat provided continued protein sources. AB was asked to eat two portions of oily fish per week.

Table 9.2 Personalized 5R programme

5Rs	Function	Key strategies
Remove	Support optimal microbiota (from dysbiosis to eubiosis)	Avoid simple sugars Use selected antimicrobial/antifungal agents
Replace	Support digestive potency, to ensure optimal assimilation	Chew thoroughly, eat mindfully, stress management Betaine HCl
Reinoculate	Support microbiota population and diversity	Provide fibre, fermented foods, probiotics
Repair	Support intestinal membrane health	Probiotics, glutamine and support for connective tissues
Rebalance	Support intestinal immune health, improve sIgA levels	Micronutrients, *Saccharomyces boulardii*

Supplements (phase 1)

The following supplements were recommended:

- Multinutrient liver support powder containing rice protein concentrate. Dose and full ingredients may be found in Appendix 9.2. Per daily serving (two scoops) contained 15 g protein, 21 g carbohydrate of which 16 g was simple carbohydrates, 2.5 g fat.
- Betaine HCl 300 mg and pepsin 5 mg with each meal to support digestion and assimilation.
- Grapefruit seed extract – 500 mg TID with meals.
- Caprylic acid – 4226 mg TID with meals.
- Garlic concentrate – 500 mg BID with meals.
- *Saccharomyces boulardii* – 1.5+ billion organisms QD.

It was recommended to introduce the new supplements one at a time and at half dose, gradually building to full dose. As bacteria die-off they can release endotoxins and sometimes a rise in cytokines, which can manifest as Jarisch–Herxheimer reactions (Pound and May, 2005). Based on the practitioner's experience, Jarisch–Herxheimer reactions may occur when antimicrobials are introduced too quickly.

AB was already taking many supplements, and although she didn't have reservations about adding more, the practitioner recommended simplifying things by stopping those products that were not contributing to the goals of the 5R protocol (such as glutamine for gut repair and turmeric for inflammation) or directly supportive of energy production (CoQ$_{10}$) or detoxification/histamine clearance (glutathione, quercetin, bromelain). AB was asked to stop the multivitamin and the multimineral (as these would overlap with the liver support multinutrient powder), the vitamin D (as her serum level was optimal), probiotics (given the antimicrobial supplements to be added) and the omega EPA and DHA (while supportive, these essential fats could be supplied by eating oily fish). Table 9.3 summarizes changes in supplements from AB's self-prescribed supplements to those recommended at this stage.

Supplement rationale

Stomach acidity is key to optimal digestion and assimilation, not only to denature protein in the stomach but also to create the right pH to stimulate digestive secretions further down, from the gallbladder and pancreas. Hypochlorhydria (low stomach acidity) has been associated with digestive symptoms including stomach pain and constipation (Iwai *et al.*, 2013). Betaine HCl was included as it has been shown to support optimal stomach acidity (Yago *et al.*, 2014).

A systematic review concluded *S. boulardii* may interfere with intestinal pathogens and could increase sIgA levels in the intestine (McFarland, 2010).

Antimicrobial supplements were included to address the yeast and commensal bacterial which are part of the overall dysbiosis as discussed above. The main active antimicrobial constituent of garlic is allicin (allyl 2-propene thiosulfinate), which is formed when the herb is crushed and alliinase (an enzyme from the bundle sheath cells) combines with the substrate alliin. Garlic has been found to interrupt quorum sensing, the communication system by which pathogenic bacteria develop biofilm and antibiotic resistance (Harjai, Kumar and Singh, 2010; Jakobsen *et al.*, 2012).

Caprylic (octanoic) acid has an antimicrobial action on yeast and bacteria species (Huang *et al.*, 2011; Pohl, Kock and Thibane, 2011). It also inhibits IL-8 secretion and hence has an anti-inflammatory action (Hoshimoto *et al.*, 2002).

Grapefruit seed extract (GSE) has been shown to have in-vitro antibacterial activity against a broad spectrum of gram-negative and gram-positive organisms at safe dilution levels (Heggers *et al.*, 2002) as well as yeasts (Cvetnić and Vladimir-Knezević, 2004). While in-vivo studies are lacking, GSE has been used in natural medicine for many years and has anecdotal clinical support for its use as an antifungal and antimicrobial agent (Martins *et al.*, 2014)

In addition to the slow introduction of antimicrobial supplements, the effect and likelihood of Jarisch–Herxheimer reactions can be minimized with the use of fibre (soluble and insoluble) and nutrients that support detoxification pathways (Martins *et al.*, 2014). The multinutrient liver support formula was recommended to provide easily available macronutrients and micronutrients that should support detoxification pathways. This included glutathione (Altomare *et al.*, 1996; Dentico *et al.*, 1995; Honda *et al.*, 2017) and green tea extract (Bernatoniene and Kopustinskiene, 2018; Kumar *et al.*, 2012). The powder was also useful as a simple meal replacement or snack, given the macronutrient levels (13 g protein, 21 g carbohydrate and 2.5 g fat). It replaced the multivitamin, multimineral and B complex that AB was previously taking.

Additional advice

AB was advised to take time to eat each meal and chew each mouthful thoroughly. Stress-management advice included the use of apps for meditation and to undertake simple breathing exercises known as deep belly breathing. Breathing exercises have been shown in primary studies to increase heartrate variability and reduce pulse rate as measures of an improved stress response (Mejía-Mejía, Torres and Restrepo, 2018). Meditation can reduce the physiological markers of stress according to a systematic review (Pascoe *et al.*, 2017).

Table 9.3 Summary of supplement recommendations compared with self-prescribed supplements

Supplement	Dose/day at initial intake	Self-prescribed	Practitioner recommended
Probiotic		✓	
L-glutamine	1000 mg	✓	✓
L-glutathione	150 mg	✓	✓
L-cysteine hydrochloride (later as N-acetyl-L-cysteine)	600 mg	✓	✓
Vitamin C (as ascorbic acid)	1500 mg	✓	✓

B complex	See Appendix 9.1	✓	
Bromelain	400 mg	✓	✓
Omega EPA/DHA	See Appendix 9.1	✓	
Ginkgo biloba	600 mg	✓	
Magnesium (from magnesium l-threonate)	144 mg	✓	✓
CoQ$_{10}$ (in C2 as ubiquinol)	200 mg	✓	✓
Quercetin	500 mg	✓	✓
Vitamin C and K complex	See Appendix 9.1	✓	
Turmeric	500 mg		✓
Vitamin D3	10000 IU	✓	
Multivitamin	See Appendix 9.1	✓	
Multimineral	See Appendix 9.1	✓	
Magnesium (as citrate)	Up to 450 mg	✓	
Multinutrient liver support	See Appendix 9.2		✓
Betain HCL	300 mg		✓
Saccharomyces boulardii	1.5 billion CFU		✓
Botanical antimicrobials (grapefruit seed extract (GSE), caprylic acid (CA), garlic)	GSE 500mg TID, CA 4226mg TID, garlic 500mg BID		✓

Patient management

Despite instructions to introduce supplements slowly, in her eagerness to get started AB had introduced all the supplements at full dose on the same day. She then felt, in her own words, 'uncoordinated, weak, dizzy and in bad shape'. The practitioner suspected this was a Jarisch–Herxheimer reaction and recommended that she reduce to a lower dose for a few days, wait for the feeling to ease and then gradually build back up to full dose, pausing at a dose if symptoms returned. AB was able to do this successfully with no return of the initial symptoms.

A few weeks later AB reported as follows:

- She had found it initially difficult to eliminate sugary foods but soon adjusted.
- She felt a 'peaceful tired' for the first few days.
- Initially, she fluctuated between constipation and diarrhea, but within a few weeks was passing a daily stool.
- There was a notable improvement to energy levels; she was now able to walk up to 700 m without any loss of strength in leg muscles.

Repair and reinoculated adjustments (phase 2)

The protocol transitioned towards 'repair and reinoculate', and the practitioner stopped some of the initial 'remove' supplements.

Supplements stopped

- Grapefruit seed extract/caprylic acid/garlic concentrate.
- Multinutrient powder.

Continued 5R supplements

- Betaine HCl.
- *S. Boulardii*.

New 5R supplements

- Multivitamin, 1 QD for four weeks, then gradual increase to TID. This was easier compliance than the powder formula; the formula can be found in Appendix 9.2. At 1 QD this is a similar dosage to the multinutrient powder.
- Multi-strain probiotic (QD):
  - *Lactobacillus plantarum* 10 billion CFUs
  - *Lactobacillus salivarius* 4 billion CFUs
  - *Lactobacillus rhamnosus* 3 billion CFUs.
- Hydrolyzed collagen 5g each morning.
- Digestive support powder containing glutamine, N-acetyl glucosamine (NAG), slippery elm and methylsulfonylmethane (MSM) – 1 tablespoon at bedtime.

Table 9.4 summarizes the new supplement recommendations and how they differ from those that AB self-prescribed and those prescribed initially by the practitioner.

The mechanisms by which probiotics are thought to exert effect are not fully understood but are thought to involve (Baugher and Klaenhammer, 2011):

- production of bacteriocins (with an antibacterial effect)
- immune system modulation
- cell adhesion factors, leading to competitive exclusion of other microbiota
- production of SCFA and other metabolites which support the native microbiota environment.

It is now widely accepted that supplementary probiotics do not colonize the GI tract for more than a few days; however, there is evidence to suggest that they do exert a balancing effect on the intestinal ecosystem and can have a restorative effect upon microbial diversity. In a murine model of intestinal permeability, *Lactobacillus rhamnosus* attenuated cytokine production and gastrointestinal leakage (Panpetch *et al.*, 2018), while in a small RCT of patients with gastrointestinal inflammation,

L. rhamnosus was shown to reduce expression of inflammation markers (Pagnini *et al.*, 2018). *L. plantarum* produced diverse and potent antimicrobial peptides and has support from clinical trials (although not conclusive) that its use leads to a reduction in irritable bowel syndrome (IBS) symptoms compared with controls (Seddik *et al.*, 2017).

Given the role of collagen as a structural protein in connective tissues, dietary intake of collagen and supplementation is proposed to support connective tissue synthesis. In an in-vitro model of increased intestinal permeability, collagen peptides were found to improve intestinal barrier function (Chen *et al.*, 2017).

Glutamine is a key substrate for cells in the intestinal wall, and dietary or supplement intake has been shown to improve intestinal barrier function (Benjamin *et al.*, 2012; Kim and Kim, 2017; Wang *et al.*, 2015).

NAG is another building block of glycoproteins and other connective tissue building blocks (Chen, Shen and Liu, 2010) and in a pilot study was shown to improve outcomes in chronic inflammatory bowel disease (IBD) (Salvatore *et al.*, 2000). While AB does not have IBD, the finding is suggestive that NAG can support gastrointestinal immune tolerance. Slippery elm (as part of the digestive support powder) has been shown to improve some symptoms of IBS (Hawrelak and Myers, 2010).

Use of previous supplements
The following supplements were reviewed from her previous list, with some adjustments to streamline and simplify – for example, use of products that contain more than one ingredient to minimize number of capsules:

- Formula containing vitamin C 900 mg, quercetin 500 mg, bromelain 100 mg. AB noticed improvements when she first started these nutrients and thus we kept them. The benefit of these, in conjunction with ongoing symptoms, later lead the practitioner to consider histamine clearance issues as a potential factor.

- Magnesium 116 mg as magnesium malate QD, replacing threonate and citrate forms. The bioavailability of different magnesium preparations is inconclusive, possibly due to the variety of factors that can increase (e.g. initial magnesium status) or decrease (e.g. phytate, oxalates) absorption (Schuchardt and Hahn, 2017). Magnesium malate may be more effective for ATP production given that malate is a metabolite of the citric acid cycle (Russell *et al.*, 1995). Magnesium malate was shown to improve pain scores in patients with fibromyalgia (FM), thought to be due to improvements in ATP synthesis (Abraham and Flechas, 1992; Russell *et al.*, 1995). While AB does not have FM, fatigue is present and hence support for ATP synthesis may be beneficial. There is some evidence that magnesium malate levels remain higher in the serum for a prolonged period compared with other magnesium compounds, which could potentially mean increased availability for cellular uptake (Uysal *et al.*, 2019).
- Ubiquinol 100 mg. CoQ_{10} acts both as an antioxidant and as a key cofactor for adenosine triphosphate (ATP) production within in the electron transport chain in the mitochondria. The brain requires high amounts of ATP. AB experienced very low energy levels and experienced brain fog after periods of physical exertion, suggesting energy production was compromised. CoQ_{10} supplementation has been demonstrated to be beneficial in supporting both fatigue and cognitive function in chronic fatigue (Werbach, 2000). High-dose CoQ_{10} supplementation (500 mg/d) improved fatigue and mood in patients with MS patients compared with control groups (Sanoobar *et al.*, 2016). There is in-vitro evidence that ubiquinol is more bioavailable than ubiquinone (Failla, Chitchumroonchokchai and Aoki, 2014) and empirically the practitioner has found that some clients do better on the ubiquinol form.
- Turmeric root extract 500 mg extract 95% curcumin. Curcumin has been shown to exhibit anti-inflammatory activity through multiple cell-signalling pathways including NFKB, COX2 and Nrf2 (Kunnumakkara *et al.*, 2017).

- N-acetyl-L-cysteine (NAC) 600 mg. In addition to supporting glutathione production through supplying the limited amino acid cysteine (Kasperczyk *et al.*, 2013), cell culture studies have shown NAC to disrupt *Candida albicans* biofilm production (Abd, Ela and Gad, 2014).
- Vitamin D 2000 IU. Vitamin D was reintroduced at a maintenance dose of 2000 IU.
- Vitamin K2 formula 2200 mg (with 10 mg vitamin C). Vitamin K2 was reintroduced alongside the vitamin D as there appears to be a synergistic action between the two nutrients (van Ballegooijen *et al.*, 2017).

Further testing

AB had never been tested for coeliac disease prior to going gluten-free and continued to experience notable symptoms if she ever accidentally consumed gluten. Having avoided gluten for so long, it was no longer possible to run a coeliac antibody profile unless she was willing to reintroduce gluten over an extended period of time in order for the relevant markers to rise. AB was given the option to check her coeliac susceptibility HLA DQ2/8 genes. AB knew gluten made her feel terrible and maintained she intended never to eat gluten again, so she felt determining susceptibility to coeliac disease was somewhat irrelevant.

The practitioner was keen to widen her dietary intake, to avoid unnecessary dietary avoidance and to support microbial diversity. Antigenic similarity or cross-reactivity can exist between gluten and other dietary proteins, which can lead to a continuation of symptoms related to gluten sensitivity, despite the avoidance of gluten-containing foods (Vojdani, 2015; Vojdani and Tarash, 2013). It was agreed to test for these potential interactions. Further information on these tests can be found in Chapter 3.

The test showed out-of-range results for cow's milk, casomorphin, milk chocolate, oats, sorghum, teff and egg. This indicated that, if consumed, these foods were initiating an immune response that could also represent a trigger or mediator of ongoing increased intestinal permeability. From this list, cow's-milk-based foods (including cheese) were the only ones frequently eaten (at that stage). All dairy-based foods were now excluded. It was also recommended that AB diligently avoid the other out-of-range foods.

Alongside rice, the grains quinoa, amaranth and millet were all negative. This gave the practitioner confidence that these foods could be reintroduced, which would increase dietary options.

The option to repeat the IgG panel that AB had carried out prior to the first consultation was discussed. It was decided not to do so, in part from a perspective of resources but also to allow sufficient time for the gastrointestinal repair to occur, as the practitioner suspected this was a factor in the previous number of IgG elevations.

Six-month follow-up

AB reported that her energy levels and stamina continued to improve and she could walk up to 1.5 km without difficulty. Her brain fog was improved to the extent she felt able to apply for a new role within her organization – a major achievement given that six months prior she had struggled to tackle anything outside her daily work routine. AB's digestion had improved and she experienced less bloating, and while episodes of constipation and loose stools still occurred, they were less frequent. The intestinal permeability test was repeated and now showed normal findings. This suggests that there was improvement in her gastrointestinal integrity (and perhaps improved microbiota balance, although this was not retested)

Some symptoms persisted, including occasional migraines, sinus congestion/post-nasal drip. The practitioner and AB discussed a follow-up with the neurologist, but this was not something AB wanted to pursue. Histamine was considered, based on 'positive' responses to previous self-prescribed supplements, and at the time of writing the case study this is being explored through support for histamine metabolism and the avoidance of high histamine-containing foods.

Table 9.4 Summary of changes in supplements from initial intake, through phase 1 (P1, page 268) and phase 2 (P2, page 272)

Supplement	Dose/day at initial intake	Self-prescribed	P1	P2
Probiotic		✓		✓
L-glutamine	1000 mg	✓	✓	
L-glutathione	150 mg	✓	✓	
L-cysteine hydrochloride (later as N-acetyl-L-cysteine)	600 mg	✓	✓	✓
Vitamin C (as ascorbic acid)	1500 mg	✓	✓	✓ 900 mg
B complex	See Appendix 9.1	✓		
Bromelain	400 mg	✓	✓	✓ 100 mg
Omega EPA/DHA	See Appendix 9.1	✓		
Ginkgo biloba	600 mg	✓		
Magnesium (from magnesium l-threonate)	144 mg	✓	✓	
CoQ$_{10}$ (in C2 as ubiquinol)	200 mg	✓	✓	✓ 100 mg
Quercetin	500 mg	✓	✓	✓
Vitamin C and K complex	See Appendix 9.1	✓		✓
Turmeric	500 mg		✓	✓
Vitamin D3	10,000 IU	✓		✓2000 IU
Multivitamin	See Appendix 9.1	✓		

Multimineral	See Appendix 9.1	✓		
Magnesium (as citrate)	Up to 450 mg	✓		
Multinutrient liver support	See Appendix 9.2		✓	
Betaine HCl	300 mg		✓	✓
Saccharomyces boulardii	1.5 billion CFU		✓	✓
Botanical antimicrobials (GSE, CA, garlic)	GSE 500mg TID, CA 4226mg TID, garlic 500mg BID		✓	
Multivitamin	See Appendix 9.2			✓
Collagen	5 g			✓
Glutamine (NAG), slippery elm and MSM	1 tablespoon			✓
Magnesium as malate	116 mg			✓

Discussion

There is a growing body of evidence for a gut, brain and microbiome axis and its involvement in neurological related conditions, which appears to have been central to this case. The structural components of the gut–brain–microbiota axis are the central nervous system, the microbiota, the autonomic nervous system, the enteric nervous system and neuroendocrine and neuroimmune systems (Dinan *et al.*, 2015).

Disturbance or imbalance in the microbial composition and intestinal permeability has been identified in MS. Le Berre and colleagues (2017) identified an altered immune response to microbial antigens in patients with MS. A comparison of 20 relapsing–remitting patients with MS with 40 healthy controls showed moderate dysbiosis in MS subjects and significant differences in 21 species of microbiota (Miyake *et al.*, 2015). Similarly, Chen and colleagues (2016) found differences in the microbiota of MS patients (increased abundance of *Pseudomonas, Mycoplasma, Haemophilus, Blautia* and *Dorea* genera) compared with controls (increased abundance of *Parabacteroides, Adlercreutzia* and *Prevotella* genera). In a study of 22 relapsing–remitting patients with multiple sclerosis, intestinal permeability (measured by lactulose/mannitol levels in the urine) was significantly higher in the MS group compared with 18 control subjects (Buscarinu *et al.*, 2017).

It is thought to be a bidirectional axis, with the composition of the gut microbiota, the integrity of the gastrointestinal barrier as well as neurotransmitters, immune signalling, hormones and neuropeptides produced in the gut, all involved in modulation of the central nervous system (Sundman *et al.*, 2017).

As the principal component of the parasympathetic nervous system, the vagus nerve is thought to be key to communication within the gut–brain–microbiota axis. The vagus nerve is able to sense the microbiota metabolites through its afferent nerves, to transfer information to the CNS where it can be processed and integrated in the central autonomic network and a response triggered (Bonaz, Bazin and Pellissier, 2018). A high stress load is thought to inhibit the vagus nerve and hence have a negative impact on the microbiota and gastrointestinal tract. Pellissier and colleagues (2014) demonstrated imbalance in vagal tone and the HPA axis in those with Crohn's disease and IBS compared with controls.

AB's initial neurological flare-up occurred after a period of high stress load and following a long period of antibiotic use. It can be hypothesized that these significantly impacted her gut–brain–microbiota axis.

The patient's journey prior to personalized nutrition

AB arrived at the practitioner's clinic having self-prescribed diet and supplements. Anecdotal and primary peer-reviewed evidence can be found for the use of a 'Palaeo-based' diet and many of the supplements in supporting intestinal permeability, digestive function or neurological conditions. AB had reached a point where it was unclear how to move forward on her own without laboratory testing and professional insight to shape a programme to suit her specific needs.

Comprehensive functional testing revealed that increased intestinal permeability was evident and the underlying factors that were likely to be contributing to it. This helped to empower the client with further steps that could be taken to support her health. Targeting the dysbiosis, alongside continued support for intestinal membrane health, led to improvements in symptoms as well as normalization of the intestinal permeability results.

To try to address increased intestinal permeability without addressing dysbiosis would be unlikely to be truly effective. To have left foods in the diet that were triggering cross-reactions and low-grade immune response would have stalled progress. The case demonstrates the value in seeking to understand the root cause, which is fundamental to a personalized nutrition approach. The solutions were not dramatic or fast, but through tracking with modest follow-up testing, the practitioner and client were able to recognize that they were making progress. This case is ongoing as both the client and practitioner believe there are still underlying factors to be addressed. These are discussed in the question-and-answer section below.

Q&A

AW: AB was taking an awful lot of supplements. I know you have discussed some of the challenges faced when a client arrives with an long list of existing supplements. Was there a 'security' she experienced from taking so many supplements, given her long period of ill health? I'm curious about sometimes the emotional connection clients can have to their supplements, while at other times I've heard them described as a sign that they aren't well and which they wish they could get rid of!

ES: AB's supplement list was longer than any client I had worked with previously, so, yes, initially I was mindful of their role – were they all necessary/helpful? Were they a 'psychological crutch'? However, as we moved forward, I could see that she had, in fact, made sound choices with the supplements she had chosen and the reasoning behind them. Although perhaps they weren't all 'essential', there was logic to each one;

AB perceived a benefit from taking them and neither the cost nor the logistics of taking them was an issue for her.

AW: How is this case evolving?

ES: AB reported a gradual but steady improvement to energy levels in the months following the 5R protocol. We actually decided to repeat the 5R protocol. I find that digestive restoration work can take a long time. The patient had been unwell for 12+ years but it is also likely these imbalances began many years previously. I am also looking at the impact of histamines as the histamine response in the gut can be a factor in intestinal permeability and this area that is being explored further with the client.

AW: Reflecting on the case so far, is there anything you would have done differently?

ES: As clinical experience and knowledge increases or I become aware of new research, theories, products or laboratory tests, it is easy to say 'I would do that differently' with hindsight. In this instance, I wouldn't now recommend the liver support multinutrient powder as it is relatively high in simple carbohydrates which contradicts my dietary recommendations to reduce simple sugars. Another thing I might now do differently is to be firmer in my recommendations around excluding dairy earlier in the process. I had my suspicions, given that dairy is such a common irritant and normally a core exclusion for someone on a Palaeo-style protocol. However, during consultations, I queried AB and she hadn't felt that dairy was an issue for her. As she had been experimenting with her diet for ten years, including periods of dairy exclusion. I trusted her experience. When dairy was later highlighted as problematic in the gluten cross-reactivity screen, it was finally removed and improvements were reported.

Appendix 9.1 Supplement formulas at initial intake

B complex used by AB at intake	2 capsules providing total
Thiamine (vitamin B1) (as thiamine HCl)	100 mg
Riboflavin (vitamin B2) (as riboflavin and riboflavin 5'-phosphate)	75 mg
Niacin (as niacinamide and niacin)	100 mg
Vitamin B6 (as pyridoxine HCl and pyridoxal 5'-phosphate)	100 mg
Folate (as L-5-methyltetrahydrofolate calcium salt)	400 mcg
Vitamin B12 (as methylcobalamin)	300 mcg
Biotin	1000 mcg
Pantothenic acid (as D-calcium pantothenate)	500 mg
Calcium (as D-calcium pantothenate, dicalcium phosphate)	90 mg
Inositol	100 mg
PABA (para-aminobenzoic acid)	50 mg
Omega EPA/DHA used by AB at intake	**2 soft gels providing total**
EPA (eicosapentaenoic acid)	202 mg
DHA (docosahexaenoic acid)	180 mg
DPA (docosapentaenoic acid)	41 mg
Other omega 3 fatty acids	77 mg
Total omega 5 fatty acids	1.9 mg
Total omega 6 fatty acids	48 mg

cont.

Omega EPA/DHA used by AB at intake	2 soft gels providing total
Total omega 7 fatty acids	192 mg
Total omega 9 fatty acids	384 mg
Astaxanthin	20 mcg
C and K2 complex used by AB at intake	**Daily dose**
Vitamin C (as ascorbyl palmitate)	10 mg
Vitamin K, from: Vitamin K1 (as phytonadione) Vitamin K2 (as menaquinone-4) Vitamin K2 (as all-*trans* menaquinone-7)	2600 mcg 1500 mcg 1000 mcg 100 mcg
Multivitamin and mineral used by AB at intake and at P2	**Taking every other day**
Vitamin A	800 mcg
Vitamin D	310 mcg
Vitamin E	24 mg
Vitamin K	75 mcg
Vitamin C	120 mg
Thiamin	5 mg
Riboflavin	4 mg
Niacin	16 mg
Vitamin B	610 mg
Folic Acid	200 mcg
Vitamin B	1250 mcg
Biotin	150 mcg
Pantothenic acid	12 mg
Calcium	800 mg

Magnesium	300 mg
Iron	7 mg
Zinc	15 mg
Copper	1 mg
Manganese	4 mg
Selenium	110 mcg
Chromium	200 mcg
Iodine	150 mcg
Choline bitartrate	5 mg
Inositol	5 mg
PABA	5 mg
Lutein	2 mg
Turmeric extract	50 mg
Green tea extract	50 mg
Grape seed extract	50 mg
Multimineral used by AB at intake	**Taking every other day**
Calcium	1000 mg
Phosphorus	200 mg
Magnesium	376 mg
Iron	14 mg
Zinc	15 mg
Copper	1 mg
Manganese	4 mg

cont.

Multimineral used by AB at intake	Taking every other day
Selenium	100 mcg
Chromium	100 mcg
Molybdenum	5 mcg
Iodine	140 mcg
Boron	2 mg

Appendix 9.2 Supplement formulas recommended at P1 and P2

Multinutrient liver support powder used at P1	Daily dose
	171 kcal 2.5 g fat 21 g carbohydrate or which 16 g sugars 13 g protein
Potassium	719 mg
Vitamin A1	501 mcg • retinyl palmitate 180 mcg • beta-carotene 1021 mcg
Vitamin B1	2 mg
Vitamin B2	1.4 mg
Niacin (Vitamin B3)	16 mg
Vitamin B	62.8 mg
Vitamin B12	25 mcg
Vitamin C	300 mg
Vitamin D (500 IU)	12.5 mcg
Vitamin E (45 IU)	30 mg

Pantothenic acid	31.7 mg
Biotin	150 mcg
Folate (metafolin)	150 mcg
Iodine	75 mcg
Magnesium	188 mg
Molybdenum	50 mcg
Calcium	150 mg
Zinc	10 mg
Copper	1000 mcg
Chromium	80 mcg
Selenium	55 mcg
L-glutathione	10 mg
L-glycine	3661 mg
L-cysteine	219 mg
L-lysine	456 mg
L-threonine	467 mg
N-acetyl-L-cysteine	20 mg
Sodium sulphate	20 mg
Taurine	100 mg
Choline	152 mg
Green tea extract	50 mg providing catechins 10 mg
Multivitamin and mineral used at P2	**1 capsule**
Vitamin A	43 mg (312 mcg from beta-carotene and 125 mcg as palmitate)

cont.

Multivitamin and mineral used at P2	1 capsule
Vitamin C (as ascorbic acid)	142 mg
Vitamin D (as vitamin D3) (166 IU)	4 mcg
Vitamin E (as d-alpha tocopheryl)	45 mg
Thiamin (as thiamin HCl)	6.6 mg
Riboflavin (as riboflavin 5'-phosphate sodium)	1.8 mg
Niacin	27 mg
Vitamin B6 (as pyridoxal 5'-phosphate)	1.6 mg
Folate	0.3 mg DFE (83 mcg as calcium folinate and 83 mcg as L-5-methyltetrahydrofolate from L-5-methyltetrahydrofolic acid, glucosamine salt)
Vitamin B12	75 mcg (37.5 mcg as adenosylcobalamin and 37.5 mcg as methylcobalamin)
Biotin	67 mcg
Pantothenic acid (as calcium pantothenate)	69 mg
Choline (as choline citrate)	5.9 mg
Calcium	35 mg (20 mg as calcium citrate and 15 mg as calcium malate)
Iron (as iron picolinate)	2.5 mg
Iodine (as potassium iodide)	37.5 mcg
Magnesium	25 mg (15 mg as magnesium citrate and 10 mg as magnesium malate)
Zinc (as zinc picolinate)	2.5 mg

Selenium (as L-selenomethionine)	33 mcg
Copper (as copper picolinate)	0.25 mg
Manganese (as manganese picolinate)	1 mg
Chromium (as TRAACS® Chromium Nicotinate Glycinate Chelate)	33.3 mcg
Molybdenum (as TRAACS® Molybdenum Glycinate Chelate)	16.7 mcg
Boron (as Bororganic™ Boron Glycinate Complex)	0.5 mg
Lutein (from Aztec marigold extract (flower) (*Tagetes erecta*))	24 mcg
Vanadium (as vanadium picolinate)	16.7 mcg

References

Abd, E.-B.R.M., Ela, D.M.M.A.E., Gad, G.F.M., 2014. N-acetylcysteine inhibits and eradicates *Candida albicans* biofilms. *American Journal of Infectious Diseases and Microbiology* 2, 122–130. https://doi.org/10.12691/ajidm-2-5-5

Abraham, G.E., Flechas, J.D., 1992. Management of fibromyalgia: Rationale for the use of magnesium and malic acid. *Journal of Nutritional Medicine* 3, 49–59. https://doi.org/10.3109/13590849208997961

Altomare, E., Colonna, P., D'Agostino, C., Castellaneta, G. *et al.*, 1996. High-dose antioxidant therapy during thrombolysis in patients with acute myocardial infarction. *Current Therapeutic Research* 57, 131–141. https://doi.org/10.1016/S0011-393X(96)80007-5

Baugher, J.L., Klaenhammer, T.R., 2011. Invited review: Application of omics tools to understanding probiotic functionality. *Journal of Dairy Science* 94, 4753–4765. https://doi.org/10.3168/jds.2011-4384

Bel, S., Pendse, M., Wang, Y., Li, Y. *et al.*, 2017. Paneth cells secrete lysozyme via secretory autophagy during bacterial infection of the intestine. *Science* 357, 1047–1052. https://doi.org/10.1126/science.aal4677

Belkaid, Y., Hand, T., 2014. Role of the microbiota in immunity and inflammation. *Cell* 157, 121–141. https://doi.org/10.1016/j.cell.2014.03.011

Benjamin, J., Makharia, G., Ahuja, V., Anand Rajan, K.D. *et al.*, 2012. Glutamine and whey protein improve intestinal permeability and morphology in patients with Crohn's disease: A randomized controlled trial. *Digestive Diseases and Sciences* 57, 1000–1012. https://doi.org/10.1007/s10620-011-1947-9

Bernatoniene, J., Kopustinskiene, D.M., 2018. The role of catechins in cellular responses to oxidative stress. *Molecules* 23. https://doi.org/10.3390/molecules23040965

Bischoff-Ferrari, H.A., Giovannucci, E., Willett, W.C., Dietrich, T., Dawson-Hughes, B., 2006. Estimation of optimal serum concentrations of 25-hydroxyvitamin D for multiple health outcomes. *American Journal of Clinical Nutrition* 84, 18–28. https://doi.org/10.1093/ajcn/84.1.18

Bonaz, B., Bazin, T., Pellissier, S., 2018. The vagus nerve at the interface of the microbiota–gut–brain axis. *Frontiers in Neuroscience* 12, 49. https://doi.org/10.3389/fnins.2018.00049

Buscarinu, M.C., Cerasoli, B., Annibali, V., Policano, C. *et al.*, 2017. Altered intestinal permeability in patients with relapsing–remitting multiple sclerosis: A pilot study. *Multiple Sclerosis Journal* 23, 442–446. https://doi.org/10.1177/1352458516652498

CDC, 2018. Diagnosis of Parasitic Diseases. Accessed on 26/05/2019 at https://www.cdc.gov/parasites/references_resources/diagnosis.html

Chen, J., Chia, N., Kalari, K.R., Yao, J.Z. *et al.*, 2016. Multiple sclerosis patients have a distinct gut microbiota compared to healthy controls. *Scientific Reports* 6, 28484. https://doi.org/10.1038/srep28484

Chen, J.-K., Shen, C.-R., Liu, C.-L., 2010. *N*-acetylglucosamine: Production and applications. *Marine Drugs* 8, 2493–2516. https://doi.org/10.3390/md8092493

Chen, Q., Chen, O., Martins, I.M., Hou, H. *et al.*, 2017. Collagen peptides ameliorate intestinal epithelial barrier dysfunction in immunostimulatory Caco-2 cell monolayers via enhancing tight junctions. *Food and Function* 8, 1144–1151. https://doi.org/10.1039/C6FO01347C

Cordain, L., Eaton, S.B., Sebastian, A., Mann, N. *et al.*, 2005. Origins and evolution of the Western diet: Health implications for the 21st century. *American Journal of Clinical Nutrition* 81, 341–354. https://doi.org/10.1093/ajcn.81.2.341

Cordain, L., Toohey, L., Smith, M.J., Hickey, M.S., 2000. Modulation of immune function by dietary lectins in rheumatoid arthritis. *British Journal of Nutrition* 83, 207–217. https://doi.org/10.1017/S0007114500000271

Cvetnić, Z., Vladimir-Knezević, S., 2004. Antimicrobial activity of grapefruit seed and pulp ethanolic extract. *Acta Pharmaceutica* 54, 243–250.

Dentico, P., Volpe, A., Buongiorno, R., Grattagliano, I. *et al.*, 1995. [Glutathione in the treatment of chronic fatty liver diseases]. *Recenti Progressi in Medicina* 86, 290–293.

Dinan, T.G., Stilling, R.M., Stanton, C., Cryan, J.F., 2015. Collective unconscious: How gut microbes shape human behavior. *Journal of Psychiatric Research* 63, 1–9. https://doi.org/10.1016/j.jpsychires.2015.02.021

Distrutti, E., Monaldi, L., Ricci, P., Fiorucci, S., 2016. Gut microbiota role in irritable bowel syndrome: New therapeutic strategies. *World Journal of Gastroenterology* 22, 2219–2241. https://doi.org/10.3748/wjg.v22.i7.2219

Failla, M.L., Chitchumroonchokchai, C., Aoki, F., 2014. Increased bioavailability of ubiquinol compared to that of ubiquinone is due to more efficient micellarization during digestion and greater GSH-dependent uptake and basolateral secretion by Caco-2 cells. *Journal of Agricultural and Food Chemistry* 62, 7174–7182. https://doi.org/10.1021/jf5017829

Foster, J.A., Rinaman, L., Cryan, J.F., 2017. Stress and the gut–brain axis: Regulation by the microbiome. *Neurobiology of Stress* 7, 124–136. https://doi.org/10.1016/j.ynstr.2017.03.001

Godoy, L.D., Rossignoli, M.T., Delfino-Pereira, P., Garcia-Cairasco, N., de Lima Umeoka, E.H., 2018. A comprehensive overview on stress neurobiology: Basic concepts and clinical implications. *Frontiers in Behavioral Neuroscience* 12, 127. https://doi.org/10.3389/fnbeh.2018.00127

Gu, Y., Nieves, J.W., Stern, Y., Luchsinger, J.A., Scarmeas, N., 2010. Food combination and Alzheimer disease risk: A protective diet. *Archives of Neurology* 67, 699–706. https://doi.org/10.1001/archneurol.2010.84

Harjai, K., Kumar, R., Singh, S., 2010. Garlic blocks quorum sensing and attenuates the virulence of *Pseudomonas aeruginosa*. *FEMS Immunology and Medical Microbiology* 58, 161–168. https://doi.org/10.1111/j.1574-695X.2009.00614.x

Hawrelak, J.A., Myers, S.P., 2010. Effects of two natural medicine formulations on irritable bowel syndrome symptoms: A pilot study. *Journal of Alternative and Complementary Medicine* 16, 1065–1071. https://doi.org/10.1089/acm.2009.0090

Heggers, J.P., Cottingham, J., Gusman, J., Reagor, L. *et al.*, 2002. The effectiveness of processed grapefruit-seed extract as an antibacterial agent: II. Mechanism of action and *in vitro* toxicity. *Journal of Alternative and Complementary Medicine* 8, 333–340. https://doi.org/10.1089/10755530260128023

Honda, Y., Kessoku, T., Sumida, Y., Kobayashi, T. *et al.*, 2017. Efficacy of glutathione for the treatment of nonalcoholic fatty liver disease: An open-label, single-arm, multicenter, pilot study. *BMC Gastroenterology* 17. https://doi.org/10.1186/s12876-017-0652-3

Hoshimoto, A., Suzuki, Y., Katsuno, T., Nakajima, H., Saito, Y., 2002. Caprylic acid and medium-chain triglycerides inhibit IL-8 gene transcription in Caco-2 cells: Comparison with the potent histone deacetylase inhibitor trichostatin A. *British Journal of Pharmacology* 136, 280–286. https://doi.org/10.1038/sj.bjp.0704719

Huang, C.B., Altimova, Y., Myers, T.M., Ebersole, J.L., 2011. Short- and medium-chain fatty acids exhibit antimicrobial activity for oral microorganisms. *Archives of Oral Biology* 56, 650–654. https://doi.org/10.1016/j.archoralbio.2011.01.011

Institute for Functional Medicine, 2011. Practitioner toolkit. Accessed on 18/06/2019 at www.ifm.org

Iwai, W., Abe, Y., Iijima, K., Koike, T. *et al.*, 2013. Gastric hypochlorhydria is associated with an exacerbation of dyspeptic symptoms in female patients. *Journal of Gastroenterology* 48, 214–221. https://doi.org/10.1007/s00535-012-0634-8

Jakobsen, T.H., van Gennip, M., Phipps, R.K., Shanmugham, M.S. *et al.*, 2012. Ajoene, a sulfur-rich molecule from garlic, inhibits genes controlled by quorum sensing. *Antimicrobial Agents and Chemotherapy* 56, 2314–2325. https://doi.org/10.1128/AAC.05919-11

Kaetzel, C.S., 2014. Cooperativity among secretory IgA, the polymeric immunoglobulin receptor, and the gut microbiota promotes host-microbial mutualism. *Immunology Letters* 162, 10–21. https://doi.org/10.1016/j.imlet.2014.05.008

Karakuła-Juchnowicz, H., Szachta, P., Opolska, A., Morylowska-Topolska, J. *et al.*, 2017. The role of IgG hypersensitivity in the pathogenesis and therapy of depressive disorders. *Nutritional Neuroscience* 20, 110–118. https://doi.org/10.1179/1476830514Y.0000000158

Karkman, A., Lehtimäki, J., Ruokolainen, L., 2017. The ecology of human microbiota: Dynamics and diversity in health and disease. *Annals of the New York Academy of Sciences* 1399, 78–92. https://doi.org/10.1111/nyas.13326

Kasperczyk, S., Dobrakowski, M., Kasperczyk, A., Ostałowska, A., Birkner, E., 2013. The administration of N-acetylcysteine reduces oxidative stress and regulates glutathione metabolism in the blood cells of workers exposed to lead. *Clinical Toxicology* 51, 480–486. https://doi.org/10.3109/15563650.2013.802797

Kim, M.-H., Kim, H., 2017. The Roles of glutamine in the intestine and its implication in intestinal diseases. *International Journal of Molecular Sciences* 18. https://doi.org/10.3390/ijms18051051

Kumar, M., Jain, M., Sehgal, A., Sharma, V.L., 2012. Modulation of CYP1A1, CYP1B1 and DNA adducts level by green and white tea in Balb/c mice. *Food and Chemical Toxicology* 50, 4375–4381. https://doi.org/10.1016/j.fct.2012.08.045

Kunnumakkara, A.B., Bordoloi, D., Padmavathi, G., Monisha, J. *et al.*, 2017. Curcumin, the golden nutraceutical: Multitargeting for multiple chronic diseases. *British Journal of Pharmacology* 174, 1325–1348. https://doi.org/10.1111/bph.13621

Le Berre, L., Rousse, J., Gourraud, P.-A., Imbert-Marcille, B.-M. *et al.*, 2017. Decrease of blood anti-α1,3 Galactose Abs levels in multiple sclerosis (MS) and clinically isolated syndrome (CIS) patients. *Clinical Immunology* 180, 128–135. https://doi.org/10.1016/j.clim.2017.05.006

Martins, N., Ferreira, I.C.F.R., Barros, L., Silva, S., Henriques, M., 2014. Candidiasis: Predisposing factors, prevention, diagnosis and alternative treatment. *Mycopathologia* 177, 223–240. https://doi.org/10.1007/s11046-014-9749-1

McFarland, L.V., 2010. Systematic review and meta-analysis of *Saccharomyces boulardii* in adult patients. *World Journal of Gastroenterology* 16, 2202–2222. https://doi.org/10.3748/wjg.v16.i18.2202

Mejía-Mejía, E., Torres, R., Restrepo, D., 2018. Physiological coherence in healthy volunteers during laboratory-induced stress and controlled breathing. *Psychophysiology* 55, e13046. https://doi.org/10.1111/psyp.13046

Miyake, S., Kim, S., Suda, W., Oshima, K. *et al.*, 2015. Dysbiosis in the gut microbiota of patients with multiple sclerosis, with a striking depletion of species belonging to Clostridia XIVa and IV clusters. *PloS ONE* 10, e0137429. https://doi.org/10.1371/journal.pone.0137429

Pagnini, C., Corleto, V.D., Martorelli, M., Lanini, C., D'Ambra, G., Di Giulio, E., Delle Fave, G., 2018. Mucosal adhesion and anti-inflammatory effects of *Lactobacillus rhamnosus* GG in the human colonic mucosa: A proof-of-concept study. *World Journal of Gastroenterology* 24, 4652–4662. https://doi.org/10.3748/wjg.v24.i41.4652

Panpetch, W., Chancharoenthana, W., Bootdee, K., Nilgate, S. *et al.*, 2018. *Lactobacillus rhamnosus* L34 attenuates gut translocation-induced bacterial sepsis in murine models of leaky gut. *Infection and Immunity* 86. https://doi.org/10.1128/IAI.00700-17

Pascoe, M.C., Thompson, D.R., Jenkins, Z.M., Ski, C.F., 2017. Mindfulness mediates the physiological markers of stress: Systematic review and meta-analysis. *Journal of Psychiatric Research* 95, 156–178. https://doi.org/10.1016/j.jpsychires.2017.08.004

Pellissier, S., Dantzer, C., Mondillon, L., Trocme, C. *et al.*, 2014. Relationship between vagal tone, cortisol, TNF-alpha, epinephrine and negative affects in Crohn's disease and irritable bowel syndrome. *PloS ONE* 9, e105328. https://doi.org/10.1371/journal.pone.0105328

Pohl, C.H., Kock, J.L.F., Thibane, V.S., 2011. Antifungal free fatty acids: A review. Accessed on 18/06/2019 at www.researchgate.net/profile/Carolina_Pohl/publication/266463207_Antifungal_free_fatty_acids_A_Review/links/54daf14b0cf261ce15ce9643.pdf

Pound, M.W., May, D.B., 2005. Proposed mechanisms and preventative options of Jarisch–Herxheimer reactions. *Journal of Clinical Pharmacy and Therapeutics* 30, 291–295. https://doi.org/10.1111/j.1365-2710.2005.00631.x

Rashtak, S., Ettore, M.W., Homburger, H.A., Murray, J.A., 2008. Comparative usefulness of deamidated gliadin antibodies in the diagnosis of celiac disease. *Clinical Gastroenterology and Hepatology* 6, 426–370. https://doi.org/10.1016/j.cgh.2007.12.030

Russell, I.J., Michalek, J.E., Flechas, J.D., Abraham, G.E., 1995. Treatment of fibromyalgia syndrome with Super Malic: A randomized, double blind, placebo controlled, crossover pilot study. *Journal of Rheumatology* 22, 953–958.

Salvatore, S., Heuschkel, R., Tomlin, S., Davies, S.E. *et al.*, 2000. A pilot study of N-acetyl glucosamine, a nutritional substrate for glycosaminoglycan synthesis, in paediatric chronic inflammatory bowel disease. *Alimentary Pharmacology and Therapeutics* 14, 1567–1579.

Sanoobar, M., Dehghan, P., Khalili, M., Azimi, A., Seifar, F., 2016. Coenzyme Q$_{10}$ as a treatment for fatigue and depression in multiple sclerosis patients: A double blind randomized clinical trial. *Nutritional Neuroscience* 19, 138–143. https://doi.org/10.1179/1476830515Y.0000000002

Schuchardt, J.P., Hahn, A., 2017. Intestinal absorption and factors influencing bioavailability of magnesium– an update. *Current Nutrition and Food Science* 13, 260–278. https://doi.org/10.2174/1573401313666170427162740

Seddik, H.A., Bendali, F., Gancel, F., Fliss, I., Spano, G., Drider, D., 2017. *Lactobacillus plantarum* and its probiotic and food potentialities. *Probiotics and Antimicrobial Proteins* 9, 111–122. https://doi.org/10.1007/s12602-017-9264-z

Sheflin, A.M., Melby, C.L., Carbonero, F., Weir, T.L., 2017. Linking dietary patterns with gut microbial composition and function. *Gut Microbes* 8, 113–129. https://doi.org/10.1080/19490976.2016.1270809

Simrén, M., Barbara, G., Flint, H.J., Spiegel, B.M.R. *et al.* (2013) Intestinal microbiota in functional bowel disorders: a Rome foundation report. *Gut* 62, 159–176. https://doi.org/10.1136/gutjnl-2012-302167

Sundman, M.H., Chen, N.-K., Subbian, V., Chou, Y.-H., 2017. The bidirectional gut–brain–microbiota axis as a potential nexus between traumatic brain injury, inflammation, and disease. *Brain, Behavior, and Immunity* 66, 31–44. https://doi.org/10.1016/j.bbi.2017.05.009

Toribio-Mateas, M., 2018. Harnessing the power of microbiome assessment tools as part of neuroprotective nutrition and lifestyle medicine interventions. *Microorganisms* 6. https://doi.org/10.3390/microorganisms6020035

Uysal, N., Kizildag, S., Yuce, Z., Guvendi, G. *et al.*, 2019. Timeline (bioavailability) of magnesium compounds in hours: Which magnesium compound works best? *Biological Trace Element Research* 187, 128–136. https://doi.org/10.1007/s12011-018-1351-9

van Ballegooijen, A.J., Pilz, S., Tomaschitz, A., Grübler, M.R., Verheyen, N., 2017. The synergistic interplay between vitamins D and K for bone and cardiovascular health: A narrative review. *International Journal of Endocrinology* 2017. https://doi.org/10.1155/2017/7454376

van der Sluys Veer, A., Brouwer, J., Biemond, I., Bohbouth, G.E., Verspaget, H.W., Lamers, C.B., 1998. Fecal lysozyme in assessment of disease activity in inflammatory bowel disease. *Digestive Diseases and Sciences* 43, 590–595.

Vanuytsel, T., van Wanrooy, S., Vanheel, H., Vanormelingen, C. *et al.*, 2014. Psychological stress and corticotropin-releasing hormone increase intestinal permeability in humans by a mast cell-dependent mechanism. *Gut* 63, 1293–1299. https://doi.org/10.1136/gutjnl-2013-305690

Vojdani, A., 2015. Molecular mimicry as a mechanism for food immune reactivities and autoimmunity. *Alternative Therapies in Health and Medicine* 21, Suppl 1, 34–45.

Vojdani, A., Tarash, I., 2013. Cross-reaction between gliadin and different food and tissue antigens. *Food and Nutrition Sciences* 4, 20. https://doi.org/10.4236/fns.2013.41005

Wahls, T., Scott, M.O., Alshare, Z., Rubenstein, L. *et al.*, 2018. Dietary approaches to treat MS-related fatigue: Comparing the modified Paleolithic (Wahls Elimination) and low saturated fat (Swank) diets on perceived fatigue in persons with relapsing-remitting multiple sclerosis: Study protocol for a randomized controlled trial. *Trials* 19, 309. https://doi.org/10.1186/s13063-018-2680-x

Wang, B., Wu, G., Zhou, Z., Dai, Z. *et al.*, 2015. Glutamine and intestinal barrier function. *Amino Acids* 47, 2143–2154. https://doi.org/10.1007/s00726-014-1773-4

Werbach, M.R., 2000. Nutritional strategies for treating chronic fatigue syndrome. *Alternative Medicine Review* 5, 93–108.

Yago, M.R., Frymoyer, A., Benet, L.Z., Smelick, G.S. *et al.*, 2014. The use of betaine HCl to enhance dasatinib absorption in healthy volunteers with rabeprazole-induced hypochlorhydria. *AAPS Journal* 16, 1358–1365. https://doi.org/10.1208/s12248-014-9673-9

10

Autoimmunity with Intestinal Permeability and Fructose Intolerance

Practitioner: Claire Sehinson

Setting the scene

The incidence and prevalence of autoimmune disorders has increased significantly over the past 30 years and it is suspected that environmental factors including diet have a strong influence (Lerner, Jeremias and Matthias, 2015; Manzel *et al.*, 2014). In autoimmune conditions the delicate balance between immune response and immune tolerance is lost (Gregersen, 2007) and the underlying factors are often multifactorial.

In complex cases the presenting symptoms can be varied, numerous and changeable. This can present frustrations for the client and practitioner alike as they attempt to pinpoint the underlying biochemical imbalances and their triggers, mediators and antecedents.

In this case we see the multiple factors which appeared to contribute to that loss of immune tolerance and the perseverance of the client and clinician in continuing to search and address those contributing factors. We will see how lifestyle, diet and genetics interplay and lead to not only physical symptoms but also anxiety patterns. It is an example of how important it is to keep looking at causal and contributing factors and to take a whole-person approach, which is at the heart of personalized nutrition.

Initial case presentation

KT is a 39-year-old woman who wanted to reduce fatigue, anxiety and panic attacks. One specific goal was to reduce her reliance on the benzodiazepine diazepam, used to treat a range of conditions including anxiety.

Recent medical history

KT was already under the care of a medical specialist who had diagnosed *Rickettsia* and *Mycoplasma* infections. She had been prescribed a rotation of antibiotic therapies for the past 14 months, which had led to gastrointestinal symptoms and chronically raised liver enzymes. KT had a diagnosis of Sjögren's syndrome (see Box 10.1) and was also positive for multiple autoimmune tissue markers with elevated antinuclear antibodies (ANA) (see Table 10.3). The severity of her symptoms (see summary below) was significantly affecting her studies, work, relationships, cognitive function and quality of life.

Previous medical history and life events

A timeline to capture the life events and medical history and symptoms prior to visiting the practitioner is shown in Table 10.1.

Table 10.1 Medical history and life events timeline

Timeline/ age	Events/activity	Symptoms/diagnosis
Birth		Jaundice (fraternal twin had no significant health problems)
Age 6–10		Irritable bowel syndrome (IBS) and chronic constipation
Age 11–15		Anaemic Chronic constipation, anxiety
Age 16–20	Gluten-free diet introduced resulting in improvements in digestive system Became a vegetarian as a health choice Recreational drug and heavy alcohol use	
Age 21–30	Vegan, vegetarian and orthorexia Gave up heavy drinking/ intoxicants Extreme exercise (yoga) Emotional stress Exposure to 'sick building'	Amenorrhoea Osteopenia Jaundice Severe anxiety
Age 31–33	Travel to India (multiple trips) Multiple dental amalgam removal in India Yoga/meditation retreat involving high amounts of papaya (fructose) consumption over a few days	Dysentery Panic attacks (GP prescribed diazepam as needed) Worsening of osteopenia and amenorrhoea

Age 34–37	Multiple medical and alternative practitioners consulted for blepharitis (an inflammatory condition of the eyelids) and other systemic inflammatory symptoms	Antibiotic and herbal creams prescribed that resulted in chronic pingueculitis Sjögren's syndrome diagnosed (see Box 10.1) Multiple food sensitivities and tissue inflammation Tested positive for *Rickettsia* (intracellular gram-negative bacteria transmitted by numerous vectors including ticks), *Mycoplasma* (small, self-replicating bacteria that lack a cell wall)
Age 38–39	Experimentation with ketogenic and Palaeolithic diets Variable improvements but generation of new symptoms (including inflammation and energy dips) Chronic laxative use	Monthly cycles of antibiotics as treatment for *Rickettsia* and *Mycoplasma* Endoscopy revealed mild reflux oesophagitis, hiatus hernia and gastritis Liver enzymes rising Diagnosed with primary biliary cirrhosis by a previous medical practitioner Raised autoantibodies Suspected diagnosis for chronic fatigue syndrome and fibromyalgia

BOX 10.1 SJÖGREN'S SYNDROME

Sjögren's syndrome is an autoimmune condition whereby the target tissues of autoimmunity are moisture-secreting glands, primarily the eyes (tear ducts) and mouth (salivary glands).

The diagnosis was made by a consultant rheumatologist. KT was offered steroid eye drops to manage her symptoms in the long term, but elected not to use this treatment at the time.

Environmental factors and live events of note

There were a number of events the practitioner suspected of being of specific note in this case. KT had worked in a building with known damp and mould exposure for a period of time. She had undertaken dental work involving amalgam removal while in India, which can involve exposure to mercury vapour (BDA, n.d.); no precaution was taken to minimize this during the procedure. KT had two body tattoos, one of which had been removed. KT had experienced and received treatment for emotional and psychological trauma for a number of years.

Current medications and supplements at initial consultation

The client was on a number of medications and supplements, which are summarized in Table 10.2.

Table 10.2 Medications and supplements at initial consultation

Supplement or medication	Dose	Duration	Prescribed by
Antibiotics: example rotations of: 1. Doxycycline and ciprofloxacin 2. Lymecycline and metronidazole 3. Doxycycline and moxifloxacin 4. Clarithromycin and amoxicillin 5. Pamaquine	Varied	14 months	Medical specialist
Diazepam	5–10 mg QD	7 months	Primary medical practitioner
Glutathione	250 mg QD	1 month	Self-prescribed
Serrapeptase (proteolytic enzyme)	80,000 IU BID	2 months	Self-prescribed
Botanical antimicrobial formula including bilberry, milk thistle, echinacea, goldenseal, white willow bark, garlic, grapeseed extract, black walnut, tea tree and oregano in liposomal form	50 mg QD	2 months	Self-prescribed

Given the presence of diagnosis and potential red flags, the practitioner ensured the client was monitored throughout by her medical practitioner. Drug–nutrient interactions were also checked. This is discussed later and shown in Appendix A.

Diet at initial consultation

KT was following a very restricted diet that eliminated all grains, refined sugar, gluten and dairy. She felt able to tolerate starchy vegetables during the periods when taken antibiotic therapy.

She had experimented with a ketogenic diet, which she described as helpful for improving 'brain fog', but her mood and energy levels felt unstable.

Summary of symptoms at initial consultation

KT described a number of current symptoms:

- persisting fatigue, regardless of rest 7/10 (10 = most severe)
- leg pains with intermittent paralysis
- yellow, burning diarrhoea if over-the-counter laxatives used
- light and noise sensitive, daily, concomitant with fatigue
- severe anxiety and panic attacks and agoraphobia, associated with tremors and thirst, daily, particularly when she has to leave the house
- severe headaches and migraines, varies from daily to weekly
- brain fog, daily, concomitant with fatigue
- disrupted sleep pattern and poor sleep quality, most nights
- unable to deviate from restricted diet without the generation of individual symptoms listed below.

In addition, the following symptoms varied depending on specific foods:

- After eating starchy foods, skin yellowed and experienced constipation.
- After eating sugar, bladder, eyes and joints felt 'irritated'.
- Coffee, pineapple and chocolate consumption led to severe pain in upper abdomen.

- Could feel shaky, anxious and experience tremors within an hour of eating, depending on foods. When eating a high-fat, low-carbohydrate (ketogenic-style diet) this did not happen.

Clinical questions

In a case such as this where the client reports a wide range of unpleasant and debilitating symptoms coupled with a myriad of medical issues past and present, the is key to create and maintain a structure to the interpretation and case management.

The first priority was to improve KT's quality of life and initiate an upward spiral towards health by making it easier for her to leave the house each day. A key clinical question was whether her debilitating anxiety had a biological or genetic trigger. The second question was to understand the underlying factors involved in KT's autoimmunity. Creating key clinical questions led the practitioner to explore gastrointestinal function, immune and toxicant reactivity and the autonomic nervous system. This systematic approach helped to reduce complexity without taking a reductionist approach.

Investigations

A number of test results were brought to the initial consultation, all carried out within the previous 12 months; Table 10.3 summarizes those that are out of range.

Table 10.3 Out-of-range tests shared at initial consultation

Test	KT's result	Reference range
Iron	7.1 umol/L	10.7–26.9 umol/L
Ferritin	8 ng/ml	15–200 ng/ml
Transferrin saturation	10%	16–50%

AST	35 U/L	< 35 U/L
ALT	36 U/L	< 32 U/L
ANA titre	1:1280	< 1:80
Bicarbonate	22 mmol/L	22–28 mmol/L
Anion gap	17 mmol/L	8–16 mmol/L
B12 (without ever supplementing)	479 pmol/L	107–443 pmol/L
25-hydroxy-vitamin D	25 nmol/L	50–200 nmol/L
Mycoplasma pneumoniae IgG	Positive	Negative
Rickettsia prowazeki *Rickettsia mooseri* Micro-agglutination Giroud method	++ +++ Levels had reduced following antibiotic therapy but were still elevated	Negative
Multiple autoimmune reactivity screen measuring autoantibodies	Equivocal: parietal cell, intrinsic factor, alpha-tubulin + beta-tubulin, synapsin Out of range: collagen	Negative
Four-point salivary cortisol	First morning and midday cortisol low	

Despite a haemoglobin count on the low end of normal range at 129 g/L (reference range 120–155 g/L), the low iron, ferritin and transferring saturation could be factors in fatigue (Vaucher *et al.*, 2012).

Table 10.4 summarizes the further investigations ordered by the practitioner and the results grouped under functional systems which relate back to the key clinical questions. Further discussion on use of functional tests can be found in Chapter 3.

**Table 10.4 Functional and genetic testing
and results after initial consultation**

Functional system	Tests	Summary of abnormal findings
Gastrointestinal	Antigenic intestinal permeability screen	• Occludin/zonulin IgG – 1.26 (equivocal/borderline) • Occludin/zonulin IgM – 3.00 (elevated) • LPS IgG 2.7 (elevated) • LPS IgA 1.79 (equivocal/ borderline) • LPS IgM 4.87 (out of range)
Gastrointestinal	SIBO breath test	Negative
Immune/toxicity	Lymphocyte reactivity	Sensitivity to nickel, benzoate and bisphenol A
Autonomic nervous system	COMT*	+/+ decreased COMT activity
Autonomic nervous system	Kryptopyrroles	Negative

* Expanded genomic profiling was used to determine the interactions between genomic SNPs; however, it is beyond the scope of the case study to discuss all significant SNPs. Consideration of the catechol-O-methyltransferase (COMT) polymorphism was a turning point in addressing the client's most problematic anxiety symptoms.

Interpretation of case

Gastrointestinal permeability
Key to this case was understanding the underlying factors that led to the autoimmune process. It is well documented that loss of effective barrier in the gastrointestinal tract, and in particular the breakdown of the tight junctions of the intestinal epithelium, can be key to the control (or loss of) immune tolerance in autoimmune disease (Gregersen, 2007; Leonard *et al.*, 2017; Lerner *et al.*, 2015; Pollard *et al.*, 2018; Sturgeon and Fasano, 2016). The antigenic intestinal permeability screen

detects elevated antibodies to intestinal barrier proteins (occludin and zonulin) which are associated with increased intestinal permeability (Sturgeon and Fasano, 2016) and macromolecules such as bacterial lipopolysaccharides which trigger the production of pro-inflammatory cytokines in the gut (Lin *et al.*, 2015; Toribio-Mateas, 2018).

The challenge for the practitioner was to identify triggering and mediating factors for the increased permeability. The symptom pattern of bloating and constipation concomitant with increased starch consumption can be a symptom of small intestinal bacterial overgrowth (SIBO) (Gabrielli *et al.*, 2013). The hydrogen and methane breath test for SIBO was negative, which was a surprise to the practitioner.

Immune/toxicity

Environmental toxins are recognized as a key factor in loss of barrier function and immune tolerance in autoimmune disease (Pollard *et al.*, 2018). The practitioner wanted to explore whether any chemicals KT may be routinely exposed to could be triggering immune reactions and therefore potentially continuing to contribute to the autoimmune process. The test measured an increase in lymphocyte intracellular calcium that accompanies exposure to the test substance (J. McLaren-Howard, 2018, personal communication).

The test highlighted sensitivity to nickel, benzoate and bisphenol A. Nickel is an alloy in stainless steel. Nickel can induce localized inflammation and act as an adjuvant (enhancing the immune response to an antigen) by increasing B and T cell response (Bonefeld *et al.*, 2015).

Bisphenol A is found in a wide range of products including plastic containers, utensils, water bottles and till receipts (Kharrazian, 2014). The implications of these findings were twofold. First, the chemicals themselves can be contributing factors to the autoimmune process (Kharrazian, 2014; Pollard *et al.*, 2018). Second, it provides guidance on what to replace problematic chemicals with – in this case, stainless-steel cooking utensils needed to be avoided as well as plastic; glass and ceramic were suitable replacements.

Benzoates are widely used as food and drink preservatives and in some pharmaceuticals. It has been detected in car exhaust gases as by-product of combustion and its benzoic acid form occurs naturally in many plants including berries (WHO, 2000).

Autonomic nervous system

A four-point salivary cortisol test completed three years previously found low normal total cortisol and low first morning and midday cortisol (see Chapter 3 for details on functional testing). This can be a factor in fatigue. Given KT's ongoing fatigue and symptom pattern, repeating that test was felt to have limited value by the practitioner. Given her history of severe anxiety, the practitioner felt it more relevant to examine underlying factors that may contribute to that.

The test referred to as the kryptopyrrole test is more accurately measuring hydroxyhaemopyrrolin-2-one (HPL). Anxiety, constipation, tremors, amenorrhea and stress intolerance are some of the signs and symptoms that are prevalent in those with high urinary HPL and are seen in this client (McGinnis *et al.*, 2008). The test was negative.

Nutrigenomic profiling can help identify genetic factors and antecedents to symptom patterns. They are also helpful in tailoring personalized nutrition programmes. Catechol-O-methyltransferase (COMT) is an enzyme involved in the metabolism of compounds such as catecholamines (Nissinen and Männistö, 2010). Functional polymorphism in the COMT gene (val158 met) is associated with up to fourfold variation in enzyme activity (Heinz and Smolka, 2006; Männistö and Kaakkola, 1999). KT is COMT +/+, meaning she is homozygous and has significantly decreased COMT activity (see Chapter 3 for an explanation of the terminology used in genetic testing). While this polymorphism may benefit attention-based activity and working memory (Heinz and Smolka, 2006), it can also lead to increased anxiety-related issues (Enoch *et al.*, 2003; Woo *et al.*, 2004, 2002).

Referring back to the key clinical question, the COMT polymorphism is suggestive that KT's debilitating anxiety had a genetic antecedent. Caution, however, is needed with nutrigenomic work. While we can ascertain polymorphisms, we don't know how the unique collection of a client's genes and environmental exposure leads to a complexity of multifactorial phenotypes, which cannot be fully understood through single tests. Van Ommen and colleagues (2017) eloquently describe a number of examples of the complexity within multifactorial phenotypes and it is clear we cannot base personalized nutrition recommendations on single polymorphism results. A single SNP, however – in this case, of a COMT-homozygous individual – may be helpful to assist the practitioner in selecting and avoiding certain supplements and foods that may inhibit or increase the workload for an enzyme.

Initial plan

The initial plan was built from three key foundations.

Autonomic nervous system

- Reduce overall stress load (part of which may be coming via inflammatory pathways or intestinal permeability).
- Ensure sufficient cofactors for methyl-transferase (COMT) enzymes.
- Use of supplements which could help the nervous system in the short term.

Increased intestinal permeability

- Provide factors which should improve the integrity of the intestinal membrane.
- Eliminate factors that are likely to be contributing to increased intestinal permeability.

Reducing toxicity load

- Given the way this can contribute to overall stress load as well as the autoimmune process.
- Given the raised liver enzymes, recurrent jaundice and biliary cirrhosis.

Lifestyle factors to address

The following were factors that, given the case interpretation, were perhaps contributing to KT's ongoing health issues:

- **Caffeine:** KT drank a small amount of caffeine from one cup of weak coffee every day. She experienced a wired feeling after drinking it, but continued to do so, because she enjoyed the taste and experience, and used it as an energy boost. Heavy coffee consumption increased acute coronary events in men who had low COMT activity compared with those with high activity (Happonen *et al.*, 2006), which is suggestive of perhaps an increased 'sensitivity' to caffeine in those with low COMT activity.
- **Environmental toxins:** Exposure to chemicals is part of normal daily life, but when someone has an overly sensitized immune system (evidenced from the elevated antibodies and lymphocyte sensitivities), the daily exposures need to be considered as mediating factors in ongoing inflammation and immune challenge.
- **Antibiotic use:** KT had been on an intensive antibiotic programme for 14 months. The microbiome is essential for immune system development and regulation of autoimmunity (Singh, Qin and Read, 2015) and it is well documented that antibiotics will reduce microbiome diversity (Karkman, Lehtimäki and Ruokolainen, 2017). The antibodies to *Rickettsia* and *Mycoplasma* were much lowered from one year ago (Table 10.3).
- **Restricted diet:** KT has self-prescribed a restricted diet based on what she felt she was able to eat without triggering symptoms. The problem with long-term dietary restrictions are the loss of phytonutrients, micronutrients and fibre, which are so vital for the microbiome and cofactors in key enzymes.

Dietary recommendations

- Follow a grain-free, dairy-free, sugar-free and processed-food-free diet, also referred to as modified Palaeolithic diet (see Box 9.1, Chapter 9), based on clinical observation and early clinical trials supporting the use of such a diet in autoimmune conditions (Bisht *et al.*, 2014; Lee *et al.*, 2017; Wahls *et al.*, 2018).
- Consume 6–8 portions (a portion is 80 g) of colourful vegetables daily to provide dietary sources of phytonutrients as well as fibre.
- Root vegetables, beans and pulses were consumed to the client's tolerance level. At this stage it was one portion 2–3 times a week.
- 70 g protein per day (based on 1.2 g/kg body weight/day and body weight of 60 kg), preferably from organic or grass-fed meat, organ meats and wild fish to optimize fatty acid profiles (Kamihiro *et al.*, 2015) and minimize toxicants (Hites *et al.*, 2004).
- Eliminate all caffeine.
- Eat foods high in mono- and polyunsaturated fats, such as avocado, almonds, walnuts and olive oil, providing a source of energy via beta oxidation given the restriction of grains. Consume a higher level of omega-3-rich foods, particularly with high EPA and DHA content (such as coldwater oily fish) which have been demonstrated to suppress LPS formation (Kaliannan *et al.*, 2015).
- A plant-based fibre supplement was recommended to see if this would alleviate KT's chronic constipation (slow bowel motility). Low-carbohydrate diets can significantly reduce fibre intake. The supplement included extracts of apple pectin, inulin, flax and prune.

Supplement recommendations

- Theanine 200 mg TID. This is the same dosage given in an eight-week double-blind, placebo-controlled trial which found that l-theanine reduced anxiety in those with schizophrenia and schizoaffective disorder (Ritsner *et al.*, 2011).
- Magnesium (as magnesium taurate) 500 mg BID. Magnesium bound to taurine can activate GABA receptors in the central

nervous system (Jia *et al.*, 2008). From this practitioner's clinical experience, anxiety may be improved with magnesium. This is partially supported in the literature (Lakhan and Vieira, 2010). Magnesium is always given bound to another molecule – in this case taurine was selected as, again based on clinical experience and some supportive evidence, the taurine can be supportive for GABA receptors (Jia *et al.*, 2008).

- DHA and phospholipids 1 g BID. This down-regulates in-flammatory prostaglandins and provides structural support for cell membranes given KT's multiple auto-inflammatory presentation (Calder, 2013).

- Methionine 500 mg BID. Primarily, this was given to provide sulfhydryl groups for toxin excretion and catecholamine clearance. There is also some in-vitro evidence it can enhance contractile action in the colon (Choe, Moon and Park, 2012) and certainly the client reported improvements in constipation after taking it.

- Vitamin D3 3000 IU QD. To address insufficient levels of serum vitamin D and immune regulation.

- Liposomal glutathione 500 mg QD. To support cellular detoxification of toxins (seen as sensitivities) and to ensure sufficient intracellular glutathione levels which often become depleted with the increased oxidative stress seen in autoimmune conditions (Perricone, De Carolis and Perricone, 2009; Pizzorno, 2014).

- Given low iron finding, short-term iron bisglycinate 25 mg QD with lactoferrin until factors affecting absorption such as gastritis and intestinal permeability resolved. Lactoferrin is added to impede the iron-sequestering properties of bacteria that promotes their own growth (given history of *Rickettsia*, *Mycoplasma* and IBS symptoms) allowing better bioavailability of iron. Iron in bisglycinate form has been demonstrated to be more bioavailable than ferrous sulphate with a tendency to be better tolerated in relation to gastrointestinal side effects (Ferrari *et al.*, 2012).

Liaison with her medical practitioner

In consultation with her medical practitioner, it was agreed to discontinue her antibiotic programme.

Drug–nutrient interactions

Drug–nutrient interactions were checked using the Natural Medicines Comprehensive Database, (see Appendix A). For due diligence, the antibiotics were included in this. No interactions were found for foods or supplements that were included in KT's recommendations.

Other advice

KT was advised how to avoid exposure to nickel, benzene and bisphenol A. Table 10.5, created for client education, provides a summary of where they are found. The practitioner ensured this was interpreted into simple positive steps the client could undertake such as:

- using ceramic and glass cookware and containers for food
- refraining from taking receipts from credit card machines
- using glass water bottles
- using gloves when filling car with petrol
- removing/avoiding plug-in air fresheners
- covering the backs of buttons, watches, zips, jewellery, which may contain nickel, with clear nail polish or masking tape.

Psychological support

The patient was referred to a qualified psychology practitioner for mind- training-based therapy allowing her to modulate her maladaptive stress response.

Table 10.5 Avoiding chemical exposure

Chemical or toxicant	Common sources in the home environment and consumer products	Alternatives or suggestion for removal
Nickel	Stainless steel, kitchen appliances, medical and dental tools, tattoo ink (nickel oxides), zips, inexpensive costume jewellery	Replace cookware with ceramic, glass, cast iron or terracotta Purchase nickel-free stainless-steel cutlery Cover backs of watches, buttons, zips and jewellery with a coating of clear nail varnish
Benzene	Cigarette smoke, fragrances (plug-in air fresheners and scented candles), exhaust fumes, glues, paints, detergents, cosmetics, furniture wax, polystyrene production, rubbers, lubricants, dyes, pesticides	Burn essential oils, not candles Choose VOC-free paints and varnishes Choose benzene-free cosmetics and body care Choose organic produce without the use of pesticides
Bisphenol A	Plastic bottles and containers, thermal paper on till receipts, tinned foods (lining)	Use glass bottles, store food in glass containers or baking parchment Use beeswax wrapping instead of clingfilm

Protocol reactions and evolutions

KT experienced an adverse reaction to the fibre supplement, intense pain in the sacrum, painful diarrhoea (she described it as acidic), yellowing of the skin, low mood and inflammation around her eyes. It was at this stage that the fructose test was ordered, which was positive (see Figure 10.1), and close examination of the fibre supplement revealed it contained inulin (a polymer of fructose) and prune (high fructose content).

Protocol: 25 gm of fructose diluted in 200ml of water
Method: Hydrogen and methane values measured every 60 minutes for 180 minutes

Basal levels: Hydrogen = 0 ppm Methane = 21 ppm

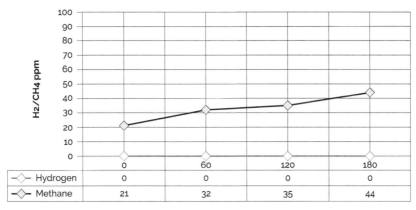

	0	60	120	180
Hydrogen	0	0	0	0
Methane	21	32	35	44

Time (minutes)

Figure 10.1 Fructose test result

At this point the practitioner re-examined the fructose content of all produce KT was consuming and established a baseline of tolerance. This turned out to be foods containing as little as 2.4 g of fructose per 100 g. Foods including watermelon or strawberries (commonly considered low-fructose fruits) were subsequently eliminated from the diet.

A low-fructose diet consists of restricting primarily the consumption of fruit – in particular those with a high fructose-to-glucose ratio. Individuals with fructose malabsorption are lacking the monosaccharide transporter GLUT5. Unabsorbed fructose in the lumen causes water to be osmotically drawn in, resulting in rapid movement of bowel contents into the colon where contents are fermented by gut microbes. This fermentation produces gas that leads to flatulence, bloating, abdominal pain or changes in bowel patterns.

Fructose is present primarily in fruit but also a variety of plant foods and sucrose (the disaccharide of glucose and fructose). Tolerance to fructose varies individually. Gastrointestinal pathologies can exacerbate the loss of monosaccharide transporters which in turn worsens the degree of fructose malabsorption. For more information on fructose sources and avoidance, see Janice Joneja's work and reference sheets

(Joneja, 2018). Appendix 10.1 includes a list of high-fructose foods created by the practitioner for client education.

Supplement additions

- L-glutamine 5 g TID. Glutamine has been shown to assist in improving permeability in the gastrointestinal tract (Maes and Leunis, 2008; Rao and Samak, 2012).

Patient follow-up

Eight weeks following the introduction of the low-fructose diet, KT reported the following improvements:

- No longer using diazepam.
- Fatigue much reduced (severity of 3/10).
- Constipation dramatically improved.
- Anxiety, agoraphobia and panic attacks were rare.
- Reduced severity in chemical/environmental reactions.
- Fewer inflammatory flare-ups, migraines and headaches (less than one a fortnight).
- Brain fog no longer present.
- Some days able to tolerate small amounts of grain and starch without subsequent leg pains, eye inflammation and constipation. However, acutely stressful events will bring on symptoms with severity scale of 10 regardless of dietary and supplement compliance.
- Laboratory results showed lowered ANA and liver enzymes with an increase in ferritin.

At the six-month follow-up, with the inclusion of low-fructose intake:

- No longer affected by fatigue, pain or bowel stasis. Considered her energy levels 'normal'.

- Anxiety was manageable and she was able to travel, work and resume her studies.
- Inflammatory symptoms were under control as long as she remained diet-compliant.
- More starches tolerated daily, but reintroduction of fruit, coffee or dairy would cause a return in initial symptoms, albeit with quicker post-flare-up recovery.
- Liver enzymes had normalized within a standard reference range. A follow-up with her medical practitioner was recommended to review her biliary cirrhosis diagnosis.

Discussion

Autoimmune disease is complex and multifactorial. It can produce a spectrum of functional impairments that can have mild to debilitating impact on the client's quality of life. It is thought that 30% of cases are due to genetic predisposition and 70% to environmental agents such as dietary factors, toxic compounds, infections and gut inflammation (Vojdani, Pollard and Campbell, 2014).

Increased intestinal permeability is thought to play a key role in some cases of autoimmune disease (Fasano and Shea-Donohue, 2005). In a 'normal' gut membrane, only a small number of large molecules will be absorbed. Increased intestinal permeability permits the entrance of a greater number of antigenic macromolecules that are normally confined to the gut lumen.

In this case, increased intestinal permeability was present. Test results (elevated IgG and IgM response to LPS and IgM response to zonulin) confirmed the suspicion based on the symptom patterns of 'gut fermentation' with starchy foods. Gram-negative bacteria contain lipopolysaccharides (LPS) in their cell walls, also known as endotoxins. When absorbed through a damaged intestinal barrier, LPS are capable of eliciting a strong immune response. In personalized nutrition, the goal is to understand why a dysfunction is present. Therefore, the practitioner tested for SIBO which could have been a trigger for LPS.

The SIBO test was negative. However, the client then responded in quite a striking and unusual way to a fibre-based supplement. The practitioner became suspicious of the fructose polymers contained in the fibre supplement. A fructose-intolerance breath test confirmed a low capacity to absorb fructose, with methane being elevated.

There are two categories of fructose absorption disorder and it is important for the practitioner to be able to distinguish between the two in order to manage expectations for recovery going forward.

- **Fructose malabsorption (FM)** is the more common condition, thought to affect up to 40% of individuals. A loss of fructose transporters (Glut5) on the enterocytes means the individual is unable to absorb large amounts of fructose which then remains in the lumen. The loss of transporters may be transient or chronic. It can be triggered by or occur alongside other gastrointestinal disorders such as coeliac disease, gastroenteritis or parasitic dysentery. In Western populations the consumption of high-fructose corn syrup (used commonly to sweeten beverages and processed foods) can lead to malabsorption in 50% of healthy adults (Beyer, Caviar and McCallum, 2005).
- **Hereditary fructose intolerance (FI)** is not a problem with absorption, but an inborn error of fructose metabolism. This is a relatively rare autosomal recessive disorder where the individual carries a defect in the liver enzyme aldolase-B that metabolizes fructose-1-phosphate into glucose. Primary clinical symptoms are abdominal pain, jaundice, biliary dysfunction, hypoglycaemia and 'shock like symptoms' (Tran, 2017). Deficiency of this enzyme results in fructose-1-phosphate accumulation and a trapping of phosphate. One of the consequences of this is diminished adenosine triphosphate regeneration (Lambertz et al., 2017). The depletion of ATP levels then contributes to low energy levels. Fructose accumulation can increase lactate in the blood that is exported to peripheral tissues. High lactate can reduce oxygen availability to organs, promoting lactic acidosis that can be experienced as muscle pain and detected as a high anion gap. This process increases the inflammatory response (Tran, 2017).

FM or FI will result in high levels of free fructose fermented by resident anaerobic flora. KT's test result showed an excess of methane gas produced by methanogenic bacteria. This dominance is more commonly found in patients with chronic constipation in epidemiological research, backed by findings in clinical research that methane slows intestinal motility (Triantafyllou, Chang and Pimentel, 2014). Although an exact mechanism of how methane slows colonic transit is yet to be elicited, translational studies have suggested neurotransmitter/modulator effects of the gas to slow down intestinal peristalsis. Preliminary evidence found that reduction of methanogenic flora with rifaximin reduced slow-transit constipation as well as methane gas on a breath test (Ghoshal *et al.*, 2011). This is consistent with KT experiencing improvements in constipation following a fructose-restricted diet as well as her ability to tolerate more starches/fibre during antibiotic therapy.

Future management

The first line of management of both types of fructose-associated disorder is strict dietary restriction. Fructose malabsorption can lead to decreased absorption and availability of nutrients including tryptophan, folate and zinc (Gibson *et al.*, 2007), all of which are key substrates (tryptophan for serotonin) or cofactors (zinc and folate) involved in the central nervous system. Since fruit is a source of vitamin C, fibre and phytonutrients, short-term supplementation may be necessary. In the longer term, we want to avoid unnecessary dietary restriction.

It was hypothesized by the practitioner that if the patient has **FM**, the threshold for absorption may improve over time as efforts are made to heal the epithelial cell lining and reduce intestinal permeability. At this stage the client can be advised to reintroduce small quantities of low-fructose fruits to gauge tolerance.

If **hereditary FI** is the case, the client will not be able to tolerate fructose even if intestinal permeability is improved. However, key symptoms (including jaundice) will only develop following ingestion of fructose, sucrose or sorbitol (which is converted to fructose by the liver).

At this stage it is unclear whether KT's fructose issues are due to hereditary fructose intolerance (and therefore unlikely to be overcome) or malabsorption (and therefore likely to resolve). Options for future management are summarized in a flowchart in Figure 10.2. Given the positive fructose-intolerance breath test, it would be best practice at this point to refer to the client's GP or consultant gastroenterologist to obtain a medical diagnosis.

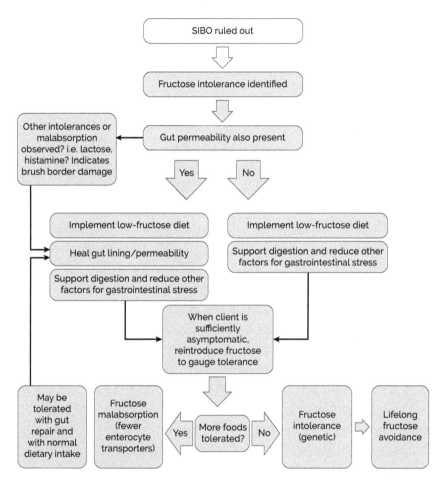

Figure 10.2 Proposed flowchart for future management, showing options and expectations of outcome

LPS, endotoxaemia and inflammation

Although it was observed that the ketogenic and Palaeolithic diet had helped some aspects of KT's complex illness initially, they had resulted in other problems when used in the longer term.

It is thus important to consider the long-term impact of such diets which are commonly practitioner-implemented or self-prescribed for various conditions such as autoimmune and chronic fatigue syndrome. These diets typically contain high levels of saturated fats (such as coconut oil, animal fats, meat drippings and butter) and can be low in fibre due to carbohydrate restriction.

It has been demonstrated that a diet high in saturated fat can result in the increased translocation of gut-derived endotoxin (LPS) into peripheral circulation and this can induce a postprandial low-grade inflammatory response through activation of NF-kB, TNF-a, IL-1 and IL-6 (Erridge *et al.*, 2007). Elevation in circulating LPS is now thought to be driving a wide range of chronic metabolic conditions such as heart disease, obesity, insulin resistance and chronic fatigue syndrome. The type of fat consumed appears to be relevant to this type of pathogenesis. Higher omega-6 fatty acid intake versus omega-3 leads to an increase in LPS-producing bacteria with pro-inflammatory effect, while a higher omega-3:omega-6 ratio mitigated inflammation and suppressed LPS-forming bacteria (Kaliannan *et al.*, 2015). The mechanism demonstrated was the increased expression of intestinal alkaline phosphatase (IAP) that was elevated in omega-3 consumption. IAP has many roles in gut barrier maintenance including detoxification of LPS, inhibition of gram-negative bacteria such as *Escherichia coli* and suppression of the inflammatory response (Jiang *et al.*, 2016).

Sugar intake is also relevant to endotoxaemia. In one study in which primates were fed a calorie-controlled high-fructose, low-fat diet compared with controls fed an isocaloric low-fructose, low-fat diet over a six-week period, significant increases in biomarkers of liver damage and endotoxemia were recorded in the high-fructose group (Kavanagh *et al.*, 2013). KT already had a number of liver-related signs, including raised liver enzymes and biliary cirrhosis.

In summary, fructose and its metabolites can directly or indirectly contribute to intestinal permeability, oxidative stress and chronic inflammation. Modifying fat intake to favour omega-3 essential fatty acids and a moderate level of saturated fat can minimize postprandial inflammation. Both interventions occurred within KT's personalized nutrition plan and will likely have assisted in effecting the significant systemic improvements seen.

Conclusion

At present the client is able to tolerate most foods (with the exception of fructose) and able to carry out a normal life. Although the journey to full recovery continues, a key stepping stone was identifying the mediators that were holding her in a chronic autoimmune state. In this case, fructose consumption was the key to personalizing her autoimmune dietary protocol to balance the microbiota, allow for intestinal barrier healing and arrest metabolic endotoxaemia (inflammation) evidenced by the dramatic improvements in the client's symptomology. The practitioner recommended a re-test for *Rickettsia*, *Mycoplasma* and ANA; however, the client elected not to do so on the basis that she felt she was no longer affected by them.

The combination of strategies addressing her emotional response (through psychological work) and supplementation of key cofactors to support COMT enzymes was likely an important step in arresting the hyper-responsive sympathetic nervous system that was proving detrimental to her capacity for recovery.

Knowledge of the environmental exposures she showed most reactivity to allowed her to live and eat in a way that was more compatible with her tendency towards autoimmunity and reduce the burden on her slow catecholamine and toxin clearance pathways.

The case demonstrates that standard autoimmune or gut-healing diet protocols will not suit every individual and that they need personalization. Following up unusual reactions to supplements or foods can give clues to the underlying mechanisms – in this case, the fructose content of a fibre supplement.

This case also highlights fructose intolerance as an underdiagnosed problem (Choi *et al.*, 2003). A key learning from this case is to consider fructose intolerance when SIBO breath tests are negative, given the strongly overlapping symptoms patterns.

Q&A

AW: This is quite a medically complex case with lots of previous diagnoses and test results. Can you give any tips on how you manage and sort that level of detail and information and avoid overwhelm?

CS: At our clinic patients typically present with a long and complex case history, having seen a string of practitioners and medical specialists, along with extensive laboratory results. Viewing all this information in the functional medicine model helps to reduce the complexity and discern a theoretical cause and effect. Drawing up a priority list of what to tackle first – for example, if there are significant gut issues co-existing with fatigue, pain and insomnia, supplementing with high-dose energy precursors or anti-inflammatory remedies would be pointless if there is a high likelihood that absorption is impaired. Instead, our first point of investigation would be to identify if malabsorption is an issue, what the root cause of this might be and work on supporting this.

It is also important to have the patient understand that to make a complete and sustained recovery from their chronic illness requires time and commitment to methodically investigate root causes and allow their body to heal at the pace it is capable of.

AW: It appears as though elements of her self-prescribed diet were a mediating factor. This theme has come up earlier in this book: that off-the-shelf therapeutic diets can be helpful to a point, and then become counter-productive for individuals. Do you think part of the issue is that they are designed as short-term therapeutic diets rather than longer-term maintenance diets?

CS: In our industry we are used to diets and supplements that polarize the research and medical/health community. The majority of the research involves short-term studies; therefore, we don't really know how this will play out in a client when applied for months to years. It is important to critically evaluate both the positive and negative sides of any diet and monitor for these negative side effects in the client. Diets that are designed to cut out an entire food group may alleviate some debilitating symptoms for the client, but they will be missing certain nutrients these food groups carry. The impact on their microbiome diversity (and downstream effects on immune status), acid–alkaline balance or energy metabolism in the long term has to be considered.

AW: What sort of signs do you look for to help you identify that a diet might be creating an acid–alkaline imbalance?

CS: With this case, I suspected that a high-protein and high-fat diet, in the absence of adequate antioxidants, fibre and vegetables, could lead to acidosis, be it metabolic, respiratory or nutrition ketoacidosis (see Box 10.2), and could be contributing to some of the client's described side effects such as muscle pain or brain fog. The anion gap is an under-utilized biomarker. It is run as part of the electrolyte panel on a standard blood panel and looks for the difference in negatively and positively charged electrolytes; if this gap is too high or low, this could indicate acidosis (higher acidity in the blood) or alkalosis – either of which are a sign of an acid–alkali imbalance.

This was carried out on request with the client's GP. Acidosis is more commonly associated with type-2 diabetes mellitus, asthma, renal problems and obesity; however, it can also be a result of chronic stress, disordered breathing patterns, insufficient mineral reserve or acid-forming diets (that deplete essential minerals) such as keto acids from a high-meat-protein and high-fat diet. Addressing all of these was an early game-changer for this client.

BOX 10.2 NUTRITIONAL KETOSIS VERSUS KETOACIDOSIS

Nutritional ketosis is the metabolic state where the body is adapted to using endogenous ketone bodies produced by fat catabolism (over carbohydrates) as the primary source of fuel. Ketoacidosis manifests where ketone levels in serum or urine become pathologically high.

Diabetic ketoacidosis is a compilation of type 1 or 2 diabetes mellitus due to abnormally low insulin secretion, which can be life-threatening if not treated medically.

Ghimire and Dhamoon (2019)

AW: It's really incredible how quickly she improved, given the long list of symptoms she had. Understanding the biochemical triggers for her anxiety seems to have been key here. Do you feel that the theanine and magnesium did the 'heavy lifting' in that area? Any tips on how to deal with COMT SNP results when we can never know the multifactored potential phenotypes?

CS: In our integrated clinic we have recognized that idiosyncratic reactions to supplements, chemicals and foods can occur when the nervous system is chronically switched on high alert. We knew that if her body was not in the parasympathetic response, there would be a likelihood that she would triage her nutrients, energy and resources into the stress response rather than growth and healing.

The client had previously noted adverse reactions to B vitamins, and could not tolerate caffeine along with some other food reactions you might see in a typical COMT polymorphism. She was made aware that although SNP panels made it possible to see a snapshot of her genetic mutations, whether they actually express or not would be down to diet and environmental influences. Where possible, we try to back up genetic SNP testing with 'functional' metabolite tests such as methylation panels which look at the relative ratio of end products. This would be the accurate way to discern if her genes and environment were out of balance. Due to a lack of funds, we were unable to utilize this test with the present client.

Magnesium taurate and theanine were selected over methyl donors in order to support her adrenaline clearance. Once this was facilitated, she was then able to tolerate methylated B vitamins (which she had previously experienced an adverse reaction to).

AW: Any tips on how you manage the therapeutic relationship, especially when there is a flare-up of symptoms (even though that eventually gave you the clue about fructose)?

CS: I aim to educate the client about potential reactions that may be expected so that it doesn't catch them by surprise. Encouraging them to listen to their bodies is important as I believe that one person's medicine is another person's poison – there really is no 'one size fits all' in our field. Our patient cohort often have multiple chemical sensitivities and very individualized reactions, so we take a gentle approach to dosing supplements, asking them to start with the smallest dose possible and titre doses to their tolerance levels. They also understand that these reactions (while being a temporary set-back) can be really informative in filling in knowledge gaps, clues to other underlying imbalances and further individualizing treatment, so it is rarely met with prolonged fear. Despondency can be an issue when flare-ups happen very regularly or there is just a lack of progress. Ultimately, flare-ups or plateaus are inevitable and usually multifactorial, even with something as seemingly black and white as fructose intolerance. Reminding them that there is always something they can do to manage one of the contributors can keep them motivated in a down period.

Personally, I chose to specialize in this field because I recovered from CFS/complex chronic illness myself; sharing my personal experiences with them or just empathizing with their feelings without judgement or having an answer helps that connection on a different level.

Appendix 10.1 List of fructose-containing foods used as client education

Food	Fructose g/100 g	Glucose g/100 g
High-fructose corn syrup	55	45
Sucrose	50	50
Honey	40.5	34.2
Raisins	29.7	27.8
Dates	23.9	24.9
Prune	15.9	30
Royal jelly	11.3	9.8
Fig	8.2	9.6
Molasses	8	8.8

Grape	7.3	8.2
Cherry	7.2	4.7
Pear	6.5	2.6
Apple	5	1.7
Gooseberry	4.1	4.4
Greengage/plum	4	5.5
Mulberry	3.6	4.4
Banana	3.5	4.5
Plum	3.4	5.2
Watermelon	3.4	1.6
Blackberry	2.9	3.2
Whitecurrant	2.6	3
Raspberry	2.4	2.3
Strawberry	2.3	2.6
Redcurrant	1.9	2.3
Orange	1.8	2.5
Peach	1.6	1.5
Melon	1.5	2.1
Lemon	1.4	1.4
Pineapple	1.4	2.3
Loganberry	1.3	1.9
Grapefruit	1.2	2
Tomato	1.2	1.6
Potato	0.1	0.1

Source: List adapted by practitioner from work by Janice Joneja (2018)

References

BDA, n.d. Dental amalgam FAQs. Accessed on 26/05/2019 at www.bda.org/about-the-bda/campaigns/amalgam/Pages/dental-amalgam-faqs.aspx

Beyer, P.L., Caviar, E.M., McCallum, R.W., 2005. Fructose intake at current levels in the United States may cause gastrointestinal distress in normal adults. *Journal of the Academy of Nutrition and Dietetics* 105, 1559–1566. https://doi.org/10.1016/j.jada.2005.07.002

Bisht, B., Darling, W.G., Grossmann, R.E., Shivapour, E.T, *et al.*, 2014. A multimodal intervention for patients with secondary progressive multiple sclerosis: Feasibility and effect on fatigue. *Alternative and Complementary Therapies* 20, 347–355. https://doi.org/10.1089/act.2014.20606

Bonefeld, C.M., Nielsen, M.M., Vennegaard, M.T., Johansen, J.D., Geisler, C., Thyssen, J.P., 2015. Nickel acts as an adjuvant during cobalt sensitization. *Experimental Dermatology* 24, 229–231. https://doi.org/10.1111/exd.12634

Calder, P.C., 2013. n-3 Fatty acids, inflammation and immunity: New mechanisms to explain old actions. *Proceedings of the Nutrition Society* 72, 326–336. https://doi.org/10.1017/S0029665113001031

Choe, E.K., Moon, J.S., Park, K.J., 2012. Methionine enhances the contractile activity of human colon circular smooth muscle *in vitro*. *Journal of Korean Medical Science* 27, 777–783. https://doi.org/10.3346/jkms.2012.27.7.777

Choi, Y.K., Johlin, F.C., Summers, R.W., Jackson, M., Rao, S.S.C., 2003. Fructose intolerance: An under-recognized problem. *American Journal of Gastroenterology* 98, 1348–1353.

Enoch, M.-A., Xu, K., Ferro, E., Harris, C.R., Goldman, D., 2003. Genetic origins of anxiety in women: A role for a functional catechol-O-methyltransferase polymorphism. *Psychiatric Genetics* 13, 33–41.

Erridge, C., Attina, T., Spickett, C.M., Webb, D.J., 2007. A high-fat meal induces low-grade endotoxemia: Evidence of a novel mechanism of postprandial inflammation. *American Journal of Clinical Nutrition* 86, 1286–1292. https://doi.org/10.1093/ajcn/86.5.1286

Fasano, A., Shea-Donohue, T., 2005. Mechanisms of disease: The role of intestinal barrier function in the pathogenesis of gastrointestinal autoimmune diseases. *Nature Clinical Practice Gastroenterology and Hepatology* 2, 416–422. https://doi.org/10.1038/ncpgasthep0259

Ferrari, P., Nicolini, A., Manca, M.L., Rossi, G. *et al.*, 2012. Treatment of mild non-chemotherapy-induced iron deficiency anemia in cancer patients: Comparison between oral ferrous bisglycinate chelate and ferrous sulfate. *Biomedicine and Pharmacotherapy* 66, 414–418. https://doi.org/10.1016/j.biopha.2012.06.003

Gabrielli, M., D'Angelo, G., Di Rienzo, T., Scarpellini, E., Ojetti, V., 2013. Diagnosis of small intestinal bacterial overgrowth in the clinical practice. *European Review for Medical and Pharmacological Sciences* 17, Suppl 2, 30–35.

Ghimire, P., Dhamoon, A.S., 2019. Ketoacidosis. In: *StatPearls*. StatPearls Publishing.

Ghoshal, U.C., Srivastava, D., Verma, A., Misra, A., 2011. Slow transit constipation associated with excess methane production and its improvement following rifaximin therapy: A case report. *Journal of Neurogastroenterology and Motility* 17, 185–188. https://doi.org/10.5056/jnm.2011.17.2.185

Gibson, P.R., Newnham, E., Barrett, J.S., Shepherd, S.J., Muir, J.G., 2007. Review article: Fructose malabsorption and the bigger picture. *Alimentary Pharmacology and Therapeutics* 25, 349–363. https://doi.org/10.1111/j.1365-2036.2006.03186.x

Gregersen, P.K., 2007. Modern genetics, ancient defenses, and potential therapies. *New England Journal of Medicine* 356, 1263–1266. https://doi.org/10.1056/NEJMe078017

Happonen, P., Voutilainen, S., Tuomainen, T.-P., Salonen, J.T., 2006. Catechol-o-methyltransferase gene polymorphism modifies the effect of coffee intake on incidence of acute coronary events. *PloS ONE* 1, e117. https://doi.org/10.1371/journal.pone.0000117

Heinz, A., Smolka, M.N., 2006. The effects of catechol O-methyltransferase genotype on brain activation elicited by affective stimuli and cognitive tasks. *Reviews in the Neurosciences* 17, 359–367.

Hites, R.A., Foran, J.A., Carpenter, D.O., Hamilton, M.C., Knuth, B.A., Schwager, S.J., 2004. Global assessment of organic contaminants in farmed salmon. *Science* 303, 226–229. https://doi.org/10.1126/science.1091447

Jia, F., Yue, M., Chandra, D., Keramidas, A. *et al.*, 2008. Taurine is a potent activator of extrasynaptic GABA(A) receptors in the thalamus. *Journal of Neuroscience* 28, 106–115. https://doi.org/10.1523/JNEUROSCI.3996-07.2008

Jiang, T., Gao, X., Wu, C., Tian, F. *et al.*, 2016. Apple-derived pectin modulates gut microbiota, improves gut barrier function, and attenuates metabolic endotoxemia in rats with diet-induced obesity. *Nutrients* 8, 126. https://doi.org/10.3390/nu8030126

Joneja, J., 2018. FAQs and Fact Sheets – Vickerstaff Health Services. Accessed on 26/05/2019 at www.allergynutrition.com/faqs-fact-sheets

Kaliannan, K., Wang, B., Li, X.-Y., Kim, K.-J., Kang, J.X., 2015. A host-microbiome interaction mediates the opposing effects of omega-6 and omega-3 fatty acids on metabolic endotoxemia. *Scientific Reports* 5, 11276. https://doi.org/10.1038/srep11276

Kamihiro, S., Stergiadis, S., Leifert, C., Eyre, M.D., Butler, G., 2015. Meat quality and health implications of organic and conventional beef production. *Meat Science* 100, 306–318. https://doi.org/10.1016/j.meatsci.2014.10.015

Karkman, A., Lehtimäki, J., Ruokolainen, L., 2017. The ecology of human microbiota: Dynamics and diversity in health and disease. *Annals of the New York Academy of Sciences* 1399, 78–92. https://doi.org/10.1111/nyas.13326

Kavanagh, K., Wylie, A.T., Tucker, K.L., Hamp, T.J. *et al.*, 2013. Dietary fructose induces endotoxemia and hepatic injury in calorically controlled primates. *American Journal of Clinical Nutrition* 98, 349–357. https://doi.org/10.3945/ajcn.112.057331

Kharrazian, D., 2014. The potential roles of bisphenol A (BPA) pathogenesis in autoimmunity. *Autoimmune Diseases* 2014. https://doi.org/10.1155/2014/743616

Lakhan, S.E., Vieira, K.F., 2010. Nutritional and herbal supplements for anxiety and anxiety-related disorders: Systematic review. *Nutrition Journal* 9, 42. https://doi.org/10.1186/1475-2891-9-42

Lambertz, J., Weiskirchen, S., Landert, S., Weiskirchen, R., 2017. Fructose: A dietary sugar in crosstalk with microbiota contributing to the development and progression of non-alcoholic liver disease. *Frontiers in Immunology* 8, 1159. https://doi.org/10.3389/fimmu.2017.01159

Lee, J.E., Bisht, B., Hall, M.J., Rubenstein, L.M. *et al.*, 2017. A multimodal, nonpharmacologic intervention improves mood and cognitive function in people with multiple sclerosis. *Journal of the American College of Nutrition* 36, 150–168. https://doi.org/10.1080/07315724.2016.1255160

Leonard, M.M., Sapone, A., Catassi, C., Fasano, A., 2017. Celiac disease and nonceliac gluten sensitivity: A review. *JAMA* 318, 647–656. https://doi.org/10.1001/jama.2017.9730

Lerner, A., Jeremias, P., Matthias, T., 2015. The world incidence and prevalence of autoimmune diseases is increasing. *International Journal of Celiac Disease* 3, 151–155. https://doi.org/10.12691/ijcd-3-4-8

Lin, R., Zhou, L., Zhang, J., Wang, B., 2015. Abnormal intestinal permeability and microbiota in patients with autoimmune hepatitis. *International Journal of Clinical and Experimental Pathology* 8, 5153–5160.

Maes, M., Leunis, J.-C., 2008. Normalization of leaky gut in chronic fatigue syndrome (CFS) is accompanied by a clinical improvement: Effects of age, duration of illness and the translocation of LPS from gram-negative bacteria. *Neuro Endocrinology Letters* 29, 902–910.

Männistö, P.T., Kaakkola, S., 1999. Catechol-O-methyltransferase (COMT): Biochemistry, molecular biology, pharmacology, and clinical efficacy of the new selective COMT inhibitors. *Pharmacological Reviews* 51, 593–628.

Manzel, A., Muller, D.N., Hafler, D.A., Erdman, S.E., Linker, R.A., Kleinewietfeld, M., 2014. Role of 'Western diet' in inflammatory autoimmune diseases. *Current Allergy and Asthma Reports* 14, 404. https://doi.org/10.1007/s11882-013-0404-6

McGinnis, W.R., Audhya, T., Walsh, W.J., Jackson, J.A. *et al.*, 2008. Discerning the mauve factor, part 1. *Alternative Therapies in Health and Medicine* 14, 40–50.

Nissinen, E., Männistö, P.T., 2010. Biochemistry and pharmacology of catechol-O-methyltransferase inhibitors. *International Review of Neurobiology* 95, 73–118. https://doi.org/10.1016/B978-0-12-381326-8.00005-3

Perricone, C., De Carolis, C., Perricone, R., 2009. Glutathione: A key player in autoimmunity. *Autoimmunity Reviews* 8, 697–701. https://doi.org/10.1016/j.autrev.2009.02.020

Pizzorno, J., 2014. Glutathione! *Integrative Medicine: A Clinician's Journal* 13, 8–12.

Pollard, K.M., Christy, J.M., Cauvi, D.M., Kono, D.H., 2018. Environmental xenobiotic exposure and autoimmunity. *Current Opinion in Toxicology* 10, 15–22. https://doi.org/10.1016/j.cotox.2017.11.009

Rao, R., Samak, G., 2012. Role of glutamine in protection of intestinal epithelial tight junctions. *Journal of Epithelial Biology and Pharmacology* 5, 47–54. https://doi.org/10.2174/1875044301205010047

Ritsner, M.S., Miodownik, C., Ratner, Y., Shleifer, T. *et al.*, 2011. L-theanine relieves positive, activation, and anxiety symptoms in patients with schizophrenia and schizoaffective disorder: An 8-week, randomized, double-blind, placebo-controlled, 2-center study. *Journal of Clinical Psychiatry* 72, 34–42. https://doi.org/10.4088/JCP.09m05324gre

Singh, B., Qin, N., Reid, G., 2015. Microbiome regulation of autoimmune, gut and liver associated diseases. *Inflammation and Allergy – Drug Targets* 14, 84–93.

Sturgeon, C., Fasano, A., 2016. Zonulin, a regulator of epithelial and endothelial barrier functions, and its involvement in chronic inflammatory diseases. *Tissue Barriers* 4, e1251384. https://doi.org/10.1080/21688370.2016.1251384

Toribio-Mateas, M., 2018. Harnessing the power of microbiome assessment tools as part of neuroprotective nutrition and lifestyle medicine interventions. *Microorganisms* 6. https://doi.org/10.3390/microorganisms6020035

Tran, C., 2017. Inborn errors of fructose metabolism. What can we learn from them? *Nutrients* 9. https://doi.org/10.3390/nu9040356

Triantafyllou, K., Chang, C., Pimentel, M., 2014. Methanogens, methane and gastrointestinal motility. *Journal of Neurogastroenterology and Motility* 20, 31–40. https://doi.org/10.5056/jnm.2014.20.1.31

van Ommen, B., van den Broek, T., de Hoogh, I., van Erk, M. *et al.*, 2017. Systems biology of personalized nutrition. *Nutrition Reviews* 75, 579–599. https://doi.org/10.1093/nutrit/nux029

Vaucher, P., Druais, P.-L., Waldvogel, S., Favrat, B., 2012. Effect of iron supplementation on fatigue in nonanemic menstruating women with low ferritin: A randomized controlled trial. *CMAJ* 184, 1247–1254. https://doi.org/10.1503/cmaj.110950

Vojdani, A., Pollard, K.M., Campbell, A.W., 2014. Environmental triggers and autoimmunity. *Autoimmune Diseases* 2014. https://doi.org/10.1155/2014/798029

Wahls, T., Scott, M.O., Alshare, Z., Rubenstein, L. *et al.*, 2018. Dietary approaches to treat MS-related fatigue: Comparing the modified Paleolithic (Wahls Elimination) and low saturated fat (Swank) diets on perceived fatigue in persons with relapsing-remitting multiple sclerosis: study protocol for a randomized control. *Trials* 19, 309. https://doi.org/10.1186/s13063-018-2680-x

WHO, 2000. 2,4-Diaminophenol. Accessed on 18/06/2019 at https://comptox.epa.gov/dashboard/dsstoxdb/results?search=DTXSID7043748

Woo, J.-M., Yoon, K.-S., Choi, Y.-H., Oh, K.-S., Lee, Y.-S., Yu, B.-H., 2004. The association between panic disorder and the L/L genotype of catechol-O-methyltransferase. *Journal of Psychiatric Research* 38, 365–370. https://doi.org/10.1016/j.jpsychires.2004.01.001

Woo, J.-M., Yoon, K.-S., Yu, B.-H., 2002. Catechol O-methyltransferase genetic polymorphism in panic disorder. *American Journal of Psychiatry* 159, 1785–1787. https://doi.org/10.1176/appi.ajp.159.10.1785

11

Endometriosis and Hormonal Health

Practitioner: Lorna Driver-Davies

Additional contribution to case write-up: Angela Walker

Introduction

Endometriosis is defined as the presence of endometrial tissue or cells outside the uterine cavity. Endometrial cells function just as those in the uterus, responding to cyclical changes in hormones and during the menstrual cycle. Growths, known as lesions, can develop, typically surrounding the female reproductive organs and, less commonly, over the surface of other organs such as the small intestines (Rogers *et al.*, 2009). It affects 6–10% of women of reproductive age (Rogers *et al.*, 2017). Those figures could easily be much higher since many women will remain undiagnosed.

It is common to experience discomfort or pain (sometimes severe) from endometrial adhesions. Sufferers may experience classic physical and mental premenstrual syndrome (PMS) symptoms as well as dysmenorrhea and menorrhagia, which can significantly impact quality of life. Endometriosis is different to classic dysmenorrhea in that pain can occur pre- and post-menstruation and in organs or tissue other than the uterus. Irritable bowel syndrome (IBS) is more likely to occur in women with endometriosis (Issa *et al.*, 2016; Schomacker *et al.*, 2018).

Definitive diagnosis is only through surgical laparoscopy, since blood tests and other types of scans are inconclusive. Endometriosis is graded depending on the severity of lesions, scar tissue and adhesions. Conventional treatment for the majority includes lasering (via laparoscopy), endometrial ablation, hysterectomy, medication and contraceptive options. Laparoscopy may be only temporary as up to 50% will develop the condition again within five years of surgery (Guo, 2009).

There is no single aetiology for endometriosis; the potential factors will be discussed during the case study.

Initial case presentation

JM is a 47-year-old woman, married with two teenage children. She was diagnosed with endometriosis age 45, classified as stage 3, meaning moderate with adhesions and possible endometrioma (ovarian cyst).

Key symptoms

- Extreme tiredness and irritability. The symptoms were not fully relieved by thyroid medication, sleep or rest. They intensified before and during menstruation and during stressful times.
- On normal days her energy was 4 or 5/10 (10 meaning fully energized).
- The day before her period, energy was 2/10. She described this as a 'crash' and would often have to go to bed on those days.
- By day 2 of her period, energy levels would begin to rise to her normal level.
- Menstrual cycle was irregular (ranging from 19 to 28 days); typically, she noticed ovulation, and menstruation would start five days after ovulation.
- Premenstrual symptoms experienced: mood swings, sweet cravings, tiredness and low mood.

- Mid-cycle pain lasting five days. This was the time of her cycle where she experienced most pain, together with mild IBS-type symptoms.
- Over the past eight years all these symptoms had worsened.
- Pressure from work had intensified over the past eight years. She had recently decided to take a work sabbatical to focus on her health.
- She suspected she was perimenopausal due to cycle irregularity and changes in her mood.

JM's main goal was to improve her energy levels, lengthen the time between future laparoscopies and avoid a hysterectomy.

Other symptoms gathered from the intake questionnaire and noted during the consultation:

- Sensitivity to stress, anxiety, irritability and feeling 'wired'.
- Sensitivity to alcohol (feeling hungover after very little alcohol).
- Sensitivity to perfumes, solvents and other chemicals.
- Exhaustion from exercise.
- Very tired after breakfast.
- Poor cognitive clarity (but not described as declining).
- Naturally slender, she weighed 51 kg; height 1.60 metres, BMI 19.9.

Digestion

Generally, JM had normal digestive function with a daily bowel movement that was easy to pass and formed. She did notice bloating and looser, more frequent stools during the mid-cycle pain phases.

Recent health history

At age 39, she was diagnosed with Hashimoto's thyroiditis and has taken levothyroxine since then (100 mcg at diagnosis and 75 mcg for the last two years). Medication had improved her overall health and energy, but had not fully resolved her current presenting symptoms.

At age 45, JM started to experience severe mid-cycle pain in the lower abdomen. During the second episode, JM was admitted to hospital and a ruptured ovarian cyst was identified and treated. The pain continued, but ultrasound, CT scan and blood tests could find no other explanation. She was discharged with no further treatment. No mention was made of endometriosis.

Shortly afterwards, JM consulted with a specialist consultant surgeon. The first diagnostic laparoscopic surgery revealed endometrial lesions on the reproductive organs, covering the ovaries and the ends of the fallopian tubes (effectively closing them), and adhesions to the large intestines and abdominal wall. Laser removal of the endometrial lesions (laparoscopy) was undertaken and the consultant anticipated this procedure would need to be repeated in the future. This was because while lasering treatment was successful, not all adhesions around her fallopian tubes and ovary were treated. He advised that a hysterectomy may be recommended in the future.

In the same year, JM had an episode of pneumonia and took six months to feel fully recovered.

JM had decided to take a sabbatical from her demanding job in order to focus on health and wellness. She was taking steps to reduce the demands on her day. She was undertaking regular sessions of female-health-specific acupuncture. She worked with a personal trainer and practised yoga when she had sufficient energy. JM was not taking any supplements.

JM's health history prior to her 40s is outlined in Table 11.1.

Table 11.1 JM's health timeline until early 40s

Age	Symptoms, health issues, lifestyle issues
Childhood	Happy childhood Active Normal childhood illnesses
Teens through 20s	Menstruation started age 14 Regular periods, no significant period pain or heavy periods No significant mood swings or PMS Only very slight mid-cycle twinge on ovulation Contraceptive pill taken for two years Physically active, keen hockey player

29–31	Stopped contraceptive pill to prepare for conception Moved to South Africa
31–35	Two full-term pregnancies, no issues with conceiving Caesarean delivery with both children No issues following delivery Three years of sleep deprivation with second baby (son had ongoing teeth and ear infections) Stressful job
35–39	Fatigue noticeable Decline in physical energy and ability to exercise; could no longer run and even walking up the stairs was tiring Various visits to GP in South Africa; no diagnosis made
39	Thyroid test, revealing abnormal results (elevated TSH and low T4) GP provided referral to endocrinologist who confirmed elevated thyroid antibodies, diagnosed Hashimoto's and prescribed levothyroxine thyroid hormone (T4)
40	Moved back to UK and continued with no changes to the initial dosage for several years Fatigue persisted Periods of very low mood

Family medical history

- Autoimmunity and thyroid conditions are present in both female siblings (referred to as 'sibling factor' below).
- Sister 1: Lupus and hypothyroidism.
- Sister 2: Reactive arthritis and recently developed Hashimoto's.
- JM's cousin (on her maternal side) has endometriosis.

Medication and supplements

- Levothyroxine thyroid hormone 75 mcg QD.

Current diet

Meals were home-cooked and freshly prepared, including meat, fish and eggs. She ate very little dairy through preference. Vegetables were eaten but not always with every meal. Wheat was avoided, a decision taken six months prior to the initial consultation. JM described feeling better with wheat avoidance; she experienced less bloating and loose stools mid-cycle.

Daily fibre intake was estimated at 15–20 g and therefore below optimal requirements (30 g per day). One portion of oily fish per week. Breakfast was oat-based, such as porridge made with a plant-based milk or water, and hence was overall relatively high in starch and low in protein. Alcohol: one glass of red wine, 2–3 days per week. Caffeine: one coffee per day in the morning.

Environment and lifestyle

JM held a successful senior position which was sedentary and involved academic work and project management. She is currently on sabbatical from work. Family home life is happy and supportive. JM had good sleep and was in bed by 10 pm and sometimes earlier.

She was a keen hockey player and enjoyed physical activity, but this was curtailed by her energy levels. She presented as a 'high' achiever. JM admitted there was a dichotomy between knowing she needed to rest but also enjoying the satisfaction of achievement and 'ticking off lists'.

Investigations

The practitioner requested a full blood count to include haemoglobin, serum iron and ferritin through JM's general practitioner (GP), to rule out these factors in fatigue. Triiodothyronine, T3 was ordered. JM had a history of stress. Animal models have suggested raised cortisol can inhibit thyroxine (T4) to T3 hormone conversion (Brtko et al., 2004). The results are shown in Table 11.2.

Table 11.2 Biochemistry results for JM after initial consultation

	JM result (reference range)
Ferritin	34 ng/ml (15–200)
Haemoglobin	140 g/L (120–155)
Iron	20 umol/L (10.7–26.9)
T3	3.4 pmol/L (3.1–6.8)

Ferritin, haemoglobin, iron and T3 were all within normal ranges. Thyroid-stimulating hormone (TSH) and T4 were already monitored by her GP and were in normal range for her medication level; these are not shown. Thyroid peroxidase antibody (TPO) was 246 kIU/L ten years previously, thyroglobulin (TGAb) had not been reported at the time of her Hashimoto's diagnosis.

In a case of endometriosis, one might anticipate ordering an oestrogen and progesterone test. This, however, was not done. The client's cycle was not regular enough to support an accurate assessment through tests such as a 'day 21' progesterone test or oestrogen markers (whether via serum, urine or saliva). These would be a later consideration. A diurnal salivary (or urine) cortisol test was also considered, but since JM did not need convincing of the need to manage stress, this was not ordered in the interest of minimizing testing expenditure.

Case interpretation and analysis

Fatigue

JM'S fatigue and irritability were not relieved by sleep or rest and continued despite medication for her thyroid. Furthermore, the full blood count and thyroid hormones (T4 and T3) were in range, so availability of iron, haemoglobin level or thyroid hormone function did not explain her fatigue. The practitioner suspected that JM's fatigue and irritation were related to hormonal imbalance and metabolism, given that symptoms intensified just before and during menstruation.

It was also possible that other nutrient depletions existed. Although diet analysis did not highlight specific areas of concern other than low fibre and protein at breakfast, fatigue could be explained by modest micronutrient deficiencies. Ames (2010) proposed the 'triage theory' in which modest micronutrient deficiencies accelerate molecular ageing and mitochondria output is affected.

Stress and sensitivity to stress

Three years of sleep deprivation may have exaggerated JM's cortisol response to stress (Minkel *et al.*, 2014) and increased her vulnerability to stressors (Schwarz *et al.*, 2018). Stress activates the immune response producing inflammatory cytokines (Godoy *et al.*, 2018). Animal models show that activation of the stress response increases the inflammatory cytokines IL-1 and IL-1R2 in the paraventricular nucleus in the hypothalamus and IL-6 and COX-2 in the adrenal glands (Hueston and Deak, 2014). So, it's possible that long-term sleep deprivation and other life events may have led to a disruption of the hypothalamus–pituitary–adrenal axis (HPA) response and hypersensitivity to normal stressors, leading to inflammation, fatigue and low mood.

Autoimmune/inflammation

A Hashimoto's diagnosis is evidence of immune dysfunction. Endometrial adhesions are a clear indicator of an inflammatory process. Increased oestrogen production in endometriotic tissue sites (lesions) creates an oestrogen–inflammation feedback loop. The enzyme aromatase P450 is highly expressed in endometriosis and is stimulated by prostaglandin E2 (PGE2); this leads to oestrogen production within endometriotic tissue which induces more PGE2 and more aromatase P450 (Ferrero *et al.*, 2014). PGE2 is associated with increased inflammation and pain.

Endometriosis is associated with an increase in the expression of the inflammatory cytokines IL-1, IL-6, IL-8, TNFa and macrophage migration inhibitory factor (MIF) (Bedaiwy and Falcone, 2004; Kats *et al.*, 2002; Malutan *et al.*, 2015; Morin *et al.*, 2005; Oku *et al.*, 2004; Rakhila *et al.*, 2014). MIF is a pluripotent cytokine that forms part of the immune response to inflammation (Calandra and Roger, 2003; Nishihira *et al.*, 2003).

Retrograde or reflux menstruation, whereby the flow of menstrual content passes into the fallopian tubes, is suspected to occur in endometriosis (Dastur and Tank, 2010). Coupled with a 'defective "immunosurveillance"' (Christodoulakos *et al.*, 2007, p.194), this may lead to a poor ability to clear the peritoneal cavity of endometrial cells and tissues. The inflammatory process is then initiated and perpetuated (Macer and Taylor, 2012).

In this practitioner's clinical experience, women with endometriosis typically have symptoms of systemic inflammation such as pain and swelling.

Endometriosis and hormone imbalance symptoms

Although no oestrogen testing was undertaken, endometriosis is a condition where oestrogen (specifically oestradiol) production is intensified, due to localized production in endometriotic lesions. PGE2 is up-regulated in the peritoneal cavity in endometriosis (Sacco *et al.*, 2012) and is known to be a potent stimulator in steroidogenesis (Wang *et al.*, 2012). Endometriotic lesions have altered hormone-metabolizing enzymes, creating an imbalance in the reduction/oxidation balance between oestrone and 17-beta-estradiol and leading to a hyper-oestrogenic situation (Delvoux *et al.*, 2009).

Two other steroid hormones – progesterone and cortisol – may be important in relation to oestrogen balance for JM. One way that oestrogen can be opposed (or balanced) is through the presence of progesterone. Although no progesterone testing was undertaken in JM, she had an irregular cycle length (usually shorter than 28 days) which can be indicative of low levels of progesterone. Progesterone (as a medication) has been shown to inhibit the endometrial process (Narin *et al.*, 2014). While prescription progesterone is not within the scope of personalized nutrition, supporting endogenous progesterone production would be a valid target.

There were two considerations:

- How is progesterone produced and how are levels managed within the hormone system?

- Was there anything unique to JM's case that could either hinder production or potential levels in general?

The steroid hormone pregnenolone is first produced by cholesterol, before forming progesterone. The main production site for progesterone is within the corpus luteum in the ovaries, and smaller amounts are produced within the ovaries themselves and in the adrenal glands. The release or stimulation of progesterone within the ovaries is controlled by the hypothalamus–pituitary–ovary (HPO) axis, involving delicate rise and falls of follicle-stimulating hormone (FSH) and luteinizing hormone (LH). Both hormones are secreted by the anterior pituitary in response to gonadotropin-releasing hormone (GnRH) released by the hypothalamus.

Cortisol is indirectly made from the progesterone metabolite 17-OH progesterone. This makes progesterone an essential precursor to glucocorticoids such as cortisol. There is the potential during a stress response for the body to prioritize cortisol production and in doing so appropriate (commandeer) progesterone for that purpose.

Helping JM to normalize her stress response (recognizing its presence through her case history) may therefore help protect progesterone, which in turn may help 'oppose' oestrogen.

Detoxification and elimination

Adequate detoxification and elimination are fundamental to the optimal handling of oestrogens. The oestrogen metabolites 2-OHE1, 4-OHE1 and 16a-OHE1, created by phase I detoxification, must be efficiently conjugated by phase II detoxification enzymes in order to minimize the risk of the metabolites oxidizing and causing cellular damage, particularly the 4-OHE1 and 16a-OHE1 metabolites (Neil, 2010).

Key phase 2 pathways for oestrogen are methylation, sulphation, glutathione conjugation and glucuronidation. Detoxification of oestrogen metabolites requires methylation – the transfer of a methyl group (CH3) from one compound to another. Diet and supplements can supply the methyl donors and thus support methylation of oestrogen metabolites. Foods rich in methyl donors include leafy green vegetables for folate and animal protein for richer sources of methylated folate, vitamin B12 and methionine. Cofactors for the methylation pathways include magnesium, vitamin B6 and vitamin B2.

Methylation and sulphation require the sulphur-containing amino acids including cysteine and methionine. Dietary sources include onions, garlic, cruciferous vegetables and animal protein. It was ideal that JM already ate animal protein to provide her with dietary sources of methionine, since vegan sources of protein (nuts and legumes) are low in methionine.

Transsulphuration, the process of breaking down homocysteine to cysteine, also requires vitamin B6. Cysteine is then synthesized to glutathione (Neil, 2010), important for global detoxification.

Glucuronidation is the main excretion pathway for oestrogens. The gut microbiome becomes involved in the regulation of circulating oestrogens through the activity of beta-glucuronidase, an enzyme produced by bacteria (see Box 5.3, Chapter 5). Low microbial diversity and dysbiosis may be associated with decreased oestrogen deconjugation and increased recirculation of oestrogen (Baker, Al-Nakkash and Herbst-Kralovetz, 2017). Optimal gastrointestinal flora balance and optimal fibre levels are therefore key.

Oestrogen detoxification also require catechol-O-methyltransferase (COMT). COMT also requires S-adenosylmethionine (SAMe) to function. COMT catalyzes the methylation of catechol oestrogens to methoxy oestrogens. This process is important to neutralize potentially harmful oestrogen metabolites. COMT is also involved in the metabolism of adrenaline and noradrenaline (Nissinen and Männistö, 2010). Under high stress, this enzyme may be overloaded. Minimizing the stress load may allow the enzyme to better support oestrogen metabolism. Indeed, symptoms related to JM's menstrual cycle worsened during times of stress, consistent with the hypothesis that resources were 'prioritized' for adrenaline and noradrenaline over oestrogen metabolism during those times.

While JM was not tested for genetic polymorphisms (SNPs) in COMT or methylation enzymes, the practitioner was mindful of supporting methylation and COMT 'globally' through dietary, supplementation and lifestyle recommendations.

Initial management plan

Figure 11.1 maps out the theoretical interaction between symptoms, history and key biochemical systems for JM. Using this 'mind map', the practitioner could hypothesize that focusing the initial management plan on the key areas below may have an overlapping effect and help to address a number of the areas of imbalance described above.

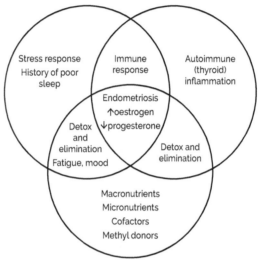

Figure 11.1 Venn diagram of the proposed interaction of the biological systems and symptoms in JM's case

This diagram helped the practitioner map out the overlaps and interactions between each aspect and helped the practitioner to organise her thinking. The cross over areas present opportunities whereby one intervention (e.g. addressing the stress response) is anticipated to have a positive effect on immune response, hormones, detoxification and elimination, fatigue and mood.

The previous section outlined the practitioner's interpretation of each section within the diagram. This diagram helped the practitioner to map out the overlaps and interactions between each aspect and organize her thinking. The crossover areas represent opportunities whereby one intervention (e.g. addressing the stress response) is anticipated to have a positive effect on immune response, hormones, detoxification and elimination, fatigue and mood.

Diet

The goal of the diet was to:

- moderate the stress response
- reduce inflammatory triggers and support the autoimmune process
- optimize resources required for metabolism, detoxification and excretion of hormones (methyl donors, cofactors, sulphur-containing amino acids)
- optimize resources for progesterone production and 'protection'
- optimize micronutrient resources for energy production.

The recommended diet was a modified Palaeolithic-style diet. The Palaeolithic-based diet (described in Box 9.1 in Chapter 9) has clinical observation and early clinical trials to support its use in autoimmune and inflammatory conditions (Bisht *et al.*, 2014; Lee *et al.*, 2017; Wahls *et al.*, 2018). It was modified to make it simple for JM to use, given her already limited energy. The practitioner did not ask JM to eliminate all grains' it was only a 'Palaeo-inspired' diet. In part, this was to avoid JM feeling too restricted by the diet, which could have increased her feeling of stress. In reality, JM included very few grains, especially when she switched from her oat-based breakfast.

Where grains were included, they were gluten-free. Gluten elimination has been shown to reduce endometriosis symptoms (Marziali *et al.*, 2012; Marziali and Capozzolo, 2015). Empirical clinical observation is that elimination of gluten may benefit autoimmune conditions. It is thought that antigens contained in food that are similar to body tissue proteins can trigger an antibody response that cross-reacts to such self-proteins. This phenomenon is known as molecular mimicry and can be a factor in autoimmunity. Wheat and dairy are foods that contain antigens with a very similar peptide sequence to some body tissues (Vojdani, 2015). A six-month gluten-free diet did reduce thyroid antibodies compared with controls in a more recent clinical trial (Krysiak, Szkróbka and Okopień, 2018). Although the clinical trial data is inconsistent, this practitioner's clinical experience is that gluten elimination can improve endometrial symptoms.

JM continued to mostly avoid dairy, as she felt better when she did; dairy is not a feature of a Palaeo-inspired diet and supply of protein from dairy was not a concern as she ate other forms of protein.

JM found legumes caused bloating and so already avoided them. The practitioner needed to ensure sufficient fibre from vegetables and fruit sources. This was achieved by recommended use of starch vegetables as a grain alternative (e.g. roasted vegetables, cooked the night before, used at breakfast) and ensuring that at each meal 50% of the plate contained vegetables. Avocados were encouraged – half an avocado contains approximately 7 g fibre or 23% of the daily target of 30 g (SACN, 2015). Breads made using flour from pseudo-grains and tuber flours were recommended, with recipe ideas provided.

Green vegetables

Green vegetables were emphasized to increase fibre, which should support microbiome diversity and support oestrogen excretion, minimizing hepatic–enteric reabsorption of conjugated oestrogens.

Phytonutrients found in vegetables, especially green, leafy and cruciferous vegetables, help to modulate CYP1 enzymes involved in metabolizing oestrogens (Hodges and Minich, 2015). Leafy green vegetables are also important sources of folates needed for optimal methylation of oestrogens.

Isothiocyanates found in cruciferous vegetables such as broccoli have been shown in clinical studies (albeit small studies) to reduce the inflammatory cytokine IL6 (Navarro *et al.*, 2014), increase detoxification of airborne pollutants (Kensler *et al.*, 2012) and increase blood concentration of glutathione (Sedlak *et al.*, 2018). Isothiocyanates upregulate the nuclear transcription factor NrF2 (Fuentes, Paredes-Gonzalez and Kong, 2015), Glucuronidation and glutathione conjugation are particularly dependent on Nrf2-regulated genes (Thimmulappa *et al.*, 2002); hence, cruciferous vegetables are thought to benefit hormone metabolism. Historically, cruciferous vegetables were avoided for those with thyroid issues due to their goitrogenic properties. It has, however, been shown that the goitrogenic effect is only evident when iodine intake is low (Truong *et al.*, 2010). This was not the case for JM, and in this practitioner's clinical experience the benefits of cruciferous vegetables far outweigh the potential impact of goitrogens, which are reduced by cooking the vegetables.

Protein sources

Each meal contained a protein source so that 25–30% of the area of the plate contained protein. Protein choices included eggs (two per portion), organic chicken, fish, organic or grass-fed beef, lamb or game. Protein contains amino acids needed for phase 2 detoxification. Oily fish was recommended three times a week (JM previously ate it once a week). In animal models, dietary fish oil inhibits endometriosis adhesions (Herington et al., 2013). Essential fats from oily fish are key substrates in the anti-inflammatory pathways (Calder, 2017). Arachidonic acid found in meat is a substrate for inflammatory eicosanoids such as PGE2 which, as seen above, is typically at high levels in endometriosis. Optimizing the fish oils EPA and DHA would be key to modulating the inflammatory eicosanoids and the fatty acid levels in cell membranes (Calder, 2017). Grass-fed beef had a higher level of EPA and DHA than grain-fed (Daley et al., 2010). Oily fish would also provide cholesterol as the raw material for the steroid hormone pregnenolone, required to produce progesterone.

Meat and fish would provide food sources of methionine vitamin B6, vitamin B12 and riboflavin (B2) necessary for oestrogen-methylation-related metabolic pathway (Hodges and Minich, 2015).

Specific breakfast recommendations

- Free-range scrambled eggs with tomato, spinach and half a sweet potato (cooked the previous night).
- Oily fish (salmon, mackerel, sardines, trout) on gluten-free toast (see gluten-free bread options below) or half an avocado.
- Two poached free-range eggs with roasted root vegetables.
- 'Treat morning': gluten-free sausages or nitrate-free bacon with roasted root vegetables (cooked the previous night) or with chestnuts (plain, pre-cooked) and wilted leafy greens. This option was to be used once a week only.

A green smoothie alongside breakfast provided a simple way to increase green vegetables. JM was given an example recipe for the smoothie: glass of water, 1 banana, 2 handfuls of any two different leafy greens (e.g. spinach, kale, chard, rocket).

Examples of gluten-free bread alternatives:

- buckwheat bread
- tiger nut bread
- coconut flour bread
- recipes with almond flour.

Coffee intake was maintained at one cup per day.

Lifestyle

JM was someone who found it hard to slow down. She had a natural inclination to be driven by her to-do list. A suppression of cortisol and HPA axis in women with endometriosis has been found (Quiñones *et al.*, 2015) similar to the pattern seen in chronic pain (Vincent *et al.*, 2011). In other words, is it the pain causing the HPA suppression or vice versa?

The practitioner coached JM on the role of the HPA axis in hormone balance and of the need to take time for herself and learn to relax. She was asked to take less on during the day, and to make proper time to sit down for lunch, eating slowly. She was also encouraged to take a short nap in the day if she felt tired, rather than trying to 'push through' the tiredness. Her bed times were already optimal – between 9.30 pm and 10 pm.

Advice was given on how to avoid exogenous xenoestrogens, such as bisphenol A (BPA) (vom Saal and Myers, 2008). BPA is also suspected as a potential trigger for autoimmunity (Kharrazian, 2014).

JM was advised to batch-cook and 'meal repeat or recycle' – meaning making extra portions for meals the following day – and provided with recipe book ideas which focused on meals that could be easily batch-cooked.

Supplements

A tailored supplement programme aimed to:

- modulate inflammation, to support the sex hormone balance
- promote oestrogen detoxification and metabolism
- support progesterone levels to oppose oestrogen
- regulate menstrual cycle for overall sex hormone balance
- support communication and signalling via the HPA axis and HPO axis.

Omega 3 fish oil providing 800 mg of EPA and 400 mg of DHA per day

The clinical rationale for omega 3 fish oils was outlined above in respect of diet. A supplement was given to support JM while she introduced more fish into her diet as her dietary intake had previously been low.

Multivitamin and mineral complex

This contained nutrients which support antioxidant pathways including vitamin C, zinc, selenium and chromium. Antioxidant vitamin and mineral supplementation has been shown to reduce pain and inflammation markers in the peritoneal fluid in women with endometriosis compared with controls in an eight-week study (Santanam *et al.*, 2013). Serum antioxidant levels are supportive of steroid hormone production (Mumford *et al.*, 2016)

The multivitamin and mineral also contained magnesium to support methylation and energy metabolism (de Baaij, Hoenderop and Bindels, 2015). In this practitioner's clinical experience, supplemental magnesium will often improve relaxation in clients.

B vitamins were included in the formula to support the methylation of oestrogens. Methylation plays an important role in mood as SAMe is involved in the activation of serotonin and dopamine. As JM experienced premenstrual low mood, this may be beneficial.

Vitamin D: 2000 IU per day

While vitamin D status was not measured, the client attended the practitioner's clinic during the winter. Vitamin D has a hormone-like action and may have a role in supporting progesterone levels (Merhi *et al.*, 2014). An association has been seen between low vitamin D levels and endometriosis (Ciavattini *et al.*, 2017). Optimal vitamin D status is well established for immune system health (Hewison, 2012).

Zinc: 30 mg per day (combined dosage from
multimineral and single supplement)

Antioxidant capacity and zinc status have both been shown to be lower in women with hormone imbalance (premenstrual syndrome) versus controls (Fathizadeh *et al.*, 2016) and in women with endometriosis (Messalli *et al.*, 2014). Zinc plays a role in influencing the production and signalling in inflammatory cytokines (Foster and Samman, 2012).

Reishi and maitake mushroom and turmeric: maitake 800 mg,
reishi 500 mg, full-spectrum turmeric 1000 mg per day

Botanical mushrooms have a long traditional use in health, and while the full molecular mechanism of their action is not yet known, there are anecdotal, case study and animal study models for their immune-modulating properties (Lull, Wichers and Savelkoul, 2005; Ma *et al.*, 2015; Rubel *et al.*, 2018; Zhang *et al.*, 2018).

Full-spectrum turmeric was chosen, which includes the three active ingredients from the turmeric plant: curcuminoids (curcumin), turmeric saccharides and turmerones. Curcumin (turmeric) has been shown to help stabilize the over-production of inflammatory cytokines (Yadav, Jee and Awasthi, 2015) and is safe and well tolerated (Kunnumakkara *et al.*, 2017). Cell-signalling studies have shown that curcumin may inhibit endometriosis endometrial cells by reducing oestradiol production (Zhang *et al.*, 2013). Although most research to date has focused on curcumin, emerging research has demonstrated the anti-inflammatory activity of the polysaccharide fractions of the whole root (turmeric saccharides) (Bethapudi *et al.*, 2017; Illuri *et al.*, 2015) and turmerones (Chen *et al.*, 2018). There is some evidence that the whole turmeric root has enhanced bioavailability compared with curcumin (Yue *et al.*, 2012).

Agnus castus (Vitex agnus castus seed): tincture 1:2, 5 ml x 1 daily (not during menstruation) (1:2 indicates the ratio of plant part to alcohol preparation in traditional herbal medicine tinctures)

While the full and exact mechanistic action of agnus castus is not yet known, it is thought to support luteinizing hormone function and progesterone production and in perimenopausal women it has been shown to reduce PMS-type symptoms (van Die *et al.*, 2009). Randomized control trials have shown Vitex agnus castus to be safe and effective in educing PMS symptoms, indicating a hormone-balancing effect (He *et al.*, 2009; Zamani, Neghab and Torabian, 2012).

Siberian ginseng (*Eleutherococcus senticosus*) tincture 1:2, 5 ml x 3 daily (1:2 indicates the ratio of plant part to alcohol preparation in traditional herbal medicine tinctures)

Eleutherococcus is the preferred name for this botanical, since its common name 'Siberian ginseng' often means it gets mistaken for 'true' ginsengs that contain ginsenosides. *Eleutherococcus* is in fact from a different botanical family and does not contain ginsenosides. Ginsenosides in some people can cause a feeling of being 'over-energized' or can be destabilizing in terms of mood for some users. *Eleutherococcus* has a traditional use in herbal medicine (in which this practitioner is trained) as an adaptogen. The beneficial stress-protective effect of adaptogens is related to regulation of homeostasis via several mechanisms of action associated with the HPA axis (Panossian and Wikman, 2009). *Eleutherococcus* may work through the melatonin-signalling system to act as a 'stress vaccine' (Panossian, Seo and Efferth, 2018). By using this adaptogenic herb it was hoped to moderate JM's stress response and therefore protect progesterone production by optimizing HPO and HPA axis signaling.

Indole-3-carbinol (I3C): 150 mg per day

I3C is one of the active phytonutrients found in cruciferous vegetables. It is used as a supplement to augment the positive benefits of cruciferous vegetables outlined above (Licznerska and Baer-Dubowska, 2016). Diindolylmethane (DIM) is a dimer of I3C and is also used as a supplement, although Marques and colleagues showed that DIM can activate the oestrogen receptor alpha inducing a more oestrogenic process (Marques *et al.*, 2014). This may be because DIM only works on the 2-OHE1 (2-hydroxyestrone) pathway.

13C has a closer relationship to the natural compounds glucosinolate and glucobrassicin, found in cruciferous vegetables. Once consumed, in the acidic environment of the stomach, 13C molecules can combine with each other to form a complex mixture of polycyclic aromatic products including DIM but also 5,11-dihydroindolo-[3,2-b] carbazole (ICZ) and a cyclic triindole, all of which are biologically beneficial to oestrogen metabolism. By providing the body with 13C, there is more possibility for 'choice' of conversion of these polycyclic aromatic compounds as determined by individual need. This practitioner therefore prefers to supplement 13C rather than DIM.

N-acetyl-L-cysteine (NAC): 150 mg

NAC provides the precursors to glutathione (Lasram *et al.*, 2015; Rushworth and Megson, 2014) which is an important conjugation route for oestrogen detoxification. The inclusion of extra cysteine was also considered to be potentially beneficial to supporting the sulphation of oestrogens.

Drug–nutrient interactions

Potential nutrient interactions with levothyroxine were checked using the Natural Medicines Comprehensive Database (see Appendix A). No interactions were found for foods or supplements that were included in JM's recommendations.

Patient management and follow-up

From two months JM reported:

- improvement in energy levels, up to 7/10 and dipping to 5/10 just before her period and the first few days of her period – an increase of 2/3 points
- mood improved and more stable
- stability in her menstrual cycle at 28 days

- by the third month her energy had risen again to 9/10 – an increase of 4/5 points
- pain much reduced (see below).

She had found it straightforward to implement the diet and lifestyle recommendations. She had found gluten-free easy to follow and found the protein additions in breakfast had made a difference to her morning energy levels and was enjoying the green smoothie. She had fewer sweet cravings before her period.

Her periods were of minimal discomfort but she had experienced some mid-cycle pain episodes. Her surgeon had said that if this was to occur again, he would like to schedule a second laparoscopy to remove the adhesions identified first time around, affecting fallopian tubes and left ovary.

Programme adjustments
Supplements were reduced so she had more of a focused supplement plan, having seen improvement. Supplements that continued to be taken in the longer term were a multivitamin and mineral containing vitamin D, magnesium and methyl donors, indole-3-carbinol, turmeric, botanical mushrooms and agnus castus. Her diet remained the same as following the first consultation.

She agreed to eliminate alcohol completely for the following month; it was felt that this, along with the dietary and supplement support, would support oestrogen metabolism, detoxification and elimination.

Twelve months after starting the personalized nutrition programme, JM had a second laparoscopy which removed existing adhesions connected to her fallopian tubes and the tubes themselves. Her surgeon confirmed the endometriosis had not worsened over nearly two years, which was a very positive sign. She recovered from surgery well in terms of energy, and her cycle remained consistent and mood stable. Since the second laparoscopy JM has not experienced any mid-cycle pain and her endometriosis diagnosis is quite unnoticeable. Since JM's cycle was now regular and many of her hormone-related symptoms relieved, it was hypothesized that JM had not yet entered into a perimenopausal phase.

Her thyroid antibodies were retested by her medical practitioner. While TPO was still elevated at 57.6 kIU/L (reference range 0–34 kIU/L), it was significantly lower than the previous 246 kIU/L. Anti-thyroglobulin antibodies was now measured and was in normal range.

She at times 'lapsed' back to oat-based breakfasts and again found this made her tired after breakfast.

JM reported that the most substantial improvement in terms of her quality of life was that she now had what she referred to as 'cognitive clarity' and felt energized enough to play hockey on a very regular basis.

Discussion

Symptoms, test results and laparoscopy findings provided the practitioner with a clear picture of the interrelationship between hormonal imbalance and inflammation. In this case there are two possible scenarios. Did endometrial lesions activate the immune system, resulting in elevated thyroid antibodies? Or did an already over-activated immune system (autoimmune Hashimoto's) and the inflammation induce and stimulate migration of endometrial cells and tissues?

The pathology of endometriosis is not fully understood. A review of literature on endometriosis pathology by Sourial, Tempest and Hapangama (2014) described eight potential mechanisms:

- retrograde menstruation
- metaplasia of extrauterine cells due to hormonal and immune factors
- imbalance of hormone metabolism, biosynthesis and signalling
- oxidative stress and inflammation
- immune dysfunction
- apoptosis suppression and alteration of endometrial cell fate
- genetics
- stem cells abnormally activated or translocated as a result of one of the factors above.

The likelihood is, as with many conditions, that the aetiology is multifactorial. There were a number of factors that were likely to have contributed to JM's endometriosis. Hormonal imbalance, oxidative stress and inflammation, and immune dysfunction are the known crossovers with the above list (Sourial *et al.*, 2014).

The involvement of autoimmunity is particularly interesting in this case, given the 'sibling factor'. Was there a genetic factor which made JM susceptible not only to Hashimoto's but also to endometriosis? Both her sisters have an autoimmune condition, and it is possible that oestrogen plays a role in autoimmune conditions such as lupus (Khan and Ansar Ahmed, 2015; Yasuda *et al.*, 2018). Genetic predispositions do not predict disease; the relevant genes need to be triggered by life experience and inputs, which can perhaps be identified in JM´s case history.

JM's response to stress is significant in this case, evidenced by her symptoms increasing during stressful times or the experience of heightened emotional pressures. It is possible that a high stress load, over time, was a trigger for defects in her immune response.

By taking a person-centred approach to the case, looking at JM's history and presenting symptoms, the practitioner implemented a diet, lifestyle and supplement programme that addressed key factors that were influencing her condition. The central impact of the programme was threefold:

1. Reduce the inflammatory load.
2. Support oestrogen metabolism, detoxification and excretion.
3. Reduce the stress load and optimize HPA and HPO axis signalling.

It was an iterative process. Reduced inflammation is likely to have improved hormone metabolism, which likely improved energy production, which likely facilitated greater adenosine triphosphate (ATP) for hormone metabolism and improved resource for immune function and anti-inflammatory systems.

This shows how an understanding of the systems biology behind the condition, and overlaying that with the client's personal case, led the practitioner to have a clear understanding of how to support the individual. The implementation of a tailored, evidence-based, integrated programme is able to address numerous factors, helping the patient to improve her health and feel empowered by doing so.

Q&A

AW: Reflecting back on the case, is there anything you would have done differently?

LDD: Ideally, I would have been able to run more testing. For example, check her vitamin D status, a four-point salivary cortisol test and a dried urine test to look at a fuller picture of the stress hormone and oestrogen metabolic pathways. Finances were the limiting factor. Genetics would have been another addition I'd have loved to have; I find with many clients that testing, especially nutrigenomic testing, can really help with motivation to change habits, especially in choices around toxicant exposure and detoxification capabilities.

AW: What is your view on the nutrigenomic factors involved in endometriosis?

LDD: Certainly, these are involved in the metabolism of oestrogens. In other cases, I have tested for genetic polymorphisms (SNPs) relating to phase I and phase II oestrogen detoxification, selecting a genetic panel that covered the entire pathway.

In just one example, the CYP1B1 gene provides instructions for producing an enzyme that is a member of the cytochrome P450 family of enzymes, and it converts oestrogens to 4-OH oestrogens. Variants (SNPs) on CYP1B1 are associated with increased production of 4-OH which is less desirable when looking at the research literature on that type of catechol oestrogen. Those kinds of insights can be valuable to a practitioner in that they can decide how to pursue supporting detoxification pathways. If a woman has a catechol-O-methyltransferase (COMT) SNP, that might mean she is less able to both activate health-promoting and inactivate harmful metabolic by-products of phase 1 oestrogen detoxification processes as efficiently. We didn't do any nutrigenomic testing with JM, so all this was unknown, but I made sure that all the other oestrogen detoxification pathways were well supported, and since COMT is involved in the metabolism of adrenaline and noradrenaline, the stress reduction should have helped to ensure no overloading of this pathway. [Editor's note: Note the need to interpret genetic testing in context with other functional tests and the wider clinical context as outlined in Chapter 3.]

AW: I know you specialize in women's health. Are there any key themes you see that link PMS, endometriosis and infertility?

LDD: For me there are two big themes in women's health. The first is issues in the HPA axis and the stress response. I describe this as causing 'signalling problems' to the rest of the endocrine and hormone system. The second is in the area of detoxification and elimination. There is so much we can do with the whole lifestyle to improve detoxification status and this is a key area I work on with my clients.

AW: Is it unusual to see so few digestive symptoms in someone with endometriosis?

LDD: Very unusual. In my clinical experience, women with endometriosis may have a weakened capacity to maintain a healthy gastrointestinal foundation, and are prone to gastrointestinal yeast symptoms, SIBO and other pathogens.

I very often use stool and breath testing to assess gut function in endometriosis clients because it is an important consideration when aiming to build a stronger foundation with which to manage the immune challenges in the condition and to optimize safe oestrogen metabolism and efficient excretion. I would then use a 5R approach to restore healthy gastrointestinal function (see Chapter 9 for a case example of the 5R approach.)

References

Ames, B.N., 2010. Optimal micronutrients delay mitochondrial decay and age-associated diseases. *Mechanisms of Ageing and Development* 131, 473–479. https://doi.org/10.1016/j.mad.2010.04.005

Baker, J.M., Al-Nakkash, L., Herbst-Kralovetz, M.M., 2017. Estrogen-gut microbiome axis: Physiological and clinical implications. *Maturitas* 103, 45–53. https://doi.org/10.1016/j.maturitas.2017.06.025

Bedaiwy, M.A., Falcone, T., 2004. Laboratory testing for endometriosis. *Clinica Chimica Acta* 340, 41–56.

Bethapudi, B., Murugan, S., Illuri, R., Mundkinajeddu, D., Velusami, C.C., 2017. Bioactive Turmerosaccharides from *Curcuma longa* extract (NR-INF-02): Potential ameliorating effect on osteoarthritis pain. *Pharmacognosy Magazine* 13, S623–S627. https://doi.org/10.4103/pm.pm_465_16

Bisht, B., Darling, W.G., Grossmann, R.E., Shivapour, E.T. *et al.*, 2014. A multimodal intervention for patients with secondary progressive multiple sclerosis: Feasibility and effect on fatigue. *Alternative and Complementary Therapies* 20, 347–355. https://doi.org/10.1089/act.2014.20606

Brtko, J., Macejová, D., Knopp, J., Kvetnanský, R., 2004. Stress is associated with inhibition of type I iodothyronine 5'-deiodinase activity in rat liver. *Annals of the New York Academy of Sciences* 1018, 219–223. https://doi.org/10.1196/annals.1296.026

Calandra, T., Roger, T., 2003. Macrophage migration inhibitory factor: A regulator of innate immunity. *Nature Reviews Immunology* 3, 791–800. https://doi.org/10.1038/nri1200

Calder, P.C., 2017. Omega-3 fatty acids and inflammatory processes: From molecules to man. *Biochemical Society Transactions* 45, 1105–1115. https://doi.org/10.1042/BST20160474

Chen, M., Chang, Y.-Y., Huang, S., Xiao, L.-H. *et al.*, 2018. Aromatic-turmerone attenuates lps-induced neuroinflammation and consequent memory impairment by targeting TLR4-dependent signaling pathway. *Molecular Nutrition and Food Research* 62. https://doi.org/10.1002/mnfr.201700281

Christodoulakos, G., Augoulea, A., Lambrinoudaki, I., Sioulas, V., Creatsas, G., 2007. Pathogenesis of endometriosis: The role of defective 'immunosurveillance'. *European Journal of Contraception and Reproductive Health Care* 12, 194–202. https://doi.org/10.1080/13625180701387266

Ciavattini, A., Serri, M., Delli Carpini, G., Morini, S., Clemente, N., 2017. Ovarian endometriosis and vitamin D serum levels. *Gynecological Endocrinology* 33, 164–167. https://doi.org/10.1080/09513590.2016.1239254

Daley, C.A., Abbott, A., Doyle, P.S., Nader, G.A., Larson, S., 2010. A review of fatty acid profiles and antioxidant content in grass-fed and grain-fed beef. *Nutrition Journal* 9, 10. https://doi.org/10.1186/1475-2891-9-10

Dastur, A.E., Tank, P.D., 2010. John A Sampson and the origins of endometriosis. *Journal of Obstetrics and Gynecology of India* 60, 299–300. https://doi.org/10.1007/s13224-010-0046-8

de Baaij, J.H.F., Hoenderop, J.G.J., Bindels, R.J.M., 2015. Magnesium in man: Implications for health and disease. *Physiological Reviews* 95, 1–46. https://doi.org/10.1152/physrev.00012.2014

Delvoux, B., Groothuis, P., D'Hooghe, T., Kyama, C., Dunselman, G., Romano, A., 2009. Increased production of 17β-estradiol in endometriosis lesions is the result of impaired metabolism. *Journal of Clinical Endocrinology and Metabolism* 94, 876–883. https://doi.org/10.1210/jc.2008-2218

Fathizadeh, S., Amani, R., Haghighizadeh, M.H., Hormozi, R., 2016. Comparison of serum zinc concentrations and body antioxidant status between young women with premenstrual syndrome and normal controls: A case-control study. *International Journal of Reproductive Biomedicine* 14, 699–704.

Ferrero, S., Remorgida, V., Maganza, C., Venturini, P.L. *et al.*, 2014. Aromatase and endometriosis: Estrogens play a role. *Annals of the New York Academy of Sciences* 1317, 17–23. https://doi.org/10.1111/nyas.12411

Foster, M., Samman, S., 2012. Zinc and regulation of inflammatory cytokines: Implications for cardiometabolic disease. *Nutrients* 4, 676–694. https://doi.org/10.3390/nu4070676

Fuentes, F., Paredes-Gonzalez, X., Kong, A.-N.T., 2015. Dietary glucosinolates sulforaphane, phenethyl isothiocyanate, indole-3-carbinol/3,3'-diindolylmethane: Anti-oxidative stress/inflammation, nrf2, epigenetics/epigenomics and *in vivo* cancer chemopreventive efficacy. *Current Pharmacology Reports* 1, 179–196. https://doi.org/10.1007/s40495-015-0017-y

Godoy, L.D., Rossignoli, M.T., Delfino-Pereira, P., Garcia-Cairasco, N., de Lima Umeoka, E.H., 2018. A comprehensive overview on stress neurobiology: Basic concepts and clinical implications. *Frontiers in Behavioral Neuroscience* 12, 127. https://doi.org/10.3389/fnbeh.2018.00127

Guo, S.-W., 2009. Recurrence of endometriosis and its control. *Human Reproduction Update* 15, 441–461. https://doi.org/10.1093/humupd/dmp007

He, Z., Chen, R., Zhou, Y., Geng, L. *et al.*, 2009. Treatment for premenstrual syndrome with Vitex agnus castus: A prospective, randomized, multi-center placebo controlled study in China. *Maturitas* 63, 99–103. https://doi.org/10.1016/j.maturitas.2009.01.006

Herington, J.L., Glore, D.R., Lucas, J.A., Osteen, K.G., Bruner-Tran, K.L., 2013. Dietary fish oil supplementation inhibits formation of endometriosis-associated adhesions in a chimeric mouse model. *Fertility and Sterility* 99, 543-550.e1. https://doi.org/10.1016/j.fertnstert.2012.10.007

Hewison, M., 2012. Vitamin D and immune function: An overview. *Proceedings of the Nutrition Society* 71, 50–61. https://doi.org/10.1017/S0029665111001650

Hodges, R.E., Minich, D.M., 2015. Modulation of metabolic detoxification pathways using foods and food-derived components: A scientific review with clinical application. *Journal of Nutrition and Metabolism* 2015. https://doi.org/10.1155/2015/760689

Hueston, C.M., Deak, T., 2014. The inflamed axis: The interaction between stress, hormones, and the expression of inflammatory-related genes within key structures comprising the hypothalamic–pituitary–adrenal axis. *Physiology and Behavior* 124, 77–91. https://doi.org/10.1016/j.physbeh.2013.10.035

Illuri, R., Bethapudi, B., Anandakumar, S., Murugan, S. *et al.*, 2015. Anti-inflammatory activity of polysaccharide fraction of *Curcuma longa* extract (NR-INF-02). *Anti-Inflammatory and Anti-Allergy Agents in Medicinal Chemistry* 14, 53–62.

Issa, B., Ormesher, L., Whorwell, P.J., Shah, M., Hamdy, S., 2016. Endometriosis and irritable bowel syndrome: A dilemma for the gynaecologist and gastroenterologist. *The Obstetrician and Gynaecologist* 18, 9–16. https://doi.org/10.1111/tog.12241

Kats, R., Collette, T., Metz, C.N., Akoum, A., 2002. Marked elevation of macrophage migration inhibitory factor in the peritoneal fluid of women with endometriosis. *Fertility and Sterility* 78, 69–76.

Kensler, T.W., Ng, D., Carmella, S.G., Chen, M. *et al.*, 2012. Modulation of the metabolism of airborne pollutants by glucoraphanin-rich and sulforaphane-rich broccoli sprout beverages in Qidong, China. *Carcinogenesis* 33, 101–107. https://doi.org/10.1093/carcin/bgr229

Khan, D., Ansar Ahmed, S., 2015. The immune system is a natural target for estrogen action: Opposing effects of estrogen in two prototypical autoimmune diseases. *Frontiers in Immunology* 6, 635. https://doi.org/10.3389/fimmu.2015.00635

Kharrazian, D., 2014. The potential roles of bisphenol a (BPA) pathogenesis in autoimmunity. *Autoimmune Diseases* 2014, 743616. https://doi.org/10.1155/2014/743616

Krysiak, R., Szkróbka, W., Okopień, B., 2018. The effect of gluten-free diet on thyroid autoimmunity in drug-naïve women with Hashimoto's thyroiditis: A pilot study. *Experimental and Clinical Endocrinology and Diabetes*. https://doi.org/10.1055/a-0653-7108

Kunnumakkara, A.B., Bordoloi, D., Padmavathi, G., Monisha, J. *et al.*, 2017. Curcumin, the golden nutraceutical: Multitargeting for multiple chronic diseases. *British Journal of Pharmacology* 174, 1325–1348. https://doi.org/10.1111/bph.13621

Lasram, M.M., Dhouib, I.B., Annabi, A., El Fazaa, S., Gharbi, N., 2015. A review on the possible molecular mechanism of action of N-acetylcysteine against insulin resistance and type-2 diabetes development. *Clinical Biochemistry* 48, 1200–1208. https://doi.org/10.1016/j.clinbiochem.2015.04.017

Lee, J.E., Bisht, B., Hall, M.J., Rubenstein, L.M. *et al.*, 2017. A multimodal, nonpharmacologic intervention improves mood and cognitive function in people with multiple sclerosis. *Journal of the American College of Nutrition* 36, 150–168. https://doi.org/10.1080/07315724.2016.1255160

Licznerska, B., Baer-Dubowska, W., 2016. Indole-3-Carbinol and its role in chronic diseases. *Anti-inflammatory Nutraceuticals and Chronic Diseases* 928, 131–154. https://doi.org/10.1007/978-3-319-41334-1_6

Lull, C., Wichers, H.J., Savelkoul, H.F.J., 2005. Antiinflammatory and immunomodulating properties of fungal metabolites. *Mediators of Inflammation* 2005, 63–80. https://doi.org/10.1155/MI.2005.63

Ma, X.-L., Meng, M., Han, L.-R., Li, Z., Cao, X.-H., Wang, C.-L., 2015. Immunomodulatory activity of macromolecular polysaccharide isolated from *Grifola frondosa*. *Chinese Journal of Natural Medicine* 13, 906–914. https://doi.org/10.1016/S1875-5364(15)30096-0

Macer, M.L., Taylor, H.S., 2012. Endometriosis and infertility: A review of the pathogenesis and treatment of endometriosis-associated infertility. *Obstetrics and Gynecology Clinics of North America* 39, 535–549. https://doi.org/10.1016/j.ogc.2012.10.002

Malutan, A.M., Drugan, T., Costin, N., Ciortea, R. *et al.*, 2015. Pro-inflammatory cytokines for evaluation of inflammatory status in endometriosis. *Central European Journal of Immunology* 40, 96–102. https://doi.org/10.5114/ceji.2015.50840

Marques, M., Laflamme, L., Benassou, I., Cissokho, C., Guillemette, B., Gaudreau, L., 2014. Low levels of 3,3'-diindolylmethane activate estrogen receptor α and induce proliferation of breast cancer cells in the absence of estradiol. *BMC Cancer* 14, 524. https://doi.org/10.1186/1471-2407-14-524

Marziali, M., Capozzolo, T., 2015. Role of gluten-free diet in the management of chronic pelvic pain of deep infiltrating endometriosis. *Journal of Minimally Invasive Gynecology* 22, S51–S52. https://doi.org/10.1016/j.jmig.2015.08.142

Marziali, M., Venza, M., Lazzaro, S., Lazzaro, A., Micossi, C., Stolfi, V.M., 2012. Gluten-free diet: A new strategy for management of painful endometriosis related symptoms? *Minerva Chirurgica* 67, 499–504.

Merhi, Z., Doswell, A., Krebs, K., Cipolla, M., 2014. Vitamin D alters genes involved in follicular development and steroidogenesis in human cumulus granulosa cells. *Journal of Clinical Endocrinology and Metabolism* 99, E1137–1145. https://doi.org/10.1210/jc.2013-4161

Messalli, E.M., Schettino, M.T., Mainini, G., Ercolano, S. *et al.*, 2014. The possible role of zinc in the etiopathogenesis of endometriosis. *Clinical and Experimental Obstetrics and Gynecology* 41, 541–546.

Minkel, J., Moreta, M., Muto, J., Htaik, O. *et al.*, 2014. Sleep deprivation potentiates HPA axis stress reactivity in healthy adults. *Health Psychology* 33, 1430–1434. https://doi.org/10.1037/a0034219

Morin, M., Bellehumeur, C., Therriault, M.-J., Metz, C., Maheux, R., Akoum, A., 2005. Elevated levels of macrophage migration inhibitory factor in the peripheral blood of women with endometriosis. *Fertility and Sterility* 83, 865–872. https://doi.org/10.1016/j.fertnstert.2004.10.039

Mumford, S.L., Browne, R.W., Schliep, K.C., Schmelzer, J. *et al.*, 2016. Serum antioxidants are associated with serum reproductive hormones and ovulation among healthy women. *Journal of Nutrition* 146, 98–106. https://doi.org/10.3945/jn.115.217620

Narin, R., Nazik, H., Aytan, H., Narin, M.A. *et al.*, 2014. Effects of natural progesterone on endometriosis in an experimental rat model: Is it effective? *Clinical and Experimental Obstetrics and Gynecology* 41, 455–459.

Navarro, S.L., Schwarz, Y., Song, X., Wang, C.-Y. et al., 2014. Cruciferous vegetables have variable effects on biomarkers of systemic inflammation in a randomized controlled trial in healthy young adults. *Journal of Nutrition* 144, 1850–1857. https://doi.org/10.3945/jn.114.197434

Neil, K., 2010. Sex Hormone Imbalances. In L. Nicolle and A. Woodriff Beirne (eds) *Biochemical Imbalances in Disease*. Singing Dragon.

Nishihira, J., Ishibashi, T., Fukushima, T., Sun, B., Sato, Y., Todo, S., 2003. Macrophage migration inhibitory factor (MIF): Its potential role in tumor growth and tumor-associated angiogenesis. *Annals of the New York Academy of Sciences* 995, 171–182.

Nissinen, E., Männistö, P.T., 2010. Biochemistry and pharmacology of catechol-O-methyltransferase inhibitors. *International Review of Neurobiology* 95, 73–118. https://doi.org/10.1016/B978-0-12-381326-8.00005-3

Oku, H., Tsuji, Y., Kashiwamura, S.-I., Adachi, S. et al., 2004. Role of IL-18 in pathogenesis of endometriosis. *Human Reproduction* 19, 709–714. https://doi.org/10.1093/humrep/deh108

Panossian, A., Seo, E.-J., Efferth, T., 2018. Novel molecular mechanisms for the adaptogenic effects of herbal extracts on isolated brain cells using systems biology. *Phytomedicine* 50, 257–284. https://doi.org/10.1016/j.phymed.2018.09.204

Panossian, A., Wikman, G., 2009. Evidence-based efficacy of adaptogens in fatigue, and molecular mechanisms related to their stress-protective activity. *Current Clinical Pharmacology* 4, 198–219.

Quiñones, M., Urrutia, R., Torres-Reverón, A., Vincent, K., Flores, I., 2015. Anxiety, coping skills and hypothalamus–pituitary–adrenal (HPA) axis in patients with endometriosis. *Journal of Reproductive Biology and Health* 3. https://doi.org/10.7243/2054-0841-3-2

Rakhila, H., Girard, K., Leboeuf, M., Lemyre, M., Akoum, A., 2014. Macrophage migration inhibitory factor is involved in ectopic endometrial tissue growth and peritoneal-endometrial tissue interaction *in vivo*: A plausible link to endometriosis development. *PLoS ONE* 9. https://doi.org/10.1371/journal.pone.0110434

Rogers, P.A.W., Adamson, G.D., Al-Jefout, M., Becker, C.M. et al., 2017. Research priorities for endometriosis. *Reproductive Sciences* 24, 202–226. https://doi.org/10.1177/1933719116654991

Rogers, P.A.W., D'Hooghe, T.M., Fazleabas, A., Gargett, C.E. et al., 2009. Priorities for endometriosis research: Recommendations from an international consensus workshop. *Reproductive Sciences* 16, 335–346. https://doi.org/10.1177/1933719108330568

Rubel, R., Santa, H.S.D., Dos Santos, L.F., Fernandes, L.C., Figueiredo, B.C., Soccol, C.R., 2018. Immunomodulatory and antitumoral properties of ganoderma lucidum and *Agaricus brasiliensis* (Agaricomycetes) medicinal mushrooms. *International Journal of Medicinal Mushrooms* 20, 393–403. https://doi.org/10.1615/IntJMedMushrooms.2018025979

Rushworth, G.F., Megson, I.L., 2014. Existing and potential therapeutic uses for N-acetylcysteine: The need for conversion to intracellular glutathione for antioxidant benefits. *Pharmacology and Therapeutics* 141, 150–159. https://doi.org/10.1016/j.pharmthera.2013.09.006

Sacco, K., Portelli, M., Pollacco, J., Schembri-Wismayer, P., Calleja-Agius, J., 2012. The role of prostaglandin E2 in endometriosis. *Gynecological Endocrinology* 28, 134–138. https://doi.org/10.3109/09513590.2011.588753

Scientific Advisory Committee on Nutrition (SACN), 2015. SACN Carbohydrates and Health Report. Accessed on 26/05/2019 at www.gov.uk/government/publications/sacn-carbohydrates-and-health-report

Santanam, N., Kavtaradze, N., Murphy, A., Dominguez, C., Parthasarathy, S., 2013. Antioxidant supplementation reduces endometriosis related pelvic pain in humans. *Translational Research* 161, 189–195. https://doi.org/10.1016/j.trsl.2012.05.001

Schomacker, M.L., Hansen, K.E., Ramlau-Hansen, C.H., Forman, A., 2018. Is endometriosis associated with irritable bowel syndrome? A cross-sectional study. *European Journal of Obstetrics and Gynecology and Reproductive Biology* 231, 65–69. https://doi.org/10.1016/j.ejogrb.2018.10.023

Schwarz, J., Gerhardsson, A., van Leeuwen, W., Lekander, M. *et al.*, 2018. Does sleep deprivation increase the vulnerability to acute psychosocial stress in young and older adults? *Psychoneuroendocrinology* 96, 155–165. https://doi.org/10.1016/j.psyneuen.2018.06.003

Sedlak, T.W., Nucifora, L.G., Koga, M., Shaffer, L.S. *et al.*, 2018. Sulforaphane augments glutathione and influences brain metabolites in human subjects: A clinical pilot study. *Molecular Neuropsychiatry* 3, 214–222. https://doi.org/10.1159/000487639

Sourial, S., Tempest, N., Hapangama, D.K., 2014. Theories on the pathogenesis of endometriosis. *International Journal of Reproductive Medicine*. https://doi.org/10.1155/2014/179515

Thimmulappa, R.K., Mai, K.H., Srisuma, S., Kensler, T.W., Yamamoto, M., Biswal, S., 2002. Identification of Nrf2-regulated genes induced by the chemopreventive agent sulforaphane by oligonucleotide microarray. *Cancer Research* 62, 5196–5203.

Truong, T., Baron-Dubourdieu, D., Rougier, Y., Guénel, P., 2010. Role of dietary iodine and cruciferous vegetables in thyroid cancer: A countrywide case-control study in New Caledonia. *Cancer Causes and Control* 21, 1183–1192. https://doi.org/10.1007/s10552-010-9545-2

van Die, M.D., Bone, K.M., Burger, H.G., Reece, J.E., Teede, H.J., 2009. Effects of a combination of *Hypericum perforatum* and *Vitex agnus-castus* on PMS-like symptoms in late-perimenopausal women: Findings from a subpopulation analysis. *Journal of Alternative and Complementary Medicine* 15, 1045–1048. https://doi.org/10.1089/acm.2008.0539

Vincent, K., Warnaby, C., Stagg, C.J., Moore, J., Kennedy, S., Tracey, I., 2011. Dysmenorrhoea is associated with central changes in otherwise healthy women. *Pain* 152, 1966–1975. https://doi.org/10.1016/j.pain.2011.03.029

Vojdani, A., 2015. Molecular mimicry as a mechanism for food immune reactivities and autoimmunity. *Alternative Therapies in Health and Medicine* 21 Suppl 1, 34–45.

vom Saal, F.S., Myers, J.P., 2008. Bisphenol A and risk of metabolic disorders. *JAMA* 300, 1353–1355. https://doi.org/10.1001/jama.300.11.1353

Wahls, T., Scott, M.O., Alshare, Z., Rubenstein, L. *et al.*, 2018. Dietary approaches to treat MS-related fatigue: Comparing the modified Paleolithic (Wahls Elimination) and low saturated fat (Swank) diets on perceived fatigue in persons with relapsing-remitting multiple sclerosis: study protocol for a randomized control. *Trials* 19, 309. https://doi.org/10.1186/s13063-018-2680-x

Wang, J., Shen, X., Huang, X., Zhao, Z., 2012. Follicular fluid levels of prostaglandin E2 and the effect of prostaglandin E2 on steroidogenesis in granulosa-lutein cells in women with moderate and severe endometriosis undergoing in vitro fertilization and embryo transfer. *Chinese Medical Journal* 125, 3985–3990.

Yadav, R., Jee, B., Awasthi, S.K., 2015. Curcumin suppresses the production of pro-inflammatory cytokine interleukin-18 in lipopolysaccharide stimulated murine macrophage-like cells. *Indian Journal of Clinical Biochemistry* 30, 109–112. https://doi.org/10.1007/s12291-014-0452-2

Yasuda, H., Sonoda, A., Yamamoto, M., Kawashima, Y. *et al.*, 2018. 17-β-estradiol enhances neutrophil extracellular trap formation by interaction with estrogen membrane receptor. *Archives of Biochemistry and Biophysics* 663, 64–70. https://doi.org/10.1016/j.abb.2018.12.028

Yue, G.G.L., Cheng, S.-W., Yu, H., Xu, Z.-S. *et al.*, 2012. The role of turmerones on curcumin transportation and P-glycoprotein activities in intestinal Caco-2 cells. *Journal of Medicinal Food* 15, 242–252. https://doi.org/10.1089/jmf.2011.1845

Zamani, M., Neghab, N., Torabian, S., 2012. Therapeutic effect of *Vitex agnus castus* in patients with premenstrual syndrome. *Acta Medica Iranica* 50, 101–106.

Zhang, K., Liu, Y., Zhao, X., Tang, Q., Dernedde, J., Zhang, J., Fan, H., 2018. Anti-inflammatory properties of GLPss58, a sulfated polysaccharide from *Ganoderma lucidum*. *International Journal of Biological Macromolecules* 107, 486–493. https://doi.org/10.1016/j.ijbiomac.2017.09.015

Zhang, Y., Cao, H., Yu, Z., Peng, H.-Y., Zhang, C., 2013. Curcumin inhibits endometriosis endometrial cells by reducing estradiol production. *Iranian Journal of Reproductive Medicine* 11, 415–422.

12

Learnings and Conclusions

Angela Walker

The goal of this book is to showcase the application of systems biology, nutritional science and the therapeutic relationship via a series of case studies. In this chapter, we will reflect on the preceding eight case chapters and identify some of their key themes, creating a summary of principles involved in best practice within a personalized nutrition clinical setting.

Critical thinking applied to evidence sources

The idea of the practitioner as a researcher was introduced in Chapter 2 when considering the evidence base for personalized nutrition. These cases demonstrate that clinically effective interventions do not need to be based solely on findings from a randomized controlled trial. Practitioners learn clinical insights from a wide range of sources including but not limited to systematic reviews, meta-analyses, clinical trials, expert opinions, experience with other cases, peer discussion groups. When *critical thinking* is applied, all of these are valid sources of evidence. In Chapter 10, for example, the practitioner wants to use magnesium. Magnesium must be bound to another molecule, and taurine is an option. Animal studies show that taurine can activate

GABA receptors which may regulate 'excitability' in the brain. A key clinical goal is to reduce the client's anxiety. Magnesium taurate makes sense as a form of magnesium to use. The practitioner is collecting insight from a number of sources to make a clinical decision. We can see similar decisions made throughout the case studies. In Chapter 7, the focus on dietary diversity to stimulate microbial diversity is based on an understanding of the gut, brain and microbiome axis in the context of the client's historical diet (very restricted) and laboratory test findings. These clinical decisions were clearly evidence-based, but they required critical thinking from the practitioner and an ability and willingness to draw from a wide range of evidence sources. What can be summarized from the above, and the other examples through this book, is perhaps a common structure to the process of critical thinking:

- What are the biochemical pathways involved? What cofactors do they need? What potential inhibitors need to be avoided?
- What is published regarding this specific intervention or the imbalance I am supporting from primary or secondary/filtered sources?
- What is my clinical experience in cases like this?
- What are the peer-group/expert opinion views?
- How does this information relate to my client?

The successful practitioner is nimble in how they apply critical thinking, and in how to review and interpret sources of evidence through the lens of their own clinical practice. While, generally, this comes from experience, for the less experienced practitioner reviewing case studies (such as these) that demonstrate the process may be useful in developing the required skills.

Use systems to manage the complexity

Clinical work in complex cases often involves working 'on the edge of chaos' as discussed in Chapter 2. In Chapter 7, the term 'wide-angled lens' is used to describe the type of focus needed for effective clinical practice. A client timeline and an organizing 'matrix' of body systems and symptoms are core principles taught to students of personalized nutrition. The learnings from these cases are about how to *apply* those tools – in particular, the organizing matrix – in practice.

In each of the cases presented, the practitioner has demonstrated non-linear thinking. Each practitioner has their own way to order that thinking – which makes sense, as we all process information in different ways. For the purposes of presenting the case studies, the critical thinking and rationale needed to be in a written form, but visuals were also included, where appropriate, to illustrate the application of the rationale. Specific examples include:

- Chapter 9 used the functional matrix template from the Institute for Functional Medicine (2011 version).
- Chapter 10 used clinical questions as well as a table format to help structure thinking in the face of complex symptom patterns and numerous data points from functional testing.
- Chapter 11 used a Venn diagram to link the case analysis with targeted interventions.

The common theme of each is that they all include a wide spectrum of biochemical systems that are involved in health and disease. Each case also included the practitioner's own version of the timeline to understand the chronology of the client's story.

The takeaway lesson from this is to find an organizing system that works for you, that is practical to use face to face with clients as well as when interpreting the case findings.

Give the client ownership of their story

Looking at a case through a wide-angled lens and plotting a client's health on a timeline are tools to help interpret the case. They have an additional role. When used to replay the 'story' back to a client, they can be very powerful tools to help the client make sense of their own health. If someone can understand their health issues, they are empowered to change the course of their health. This is a subtle but vital skill that all the practitioners used in their work with the clients. Chapter 9 includes a great example of this, where the practitioner was able to hypothesize that AB's stress response systems have been 'primed' by early psychological stresses, helping AB understand her situation more completely. In Chapter 8, SD was empowered to take positive steps to address her sleep patterns with the understanding of how this could have an impact on insulin resistance. In Chapter 6, the insight from extensive functional testing helped AR to understand why weight loss had previously been so difficult and to feel motivated that it could now be achieved. This is also an example of how functional laboratory testing can help by providing information that informs the client's story.

Engage clients in the process, focus on education

The work of personalized nutrition doesn't happen during the one-to-one consultation time with the client; it happens when the client is in their daily life, cooking, shopping, eating, meditating, breathing, exercising. There are numerous examples from the case study chapters of education and engagement tools, including TED talk videos, meditation apps and various handouts. Two examples are worth a particular mention here. In Chapter 6, the practitioner used his '50 food chart' as a simple yet practical way to educate and support the client to increase diet diversity from the supermarket through to the dining table. In Chapter 4, we see how a 24-hour dietary recall helped to identify that the client had inadvertently added refined sugars and lowered vegetables. Sometimes these apparent 'mistakes' can actually be very helpful as education in exactly how to personalize the diet for that individual. Functional laboratory testing can be seen in some of the cases to have played an education and engagement role. In Chapter 5, testing and follow-up helped MA to have confidence in her new energy levels.

The takeaway here is that such tools help the client to educate themselves – to learn new ways to shop for food, to prepare food, to think about food, to manage their lifestyle – which is key to long-term habit changes.

Have a growth mindset for each case

Dealing with complexity can be a genuine challenge in clinical work. It is unrealistic for a practitioner to expect to know *every* potential imbalance and interaction within a case. A practitioner with a growth mindset can embrace the unknown and be comfortable it, knowing they will learn from the process. Sometimes an adverse reaction leads to new insights. In Chapter 10 there is a perfect example of this: a reaction to a fibre supplement led the practitioner to new insight (fructose intolerance) that ultimately unlocked the case. That is not, of course, to say that a practitioner wants to create an adverse reaction, but the lesson learned is not to be afraid to start somewhere, based on the interpretation of the case with the best information held at that point. Remaining open to learning from every response, or lack of response, to an intervention that a client shares will potentially help to gain further insight on underlying factors and help deepen the therapeutic relationship with the client.

Most paths lead to or from the gut

The Q&A sections of each chapter were designed to bring out an aspect of reflective practice in each case. What is often addressed in these sections is the practitioners' reflections that there were other potential routes they could theoretically have taken to address the case. Most practitioners would agree that if ever there is a question on exactly where to start in a case, the answer is usually to begin with the gut. The reason is based on systems biology. Change in the microbiome will impact many different systems in the body. In Chapter 4, addressing small intestinal bacterial overgrowth (SIBO) was a key factor in addressing recurring urinary tract infections. In Chapter 7, the gut was key to improving cognitive function. The takeaway is 'when in doubt, think gut'; personalized nutrition interventions will always act through the gut (as the location for digestion and absorption of diet) and that, via manipulation of the microbiome, has the potential for wide-reaching effects on health and disease.

Diet, diet, diet

While the cases include a number of functional tests and in-depth biochemistry, in the end, the primary driver for positive change in each case was the diet.

Dietary change involves including some foods and excluding others and it is both inclusions and exclusions that drive the impact of diet on an individual. Some cases have a lot of supplements, some very few, but ALL feature fundamental dietary change that is the foundation for effecting change in that individual. While a lot of the focus in professional development in the personalized nutrition field can focus on supplementation, it is crucial to focus on the foundations of diet in successful clinical practice. The message here is that although the systems biology and nutritional science can at times appear complex, dietary changes (especially when tailored and personalized) are the foundation of an effective personalized nutrition programme. Always remember that clients will require specific and precise examples: number of portions of a food, how much is in a portion, practical ideas on preparing that type of food. We attempted to provide examples of exactly how the practitioners communicated that to the clients in each of the case chapters.

Personalizing an off-the-shelf diet

This is a theme that arose in virtually every case. The recommended diets are typically based on an existing diet such as Mediterranean, Palaeolithic, low-FODMAP or ketogenic, but they were personalized to suit individual requirements. This is vital. First, the off-the-shelf diets are not always well defined. Second, everyone is an individual and has a specific set of needs, especially when their health is compromised. In Chapter 6, the ketogenic diet was used to initiate weight loss and tackle cravings, but it was monitored closely, qualitatively (interaction with practitioner) and quantitatively (monitoring of blood lipids) to tailor its use and time frame. Third, long-term use of these diets can lead to issues if they are not closely monitored. We saw examples in Chapters 7, 9 and 10, where a self-prescribed restricted diet had been used for a long period and potentially had contributed to later issues. Fourth, when the off-the-shelf diet is well described, it may not be ideally suitable in that form for an individual. In Chapter 4, TT was advised to reduce high-FODMAP foods but initially this led to an increased intake of refined sugar and starches and a reduction in vegetables, which was in alignment with an off-the-shelf low-FODMAP diet, but was not the intention in this case. This was quickly adjusted, and TT was guided on how to personalize the diet. The systems biology and nutritional science give us the rationale for how to *tailor* each diet to the individual.

Personalizing means meeting clients where they are

The therapeutic relationship is key to personalized nutrition. The practitioner's role is to coach the client and to build their confidence and trust. This requires creating recommendations that are achievable and developing those over time. Examples of this can be seen throughout the cases: varying the colour of vegetables selected in the supermarket each week and introducing fermented drinks (Chapter 7); replacing fruit juice with whole fruit, increasing vegetable portions, switching breakfast cereal with an improved protein-to-carbohydrate ratio (Chapter 5); adjusting the timing of meals (increasing overnight fast) (Chapter 8). In Chapter 6, the practitioner recommended interventions to provide 'quick wins' through palliative support for mood and oestrogen symptoms, to help motivate AR and build her confidence that she could make the more fundamental diet and lifestyle changes. In Chapter 11, the client was coached on batch-cooking to simplify the diet changes. Those first steps might not have been enough to achieve the end result, but they built the client's confidence in the practitioner and in themselves and started the process.

Never underestimate the stress effect

The impact of stress is well understood but not always clearly identified. In every case there was an impact on the autonomic nervous system response, whether it was measured with a functional test or identified through thorough case history taking, often appearing early in the client's timeline. Diet cannot work in isolation; the practitioner needs to use the therapeutic skills and the art of retelling the client story to drive home the importance of sleep routine, relaxation tools, exercise and mindfulness tools. In Chapter 11, addressing stress through lifestyle and botanical-based supplements was key to supporting a more optimal balance between oestrogen and progesterone levels. This insight explained to JM *why* the lifestyle changes were recommended, which helped with motivation. In some cases, clients were referred on for specialist psychology support in this area (Chapter 10); in others, the practitioner provided specific recommendations of apps, digital tools, local classes or via client handouts.

Listen and keep asking questions, then listen some more

What the client has come to recognize as normal could give the practitioner a big clue to the case. A key to successful personalized nutrition practice is to keep digging and asking, 'Why is that happening?' This can sometimes lead to a big clue that unlocks the case. In Chapter 10, we saw how an adverse reaction to a fibre supplement led to a key insight regarding fructose intolerance. In Chapter 5, although digestion was not an initial concern for the client, as her energy improved and her focus turned to fertility, the practitioner's continued investigations revealed microbiome and digestive function imbalances (via stool testing) that appear to have helped resolve the remaining issues and led to MA achieving full and optimal health. In Chapter 9, continued investigations revealed issues with dairy which the client had initially thought she tolerated well. The lesson to be learned is that practitioners need to nurture the therapeutic relationship so that the client gains confidence that these insights are useful and vital to the process.

A final point on 'closure'

All these cases are successfully resolved. In clinical practice, we don't always receive that 'closure' to a case. Sometimes clients are lost to follow-up. For practitioners, it can be disheartening not to know why this happened and the eventual outcome. Perhaps the client did receive a benefit, they received what they needed at that time, or their issues resolved either partially or fully. Or perhaps it was the wrong time for them, but they came back to look at their lifestyle at some point in the future. As practitioners, we have to remain confident and believe in what we do. These cases demonstrate that personalized nutrition can be powerful and have a very positive impact on an individual's quality of life and on those around them.

In conclusion, it is hoped that this book stimulates reflection and provides insight for new and experienced personalized nutrition practitioners on the art and science of their own clinical practice – to appreciate that while there are foundation principles for effective clinical practice, there is not one single approach that suits all situations. It is hoped that through these cases practitioners can continue to learn and to deepen their own style, approach and confidence in their clinical practice.

For other health care professionals, it is hoped that this book helps to explain the depth of personalized nutrition: that it involves so much more than following standard guidelines for a 'healthy diet'; that it is rooted in the application of systems biology, nutritional science and therapeutic relationship and can be very effective in resolving complex health issues.

Drug–Nutrient Interaction Checker

In cases where clients are already taking prescription medications, checks for drug–nutrient interactions must be undertaken. The following tables outline the checks undertaken, which are primarily taken from the Natural Medicines Database: https://naturalmedicines. therapeuticresearch.com.

Chapter 6

Potential interactions exist for the drug and supplement (St John's Wort) recommendations in Chapter 6. A summary of the findings from the interaction checker are outlined below.

Drug	Known interactions (major)	Potential interactions (focus on supplements used/ considered)	Notes
Losartan potassium (anti hypertensive angiotensin-receptor blocker)	Grapefruit inhibits CYP3A4 St John's Wort (SJW) induces CYP3A4	Grapefruit may inhibit CYP 2C9 SJW may induce CYP2C9	CYP 3A4 and CYP 2C9 are two of the metabolic pathways used by losartan. It is possible that taking SJW, which induces both, may reduce the half-life of losartan. Given that the diet and lifestyle programme was designed to support weight loss and that AR had already self-prescribed the combination for four months, the case physician was satisfied that AR could continue with SJW. Within three months her BP had improved and her cardiologist reduced dose by 50%, and by six months she was no longer on the medication. Grapefruit juice was not included in her diet.

cont.

Drug	Known interactions (major)	Potential interactions (focus on supplements used/ considered)	Notes
Progesterone (topical)	Grapefruit inhibits CYP3A4 SJW induces CYP3A4	SJW may induce CYP2C19	Topical delivery of progesterone eliminates first-pass metabolism; hence, interactions with substances (food or supplement) that inhibit or induce drug metabolism in liver and small intestine will be avoided.
Levothyroxine and liothyronine (T3 and T4)	None		
Melatonin	None		

Additional sources for the above table

Sica, D.A., Gehr, T.W.B., Ghosh, S., 2005. Clinical pharmacokinetics of losartan. *Clinical Pharmacokinetics* 44, 797–814. https://doi.org/10.2165/00003088-200544080-00003

Zaidenstein, R., Soback, S., Gips, M., Avni, B. *et al.*, 2001. Effect of grapefruit juice on the pharmacokinetics of losartan and its active metabolite E3174 in healthy volunteers. *Therapeutic Drug Monitoring* 23, 369.

Zanger, U.M., Schwab, M., 2013. Cytochrome P450 enzymes in drug metabolism: Regulation of gene expression, enzyme activities, and impact of genetic variation. *Pharmacology and Therapeutics* 138, 103–141. https://doi.org/10.1016/j.pharmthera.2012.12.007

Chapter 10

No potential interactions were found for the medications and supplements/foods used in the case in Chapter 10. A summary of the findings from the interaction checker is shown below.

Drug	Known interactions (major)	Notes
Doxycycline	Beer, oleander, St John's Wort, wine	No interaction concerns with recommended programme of food or supplements
Ciprofloxacin	Beer, grapefruit, sweet orange, wine	
Lymecycline (tetracycline)	Beer, oleander, St John's Wort, wine	
Metronidazole	Wine	
Moxifloxacin	Beer, grapefruit, sweet orange, wine, ephedra	
Clarithromycin	Ephedra, grapefruit, oleander, St John's Wort	
Amoxicillin	Acacia, beer, wine	
Diazepam	Beer, cannabidol, grapefruit, kava, l-tryptophan, St John's Wort, wine	

Chapter 11

No potential interactions were found for the medications and supplements/foods used in the case in Chapter 11. A summary of the findings from the interaction checker is shown below.

Drug	Known interactions (major)	Notes
Levothyroxine and liothyronine (T3 and T4)	None	

Useful Resources

Further reading and training on personalized nutrition

Biochemical Imbalances in Disease is a comprehensive reference for the systems biology and nutritional science discussed within the cases: Lorraine Nicolle and Ann Woodriff Beirne (eds) (2010) *Biochemical Imbalances in Disease: A Practitioner's Handbook*. London: Singing Dragon.

The British Association for Nutrition and Lifestyle Medicine – http://bant.org.uk – provides training and clinical tools for members. It also provides a list of practitioners trained in this approach

The Nutrition Evidence Database a database created to support evidence-based practice in nutrition and lifestyle medicine. It is produced by BANT and it is open access – www.nutrition-evidence.com.

The Institute for Functional Medicine – www.ifm.org – provides training for healthcare professionals and provides clinical tools for member practitioners. The IFM Functional Medicine matrix (Figure 9.4) is a valuable tool for organizing the client case history. The matrix is reproduced with permission from the Institute for Functional Medicine.

TAP Integrative – www.tapintegrative.org – is a resource for clinical protocols, case studies and evidence-based clinical information for integrative health care professionals. Membership subscription.

Questionnaires used to track client progress (PROMS)

These are discussed in Chapter 2 and used in Chapter 7 (MYMOP) and Chapter 6 (MSQ).

- MYMOP – www.bris.ac.uk/primaryhealthcare/resources/mymop.
- MSQ: Members of the Institute of Functional Medicine can download a copy from via the members' toolkit section of the website. A freely available version can also be found here: https://drhyman.com/downloads/MSQ_Fillable.pdf.

Functional testing laboratories

- Biolab Medical Unit London – www.biolab.co.uk
- Genova Diagnostics – www.gdx.net/uk
- Invivo Clinical – www.invivoclinical.co.uk
- Regenerus Laboratories – http://regeneruslabs.com
- Diagnostic Solutions – www.diagnosticsolutionslab.com
- Cyrex Laboratories – www.cyrexlabs.com

About the Contributors

Angela Walker MSc mBANT is a registered nutritional therapist with 12 years clinical experience, including seven years with the award-winning Optimum Health Clinic. She holds an MSc in Nutritional Medicine from University of Surrey and has trained with the Institute of Functional Medicine. She has lectured and mentored at under- and post-graduate level and developed practitioner programmes on the clinical application of functional laboratory testing. She is also a performance coach and works with leaders and executives helping them optimize and sustain cognitive function for peak performances. Her experience brings a unique perspective and her focus is now to develop and showcase new models and best practices for clinicians in personalized nutrition and lifestyle medicine.

Miguel Toribio-Mateas DProf (c) MSc BSc (Hons) is practitioner researcher with extensive experience in gut and brain health and a unique background in nutritional medicine, clinical neuroscience and environmental science. Relevant to this book is Miguel's research interest in patient-reported outcome measures (PROMs), the subject of his doctoral research at the School of Health and Education of Middlesex University. Miguel is a visiting research fellow in brain–gut–microbiota axis and mental health at the School of Applied Sciences, London South Bank University. He continues to run a clinical practice and works as a scientific advisor in research technology and biotechnology.

Lorraine Nicolle MSc is a registered nutritionist (MBANT) and nutritional therapist (CNHC) with over 16 years of clinical experience in helping individuals to age well. She is passionate about using personalized nutrition and lifestyle medicine to help patients to reach their full health potential. She has a track record of helping individuals who have a broad range of health conditions, including gastrointestinal problems, autoimmune diseases, musculoskeletal issues and cardio-metabolic disorders.

Lorraine has an MSc in Personalised Nutrition and Chronic Illness (distinction) and a higher education teaching qualification. She has also trained with the Institute of Functional Medicine. She teaches undergraduates, postgraduates and healthcare practitioners in the application of nutrition science to real-world clinical situations.

Lorraine has author-edited three books on personalized nutrition (*Biochemical Imbalances in Disease, The Functional Nutrition Cookbook and Eat to Get Younger*) and she is the series editor for the set of practitioner texts of which this book is a part.

Helen Lynam BSc (Hons), PGChE, NTCC, MBANT is a nutritional therapist with a clinic in Ascot. She has also been Director of Nutrition for the Optimum Health Clinic, a specialist clinic for chronic fatigue, myalgic encephalomyelitis and fibromyalgia, where she also sees clients.

Helen worked at CNELM (Centre for Nutrition Education and Lifestyle Management) for six years where she led modules and lectured on the Nutritional Therapy course as well as supervising the student clinic, she also wrote for and sub-edited the professional journal *The Nutrition Practitioner* at that time. Helen is now turning her attention the preservation and enhancement of health through nutrition and lifestyle, hoping she can help people to avoid the ill health she sees on a day-to-day basis.

Romilly Hodges MS CNS CN is trained and certified through the Institute for Functional Medicine (IFM) and Board for the Certification of Nutrition Specialists (BCNS) in the United States. She holds a Masters degree in Human Nutrition from the University of Bridgeport CT.

Romilly also serves on the Board for the Accreditation Council for Nutrition Professional Education and is an approved supervisor for prospective CNS candidates seeking experience hours.

Romilly has contributed to advancing professional understanding of food and health through various publications including for peer-reviewed journals and educational initiatives.

For the past four years, Romilly has served as Nutrition Programs Director for Dr Kara Fitzgerald's Functional Medicine Clinic during which time she developed a highly-personalized nutrition delivery model, built a high-calibre nutrition team, and played an instrumental role in establishing the group as a virtual teaching clinic.

Kara Fitzgerald ND completed post-doctorate training in nutritional biochemistry and laboratory science under the direction of Richard Lord, PhD at Metametrix Laboratory. She authored/edited *Case Studies in Integrative and Functional Medicine*, and was a contributing author to *Laboratory Evaluations for Integrative and Functional Medicine*, The Institute for Functional Medicine's *Textbook for Functional Medicine*, and co-authored the eBook *The Methylation Diet and Lifestyle*. Dr Fitzgerald runs a Clinic Emersion Program for professionals and maintains an active blog and podcast series on her website,www.drkarafitzgerald. com. She is on faculty at The Institute for Functional Medicine and maintains a functional medicine practice in Sandy Hook, Connecticut.

Jo Gamble BA (Hons) DIP CNM cFMP ABAAHP fellow ICT graduated from the prestigious Institute for Functional Medicine in 2013 as part of the first cohort of certified practitioners. Jo runs a busy functional medicine clinic where she specializes in complex cases and enjoys taking her clients on a journey to dig deep into their symptoms.

Jo furthered her career with a fellowship in Integrative Cancer from the American Board of Anti-Aging Practitioners. Jo has been lecturing at an under- and post-graduate level for the last 10 years where she shares her passion to inspire practitioners to further develop their own knowledge and confidence and to bring alive her skills and experience to empower others.

Elspeth Stewart BSc (Hons) MBANT ANTA is a registered nutritional therapist and Bredesen ReCode Practitioner. Elspeth received a first class degree in nutritional therapy from CNELM and after eight years of clinical practice in the UK, most recently with the Optimum Health Clinic specializing in CFS/ME, she relocated to her home town of Perth and has since joined Metagenics Australia where she provides product support and training to naturopaths, nutritionists and integrated GPs.

Claire Sehinson MSc, mBANT gained a Masters in personalized nutrition at CNELM after leaving a career in classical music. She currently practises nutritional therapy using a functional medicine approach, with a focus in chronic fatigue syndrome and fibromyalgia. She lectures in biomedicine and chronic fatigue nutritional therapeutics in various nutritional therapy colleges. Her specialist areas of interest and research include autoimmunity, neuroscience and environmental medicine.

Lorna Driver-Davies BA (Hons) HD DHNP CNHC mNNA has worked for a decade as a registered naturopathic nutritional therapist, integrating functional medicine and her knowledge of botanicals as a herbal medicine dispenser. She has expertise in endocrine and gynaecological nutrition, with a particular focus on endometriosis, PCOS, menstrual irregularities, pre-conception, menopause and thyroid conditions – using both nutrition and herbs in clinical protocols. As senior practitioner at specialist women's clinic 'Wild Clinics'; more than 70% of her weekly clients have an endometriosis or PCOS diagnosis – which has provided her with deep clinical experience to develop highly specific protocols for these complex conditions. She regularly lectures to members of the public, medical and nutritional professionals and mentors nutrition students.

Subject Index

Author Index